The potential for investigating and diagnosing psychiatric illness in later life has been greatly enhanced by developments in neuroimaging, yet for many clinicians both the technology and its applications remain hard to grasp. This book provides them with a reliable reference, written by prominent figures in neuroradiology and old age psychiatry, which draws together current knowledge of late life mental disorders as revealed by neuroimaging.

A highly illustrated introductory chapter provides a useful overview of the various techniques of neuroimaging now available. The following chapters, also extensively illustrated, survey the contribution of neuroimaging to understanding the specific psychiatric disorders of late life, and the book concludes with guidelines for clinicians on the choice of imaging for the investigation of their patients.

For researchers, this is a useful and authoritative review of current knowledge regarding neuroimaging and the older psychiatric patient. Its primary aim, however, is to educate and advise clinicians dealing with the protean manifestations of psychiatric disorder in later life.

'A significant service to the clinical and scientific community . . . this compendium must be considered an important landmark in the growing discipline of the psychiatry of old age.' From the Foreword by Raymond Levy, Institute of Psychiatry, University of London.

NEUROIMAGING AND THE PSYCHIATRY OF LATE LIFE

Neuroimaging and the psychiatry of late life

Edited by

David Ames and Edmond Chiu
Academic Unit in Psychiatry of Old Age,
University of Melbourne, Victoria, Australia

Foreword by Raymond Levy

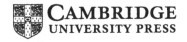

CAMBRIDGE
UNIVERSITY PRESS

CAMBRIDGE UNIVERSITY PRESS
Cambridge, New York, Melbourne, Madrid, Cape Town, Singapore, São Paulo, Delhi

Cambridge University Press
The Edinburgh Building, Cambridge CB2 8RU, UK

Published in the United States of America by Cambridge University Press, New York

www.cambridge.org
Information on this title: www.cambridge.org/9780521112475

First published 1997
This digitally printed version 2009

A catalogue record for this publication is available from the British Library

Library of Congress Cataloguing in Publication data

Neuroimaging in the psychiatry of late life / edited by David Ames and
Edmond Chiu.
    p. cm.
  Includes bibliographical references and index.
  ISBN 0 521 49505 9 (hbk)
  1. Brain – Imaging. 2. Geriatric neuropsychiatry. I. Ames,
David, 1954– . II. Chiu, Edmond.
  [DNLM: 1. Mental Disorders – in old age. 2. Mental Disorders –
diagnosis. 3. Diagnostic Imaging – methods.   4. Brain –
physiopathology.   WT 150 N4933 1997]
RC473.B7N48   1997
618.97′6890754–dc21   96-52958 CIP
DNLM/DLC
for Library of Congress

ISBN 978-0-521-49505-9 hardback
ISBN 978-0-521-11247-5 paperback

Additional resources for this publication at www.cambridge.org/9780521112475

Contents

Contributors

David Ames
Academic Unit in Psychiatry of Old Age, University of Melbourne, Parkville, Victoria 3052, Australia

Christopher Ball
Division of Psychiatry and Psychological Medicine, United Medical and Dental Schools, Guy's Hospital, St Thomas St, London SE1 9RT and Lewisham and Guy's Mental Health Trust, Community Team B, Hither Green Hospital, Hither Green Lane, London SE13 6RU, UK

Alistair Burns
School of Psychiatry and Behavioural Sciences, Department of Old Age Psychiatry, University of Manchester, Withington Hospital, Manchester M20 8LR, UK

E. Jane Byrne
Department of Old Age Psychiatry, University of Manchester, Withington Hospital, Manchester M20 8LR, UK

Edmond Chiu
Academic Unit in Psychiatry of Old Age, University of Melbourne, St George's Hospital, Kew, Victoria 3101, Australia

Ian Cook
UCLA School of Medicine, UCLA Neuropsychiatric Institute and Hospital, Los Angeles, CA 90024-1759, USA

Patricia Desmond
Department of Radiology, University of Melbourne, Royal Melbourne, Parkville, Victoria 3052 and Royal Melbourne Hospital, Victoria 3050, Australia

Marshal Folstein
Department of Psychiatry, Tufts University School of Medicine, Boston, MA 02111, USA

Hans Förstl
Department of Psychiatry and Behavioural Science, The University of Western Australia, Queen Elizabeth II Medical Centre, Nedlands, Western Australia 6009, Australia

Hillel Grossman
Department of Psychiatry, Tufts University School of Medicine, Boston, MA 02111, USA

Gordon Harris
Department of Psychiatry, Tufts University School of Medicine, Boston, MA 02111, USA

Kazuo Hasegawa
St Marianna University School of Medicine, Kawasaki 216, Japan

Rob Howard
Maudsley Hospital and the Institute of Psychiatry, Denmark Hill, London SE5 8AZ, UK

Sandra Jacobson
Department of Psychiatry, Tufts University School of Medicine, Boston, MA 02111, USA

Robin Jacoby
Department of Psychiatry, The Warneford Hospital, Oxford OX3 7JX, UK

Kim Jobst
University Department of Medicine and Therapeutics, Gardiner Institute, Western Infirmary, Glasgow G11 6NT, UK

Hiroo Kasahara
Jikei University School of Medicine, Kashiwa Hospital, Kashiwa 277, Japan

Andrew Leuchter
UCLA School of Medicine, UCLA Neuropsychiatric Institute and Hospital, Los Angeles, CA 90024-1759, USA

James Lindesay
Department of Psychiatry, University of Leicester, Leicester General Hospital, Gwendolan Road, Leicester LE5 4PW, UK

Alastair Macdonald
Hither Green Hospital, Hither Green Lane, London
SE13 6RU, UK

John O'Brien
Brighton Clinic, Newcastle General Hospital,
Westgate Road, Newcastle upon Tyne NE4 6BE UK

Michael Philpot
Maudsley Hospital and the Institute of Psychiatry,
Denmark Hill, London SE5 8AF, UK

Basil Shepstone
Oxford University Department of Radiology,
Radcliffe Infirmary NHS Trust, Woodstock Road,
Oxford OX2 6HE, UK

Stephen Simpson
Department of Psychiatry, Withington Hospital,
Manchester M20 8LR, UK

Brian Tress
Department of Radiology, University of Melbourne,
Parkville, Victoria 3052 and Royal Melbourne
Hospital, Victoria 3050, Australia

Preface

The occasional iconoclastic contribution excepted (Burns *et al.*, 1992), recent times have been characterized by an historically remarkable consensus that the brain is the chief bodily organ of relevance in the study of behavioral disturbances exhibited by older people. The last 25 years have seen tremendous advances in our ability to examine the brain during life. The younger of the two editors was issued a card at the start of his clinical training on which he was required to document his attendance at a variety of radiological procedures. When he qualified 31 months later the box for the pneumoencephalogram was still unsigned, the Royal Melbourne Hospital's first computerized tomographic brain scanner having rendered such procedures redundant within a few days of his arrival. Today, with the ubiquitous availability of computed X-ray tomography (CT), easy access to magnetic resonance imaging, single photon emission tomography and brain electrical activity mapping together with the increasing research use of positron emission tomography, that first scanner seems like a 78r.p.m. acoustic phonogram in comparison to a state of the art CD player.

Just as improvements in musical recording technology have not always been accompanied by a corresponding rise in the quality of performances to preserve for posterity, successive refinements of imaging technology have not necessarily marched in step with an increase in the sophistication of clinicians' use of such machinery. Most of us have long since ceased to expect a definitive diagnosis of dementia to be made from the result of a CT scan alone, the overlap between the normal aging brain and that of the patient with Alzheimer's disease being too great to allow easy discrimination between two isolated examples of each. However, we suspect that very few clinicians could give a confident evidence-based account of the exact place of each of the currently available neuroimaging techniques in the investigation of the elderly psychiatric patient. Our own uncertainties in this area led us directly to the compilation of this book, which should fill an irritating gap in the current literature. While researchers will find it a useful compendium of current knowledge regarding neuroimaging and the older psychiatric patient, its prime aim is to educate and advise the clinician who must deal with the protean manifestations of psychiatric disorder in late life. To counter the 'geewhiz' response to technology, the limitations as well as the contributions of neuroimaging should be presented with balance and we feel this is exactly what our distinguished contributors have achieved.

Part 1 of this book is intended to provide a succinct, illustrated account of modern methods of neuroimaging, to indicate what they can and cannot offer, and to provide some illustrative examples of the varied pathologies that they may reveal. The seven chapters of Part 2 summarize current knowledge in the neuroimaging of specific psychiatric disorders of late life (dementias, delirium, affective, schizophrenic and related paranoid disorders) as well as findings in that most ambiguous and elusive condition 'normal aging'. The final part offers one perspective from each side of the Atlantic to help the clinician decide which scan to order for which patient, when and why.

The acknowledgements that follow provide a list of those to whom the editors and chapter authors are most indebted, but we would like to emphasize our gratitude towards our contributors, whose expertise in their individual areas greatly outweighs our own and whose cheerful enthusiasm made the compilation of this text a recurring pleasure over more than two years. Last, this work would never have been started, much less finished, without the encouragement of Richard Barling of Cambridge University Press, to whom we owe a lasting debt.

David Ames
Edmond Chiu
Melbourne, June 1996

Burns, A., Howard, R., Förstl, H. & Levy, R. (1992). False teeth and Alzheimer's disease. *Psychiatric Bulletin*, 16, 227–228.

Foreword

Advances in the psychiatry of late life have increasingly been based on technological developments that are often remote from the concerns of clinicians. This has led to difficulties both in understanding what is being offered and in evaluating potential risks and benefits of the new technologies. Nowhere has this been more evident than in neuroimaging. The uncritical enthusiasm that followed the introduction of every new procedure since Hounsfield's development of computed tomography has often made way for equally uncritical negative attitudes. The problem has been aggravated by the fact that relevant data have been dispersed in a variety of different journals relating to cognate disciplines.

Associate Professors Ames and Chiu have rendered a significant service to the clinical and scientific community by bringing together the important contributions that make up this book. The technological background of the different approaches involved has been explained by relevant experts and for the first time a detailed evaluation has been produced on what each technique has to offer to the investigating and treatment of different disorders of old age. Equally important is the light cast on what neuroimaging has taught us about the possible etiology of these disorders. This compendium must be considered as an important landmark in the growing discipline of the psychiatry of old age.

Raymond Levy

Acknowledgements

Yvonne Liddicoat typed many drafts of the manuscript, searched out dozens of references and saw to it that the book was finally completed and despatched. Without her the project would have been impossible. Roz Seath provided excellent secretarial support to EC. Alistair Burns gave much valuable help in the planning stages.

Jennifer Coxson and Angela Seo helped to prepare the manuscript, figures and tables for Chapters 1(d) and 9(a) and these chapters were supported by research grants from the National Institute of Mental Health, UCLA Alzheimer Disease Center, Medication Development Division, National Institute on Drug Abuse and the US Department of Veterans Affairs. The views in these chapters represent those of the authors and do not necessarily represent those of the US Department of Veterans Affairs. Figure 3.2 was provided by courtesy of F. Hentschel, Department of Neuroradiology, Central Institute of Mental Health, the PET pictures for chapter 4 were provided by Michio Senda, Figs. 5.1 and 5.2 were reproduced with kind permission from Manchester Royal Infirmary Department of Nuclear Medicine and Neuroradiology and Kim Jobst supplied the scans in Figs. 9.5 and 9.6. Catherine Oppenheimer and Nick Hindley made helpful comments on the manuscript of Chapter 9(b).

Part 1
Modern methods
of neuroimaging

1(a) Computed tomography

Brian Tress and Patricia Desmond

Computed tomography (CT), also known as computerized axial tomography (CAT) and CAT scanning, was developed between 1967 and 1970 by the English scientist Godfrey Hounsfield. The first clinical results were reported in 1972 (Ambrose & Hounsfield, 1972a,b). Hounsfield successfully harnessed conventional X-rays and a computer to produce cross-sectional brain images of unprecedented clarity (Hounsfield, 1973).

All CT scanners share a number of key features. A finely collimated X-ray beam moves around the patient's head within a metallic shell called a gantry. The extent of X-ray absorption by the tissues is measured by detectors which fluoresce or ionize in direct proportion to the intensity of the X-ray beam striking them after traversing the patient's head. The degree of fluorescence or ionization is converted into digital information by a computer. Using one of several suitable computer algorithms, cross-sectional images of the irradiated slices of brain are constructed in which each of the individual elements of the image, called 'pixels' (shorthand for picture elements), is allocated a level of brightness somewhere between black and white. Approximately 256 shades of gray are available for use in modern CT scanners. Low-density structures such as fat and water appear black and high-density structures such as bone and calcium appear white.

CT scanner types

The original CT scanners were of the 'translate–rotate' type. While continuously emitting a finely collimated, pencil shaped X-ray beam, the tube and detectors traversed (translated) across the head in a straight line. At the completion of each traverse, the tube and detectors rotated through 1° and the traverse was repeated in the opposite direction (Fig. 1.1). The translate–rotate combination was performed at least 180 times, the whole process taking between four and five minutes. Two contiguous 13mm slices of brain could be reconstructed from the data accumulated in each completed cycle.

The second generation of CT scanners were again of the translate–rotate type but utilized a fan-shaped collimated beam and an arc of detectors, which allowed a rotation of

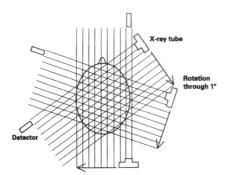

Figure 1.1 *Diagram of first-generation CT. An X-ray tube and a fixed detector moves (translates) linearly across the head being scanned while emitting a pencil beam of X-rays; it then rotates one degree and repeats the translation in the opposite direction.*

10° after each translation. This design modification reduced the time of scanning each pair of slices to 10–20 seconds. A larger gantry opening also permitted other parts of the body to be scanned.

The next advance was major and forms the basis of virtually all scanners used today. Sophisticated mechanical modifications allowed both tube and detector arc to rotate smoothly through 360° in one to two seconds. The tube and detectors were articulated together so that both rotated around the patient in tandem. These scanners were called third-generation, or rotate–rotate scanners (Fig. 1.2). A minority of the rotating scanners were constructed such that the tube rotated around the patient, exposing a fixed ring of detectors around the periphery of the gantry (Fig. 1.3). These fourth-generation scanners required a greater X-ray dose to stimulate the relatively distant ring of fixed detectors and were limited in spatial resolution by how closely the expensive solid-state detectors could be spaced. For these and other reasons, virtually all the CT scanners in current use are of the third-generation type. Consequently, the 'generation' nomenclature lacks intuitive logic and is of little practical use.

Initially, the tube and detectors in the rotate–rotate scanners had to rotate through 360° in one direction then reverse and rotate through 360° in the opposite direction, a process that demanded a minimum interscan interval of at least two to three seconds. Modern slip-ring engineering now allows continuous rotation in a single direction, allowing one second scans with one second interscan gaps for table incrementation. Contemporary top of the line CT scanners with heavy duty X-ray tubes also allow table incrementation while tube and detectors rotate and emit a continuous X-ray beam, resulting in acquisition of a three-dimensional body of data at approximately the rate of one second per centimetre of table incrementation. In restless or uncooperative patients, data from half or two thirds of the 360° excursion can be used to construct an image, reducing scan time to as little as half a second.

The three-dimensional body of acquired data is actually spiral in shape (Fig. 1.4), which is why these CT scanners are called 'spiral' or 'helical' scanners. The spiral shape of the acquired data requires the computer to interpolate data into the gaps to produce the final image. Because of this mandatory interpolation, the signal-to-noise ratio (ratio of the signal intensity detected divided by the intensity of the background noise that is

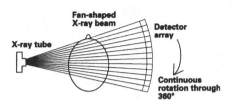

Figure 1.2 *Diagram of third-generation CT. The X-ray tube and an arc-shaped, fixed array of detectors rotate 360° around the head, while the tube emits a fan-shaped X-ray beam.*

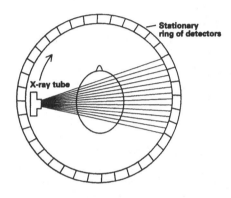

Figure 1.3 *Diagram of fourth-generation CT. While emitting a fan-shaped X-raybeam, the X-ray tube rotates around the head inside a fixed, stationary ring of detectors, only a small proportion of which are irradiated at any one time.*

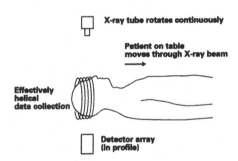

Figure 1.4 *Diagrammatic representation of helical CT scanning. While the X-ray tube and array of fixed detectors rotate continuously, the patient on the table is gently moved through the scanner gantry, resulting in a helical pattern of exposure.*

also detected) of scans acquired in this fashion is less than that for those scans acquired via a complete 360° rotation at each level and table incrementation between scans. However, the scan time is markedly reduced and it is now possible to complete a whole brain scan in 10–14 seconds in restless or uncooperative patients.

Basic physics of CT

Absorption data are acquired as individual two-dimensional bodies of data from a full 360° rotation scan, or as a three-dimensional block of data from helical CT (Fig. 1.5). The

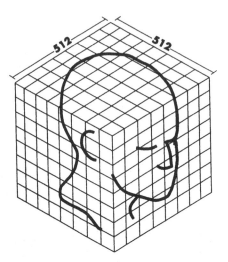

Figure 1.5 *The acquired data can be represented as a stack of tissue slices, each of which is divided into 512 × 512 volume elements (voxels), allowing reconstruction in any plane.*

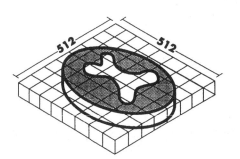

Figure 1.6 *Diagram to demonstrate that the image finally recorded represents a two-dimensional collection of voxels.*

three-dimensional data can be retrospectively reconstructed as a series of two-dimensional slices in any plane, but best resolution is achieved with transverse axial reconstructions. The transverse axial scans when photographed from the cathode ray tube image appear two dimensional, but it is important to realise that they actually represent a three-dimensional body of data (Fig. 1.6). Each scan slice is usually made up of a matrix of 512 × 512 volume elements ('voxels'), the size of which is determined by the chosen slice thickness (the thickness of the irradiated brain) in the z axis and the chosen 'field of view' in the x and y axes. For instance, when a patient is scanned using a standard brain scan slice thickness of 10mm, a square 25.6cm field of view and a 512 × 512 matrix, each voxel can be represented as a rectangular box 10mm × 0.5mm × 0.5mm (Fig. 1.7).

The average density of each voxel is calculated by the computer applying one of a number of different algorithms to the hundreds of thousands of absorption readings obtained during each scan. The density measurements are presented in arbitrary units known as 'Hounsfield units'. It is important to note that these absolute numbers can be reproduced accurately only if the CT scanner is calibrated daily and that the actual numbers may vary quite markedly from one brand of scanner to another.

If a voxel is composed entirely of one type of tissue, the calculated density will rea-

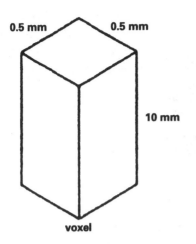

Figure 1.7 *Each individual voxel has dimensions that are dependent on the field of view and slice thickness chosen. For a 25.6cm field of view and slice thickness of 10mm, the voxel dimensions are 0.5mm × 0.5mm × 10mm.*

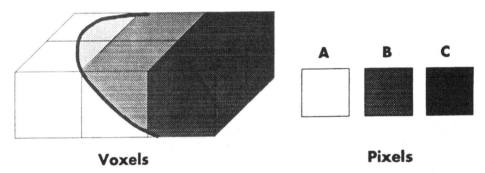

Voxels   **Pixels**

Figure 1.8 *Enlargement of three adjacent voxels containing varying proportions of CSF and brain tissue and the relative brightness of the resulting picture elements (pixels).*

sonably accurately represent the true tissue density. If, however, the voxel contains more than one tissue type, the calculated density will be somewhere between the true densities of the two tissues. For instance, if a voxel contains 50% cerebrospinal fluid (CSF) and 50% brain tissue, the average density will be below that of normal brain tissue and above that of pure CSF (Fig. 1.8). The imprudent interpreter may report that the voxel contains brain tissue of pathologically reduced density and no CSF. This pitfall is sometimes labeled the 'partial volume phenomenon' and is of particular significance when areas and volumes of tissues, or of CSF, are being calculated. The potential error can be reduced by reducing the scan slice width, ensuring that the voxels are more likely to contain only one tissue type.

The average density of each voxel is represented on the cathode ray tube image as a two-dimensional pixel with a brightness directly proportional to the calculated density. Very dense materials such as bone and calcium are very bright (white), while low-density

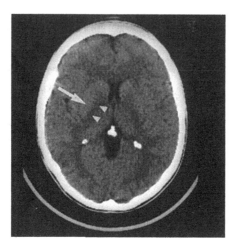

Figure 1.9 *Normal axial CT scan of brain. Note the slight but definite decrease in the density of the internal capsule (arrowheads) compared with the gray matter within the adjacent lentiform nucleus (arrow).*

materials such as CSF and fat are black. Gray matter is more cellular dense than white matter so is represented as lighter shades of gray than white matter. Gray– white differentiation should be clearly seen in normal patients on all modern CT scanners (Fig. 1.9).

By convention, images are presented as if the viewer is looking at the brain from below, so that the right side of the brain is on the viewer's left.

Most pathological processes are associated with the abnormal accumulation of extravascular fluid, so that the abnormal tissue appears less dense (blacker) than normal brain. Infarction, demyelination, inflammation, gliosis, most neoplasms and cyst formation are pathological processes that obey this general rule (Fig. 1.10). Tissues that appear hyperdense (whiter) relative to normal brain tissue include calcified gliomas and metastases, calcified tubers, most meningiomas, colloid cysts, some primary lymphomas, thrombosis and acute hemorrhage (Fig. 1.11).

Contrast enhancement

The difference between the densities of normal and abnormal tissues can be exaggerated, or 'enhanced', by the use of iodinated intravenous contrast media. Iodine has a high atomic number so is an efficient absorber of X-rays. Brain and spinal cord capillaries are unique in the body in that under normal circumstances they do not leak small molecules such as proteins and contrast media. This characteristic appears to be the result of a number of factors, chief of which are tight intercellular junctions and thickened basement membranes of the endothelial cells (Sage & Wilson, 1994). This combination of factors constitutes the 'blood brain barrier'. Breakdown of this barrier is a characteristic feature of a number of pathological conditions, including many tumors, abscesses, subacute infarcts and demyelination. Blood brain barrier breakdown permits leakage of intravascularly administered contrast media into the extravascular space, resulting in locally increased density. This phenomenon is commonly referred to as 'contrast enhancement' (Fig. 1.12).

Some normal tissues are also 'enhanced' after the administration of intravenous contrast media. Blood vessels appear dense because they contain considerably more contrast medium than extravascular tissues. The falx, petroclinoid ligaments, tentorium cerebelli, pituitary gland and the choroid plexus normally enhance vividly, as their parent tissues are not derived from neural tissue and their capillaries contain endothelial cells with fenestrated intercellular junctions (Fig. 1.13).

Indications for intravenous contrast medium

Intravenous contrast medium should be used when there is any clinical suspicion that one of the pathological processes associated with blood brain barrier breakdown is present. Therefore, patients presenting with seizures of late onset, progressive neurological deficit, symptoms and signs of raised intracranial pressure and symptoms or signs suggesting encephalitis or meningitis all should have contrast-enhanced studies in addition to a plain or precontrast study. Assessment for possible cerebral atrophy, acute trauma and acute stroke, however, are indications for plain studies alone.

Physiological studies with CT

Limited information regarding cerebral blood flow (CBF) can be obtained from any CT scanner capable of repeating scans at intervals of between one and five seconds after an intravenous bolus of iodinated contrast medium (Davis et al., 1987). Multiple 'regions of interest' may be selected electronically at the CT scanner workstation and the average density of the pixels in that region of interest plotted against time before, during and after the bolus injection. Standard software packages permit the values to be graphically represented, comparing similar regions on each side of the brain (Fig. 1.14). A more accurate representation of blood transit time can be obtained by constructing a gamma variate curve from the raw data (Hopper et al., 1987). Drawbacks of the technique are that true blood flow cannot be measured, as iodinated contrast medium does not constitute

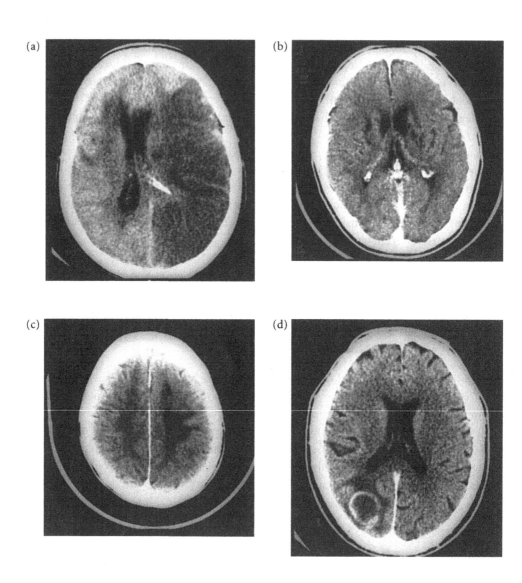

a truly diffusible tracer, and that it relies on comparison with the other side of the brain rather than being able to produce absolute measures of blood transit time.

    True blood flow can be measured by CT when diluted gaseous, nonradioactive xenon is administered by mask to the patient during dynamic scanning (Johnson *et al.*, 1991). A major advantage of this technique is that it provides accurate spatial representation and resolution in the transverse axial plane. Disadvantages include the need to administer the gas in near anesthetic doses, adding a degree of invasiveness and morbidity not shared by other techniques of CBF estimation. There is some evidence that xenon itself may increase or decrease the blood flow by as much as 30% and both the iodinated contrast medium and xenon methods are limited to only one axial slice of brain.

(e)

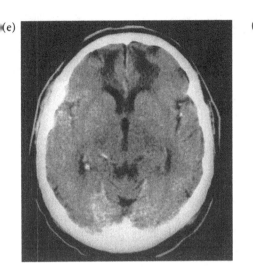

(f)

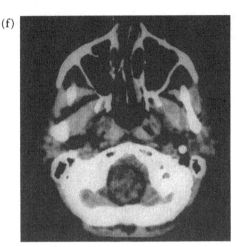

(g)

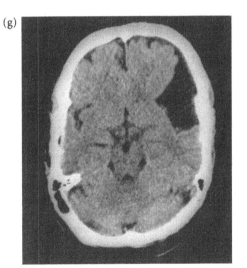

Figure 1.10 *Pathological processes associated with the abnormal accumulation of extravascular fluid (tissue appears blacker than normal tissue). (a) Large, acute left middle and posterior cerebral territory infarct, with marked mass effect. (b) Multiple lacunar infarcts in the basal ganglia and internal capsules bilaterally. (c) Irregular, low-density foci of demyelination in the left centrum semiovale in a patient with clinically definite multiple sclerosis. (d) Right parietooccipital abscess with low-density center and enhancing margin after intravenous contrast medium and surrounding vasogenic edema. (e) Bilateral frontal white matter zones of posttraumatic gliosis, following severe head injury. (f) Rounded ependymoma at foramen magnum contains areas of mixed low and normal density. (g) Sharply defined left frontal extraaxial arachnoid cyst.*

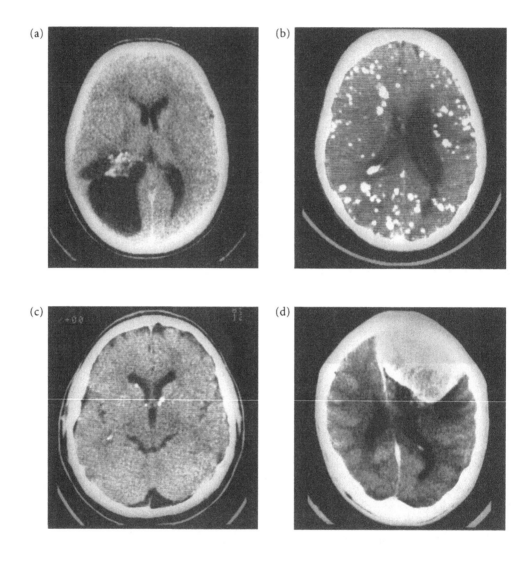

Figure 1.11 *Pathological conditions in which tissues appear hyperdense (whiter) relative to normal brain tissue. (a) Partially cystic, calcified subependymoma immediately adjacent to the trigone of the right lateral ventricle. (b) Multiple, heavily calcified breast metastases scattered throughout the whole brain. (c) Several calcified tubers in characteristic subependymal position in a patient with tuberose sclerosis. (d) Large, dense left frontal convexity meningioma. (e) Ovoid, uniformly dense colloid cyst of the third ventricle, causing marked dilatation of the lateral ventricles. (f) Slightly dense lymphoma infiltrating the lateral wall of the left lateral ventricle (arrow). (g) Hyperdense tip of basilar artery (arrow) caused by thrombus in patient with an acute brain stem stroke. (h) Acute hemorrhage in the genu of the corpus callosum (arrowheads). Note old gliotic scar in the right frontal white matter (arrow) after previous hemorrhage.*

(e)

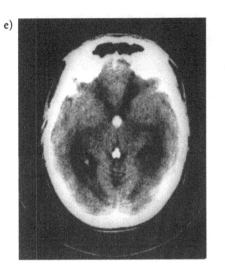

(f)

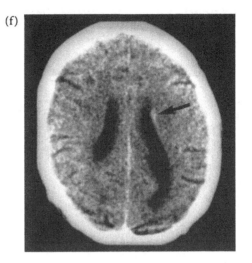

(g)

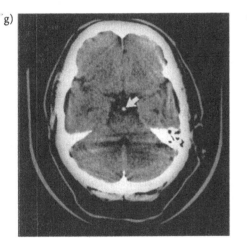

(h)

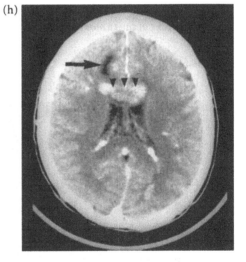

(a) (b)

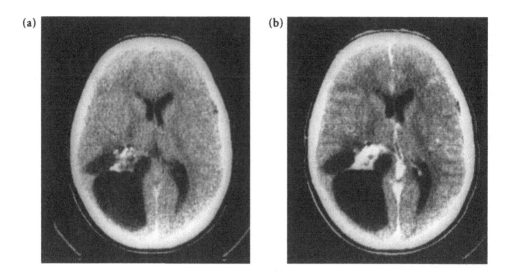

Figure 1.12 *Calcified subependymoma (same as Fig. 11a) before (a) and after (b) intravenous contrast medium, showing increase in density of the central portion of the tumor mass.*

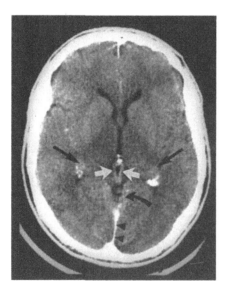

Figure 1.13 *Normal axial CT scan after intravenous contrast medium. Note increased density (enhancement) of the falx (arrowheads), the tentorium cerebelli (curved arrow), the choroid plexus (arrows) and normal vessels, such as the internal cerebral veins (short thick arrows).*

CT angiography

If scans are performed rapidly during the intravenous infusion of iodinated contrast media, intraluminal blood can be rendered very dense relative to extravascular tissue. If the scan table is incremented rapidly between scans, a three-dimensional data set can be accumulated in which blood vessels appear white (Tress *et al.*, 1986). Applying the same computer reconstruction algorithm used for magnetic resonance angiography ('maximal pixel intensity algorithm'), blood vessels can be viewed as two-dimensional images in any plane or can be shaded to give a three-dimensional appearance (Fig. 1.15).

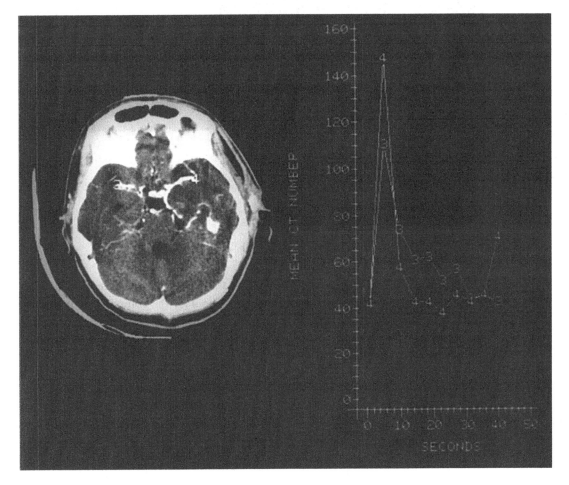

Figure 1.14 *Axial CT scan from a series taken during and immediately after a rapid intravenous bolus of contrast medium, and a graph of average Hounsfield units (density readings) from the selected regions of interest plotted against time.*

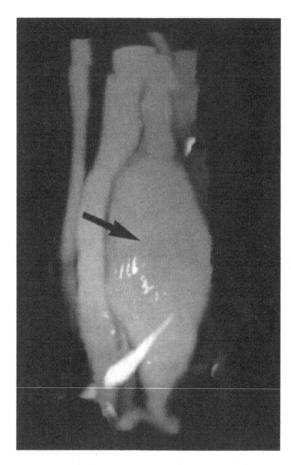

Figure 1.15 *Three-dimensional reconstruction of a carotid bifurcation obtained from a helical scan of the neck during a slow intravenous injection of contrast medium. Note the fusiform aneurysm of the proximal portion of the internal carotid artery (arrow).*

The only real drawback of the technique is that the dense calcium of heavily calcified plaques may be incorporated within the 'lumen', because the computer is unable to differentiate between the density of calcium and that of contrast medium. Nevertheless, this technique provides another method of viewing the carotid bifurcation in the neck and of evaluating the circle of Willis.

CT linear measurements and ratios

Using an electronic cursor supplied with the CT scanner workstation, point-to-point measurements can be performed simply and ratios calculated. Ratios commonly used in

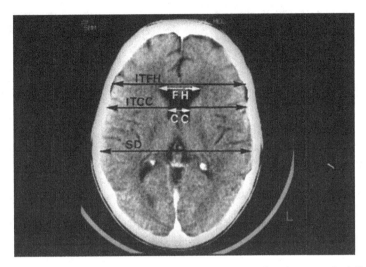

Figure 1.16 *Commonly used linear measures and ratios. FH, the bifrontal distance i.e. the maximum width of the frontal horns; ITFH, the distance between the outer tables of the skull in the transverse plane at the level of maximum width of the frontal horns; CC, the intercaudate distance, the minimum distance between the caudate heads in the transverse plane at the level of the foramina of Monro; ITCC, the distance between the inner tables of the skull at the level of the minimum intercaudate distance; SD, the maximum distance between the inner tables of the skull in the transverse plane. CC/ITCC (the bicaudate ratio) is normally 0.09± 0.02. FH/SD (Evans' ratio) is normally < 0.30. FH/ITFH (the bifrontal ratio) is normally 0.30± 0.02. FH/CC (bifrontal distance divided by the intercaudate distance) is normally 3.11± 0.68.*

the estimation of lateral ventricular size are the bifrontal ratio, the bicaudate ratio and Evans' ratio (Fig. 1.16).

It must be kept in mind that the size of normal ventricles and sulci increase very gradually during the first four decades of life. They then increase more rapidly until the age of 60, after which the increase is almost exponential (Fig. 1.17). This is clearly relevant to the diagnosis of hydrocephalus and atrophy. A very useful distinction between the two is the relative size of the temporal horns. In obstructive hydrocephalus, whatever its cause, the temporal horns are increased in size at least as much as the remainder of the lateral ventricles, while in atrophy the temporal horns are usually less prominent relative to the remainder of the ventricular system (Fig. 1.18).

(a)

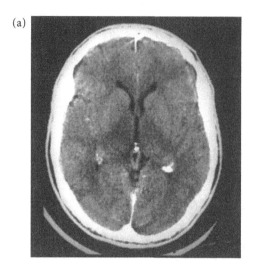

(b)

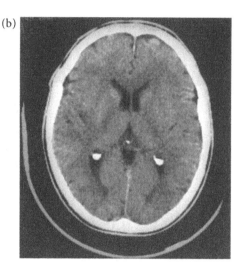

(c)

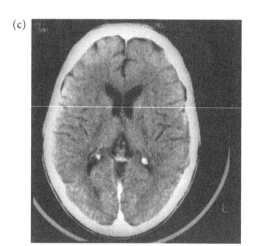

Figure 1.17 *Normal lateral ventricular size at (a) 20, (b) 40 and (c) 70 years of age.*

CT volumetrics

Because CSF has a significantly lower density than brain tissue, it is possible to calculate the number of pixels in each slice corresponding to CSF and brain tissue. These numbers are then multiplied by the slice thickness to obtain volumetric estimations. The calculated volumes from each slice can be added to obtain whole brain values. Ventricular volumes are more accurately calculated than are those of sulci and subarachnoid space, because of 'partial volume artefacts' near the inner aspect of the skull vault. Relative volumes of gray and white matter cannot be calculated accurately by CT because the density differences between them are too small.

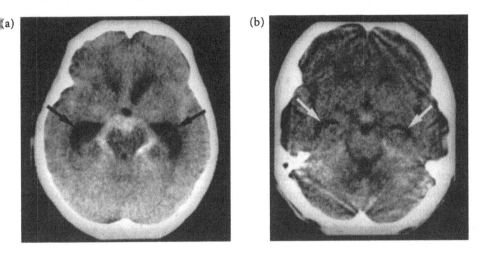

Figure 1.18 *Using a CT scan to distinguish hydrocephalus and atrophy. Note the prominent temporal horns (arrows) in communicating hydrocephalus caused by subarachnoid hemorrhage (a) compared with their size (arrows) relative to the remainder of the lateral ventricles in cerebral atrophy (b).*

Risks and adverse reactions

The risks associated with CT are threefold.

1. Radiation

CT uses ionizing radiation in the form of X-rays. Even though the beam is carefully collimated, the radiation dose can be large. The maximum skin dose for any single scan is of the order of 30–50 milligray (3–5 rad), or 30–50 times the annual natural background radiation exposure. However, scatter from the irradiation of adjacent slices increases this by a factor of about 1.4 and the total dose is again doubled if scans are repeated after intravenous contrast is administered. The minimal radiation dose required to produce lens cataracts is 2 gray (200 rad). As the dose is cumulative, this dose can be quickly reached if multiple repeat CT scans are added to by cerebral angiography and other X-rays of the cranium. It has been shown that the lens dose during head scans can be reduced by a factor of eight by angling the plane of scanning along the supraorbito–meatal line (the line between the superior margin of the orbit and the center of the external meatus) instead of the orbito–meatal line (the line between the outer canthus of the eye and the center of the external meatus). In the latter case, the lenses are in the direct path of the incident X-ray beam.

2. Contrast medium reactions

The risk of reactions varies with the contrast medium used. The older, considerably cheaper ionic contrast media have a four to six times greater adverse reaction rate than modern, nonionic contrast media. The more severe reactions include anaphylaxis, bronchospasm, severe hypotension and death. The death rate with ionic, high osmolar contrast media is about 1 in 40000, compared with approximately 1 in 250000 for the low osmolar, nonionic contrast media. The risks are greatest in those who have had previous reactions to contrast media, the elderly, those with cardiac or renal disease and asthmatics.

Nonionic contrast media are almost exclusively used in the UK, Australia and New Zealand, but in the USA, where ionic contrast media are a factor of 20 times cheaper than nonionic contrast media, intravenous ionic contrast media are still widely used.

3. Sedation

Sedation is often used for confused, uncooperative patients, many of whom are elderly and particularly sensitive to even small doses of benzodiazapines. Confused patients sedated in the wards prior to transfer to the radiology department often appear adequately sedated while lying undisturbed in bed or on a trolley but become agitated when restrained in the head holder of the CT scanner. Half revolution scans (data acquired over only half a full revolution in as little as half a second) can be tried in conjunction with sedation, but they are even more sensitive to movement-induced artefacts. It is frequently more appropriate to have the scan performed with the patient anesthetized, rather than run the risk of obtaining a suboptimal scan from movement-induced artefact, or the induction of a respiratory arrest.

CT versus magnetic resonance imaging

Although magnetic resonance imaging (MRI) is superior to CT in a number of physical and technical aspects (see Chapter 1(b)), CT still has several significant advantages compared with MRI. It is cheaper, more widely available, less claustrophobic and faster. Because scans of single slices can be performed in one second or less and a whole brain can be scanned in 20 seconds, even cerebrally irritated or confused patients can often be

a)
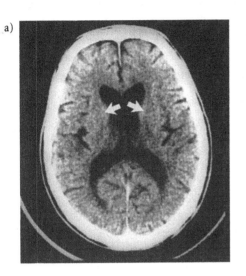
(b)
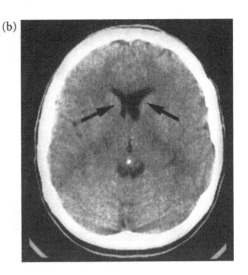

Figure 1.19 *In Huntington's disease, the caudate heads (arrows) are relatively flattened (a) compared with a normal subject of the same age (b).*

scanned without general anesthesia. Acute hematomas are easily distinguishable from acute infarcts because of their increased density (Figs. 1.11*h* and 1.18*a*) as opposed to the characteristic hypodensity of ischemic, nonhemorrhagic infarcts (Figs. 1.10*a,b*) and even subarachnoid hemorrhage can be diagnosed in 90% of patients (Fig. 1.18*a*). For these reasons, CT remains the modality of choice in acute stroke and acute head trauma.

However, CT is incapable of diagnosing hippocampal sclerosis, the most common cause of partial complex seizures, and is less sensitive to tumors, white matter diseases and inflammatory disease. MRI is, therefore, the preferred first imaging investigation for seizures.

CT has been cited as a sensitive method of diagnosing Alzheimer's disease (AD) in severe cases by simply measuring the interuncal distance (Dahlbeck *et al.*, 1991) or the minimum thickness of the medial temporal lobe (Jobst *et al.*, 1992), but the best method for mild and moderate cases is MRI, using both experienced observers (O'Brien *et al.*, 1994) and volumetric analysis (Desmond *et al.*, 1994). These methods take advantage of the ability of MRI to detect preferential shrinkage of hippocampal structures, the amygdaloid bodies and the entorhinal segments of the parahippocampal gyri. MRI is also more sensitive to chronic ischemic changes so is more effective in the diagnosis of vascular dementia, although it must be remembered that up to 60% of psychometrically normal people over the age of 60 will have some white matter changes on MRI. CT has been used to distinguish between other causes of dementia, such as normal pressure hydrocephalus, which shows the changes of communicating hydrocephalus on imaging studies (Fig. 1.18*a*), Huntington's disease (Fig. 1.19) and chronic subdural hematomas

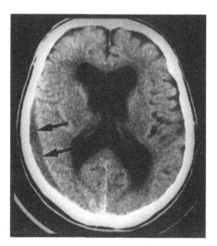

Figure 1.20 *A right parietal extracerebral low-density fluid collection (arrows) represents a chronic subdural hematoma.*

(Fig. 1.20). However, volumetric measurement of the caudate heads in Huntington's disease is more accurate using MRI, and CSF flow measurements obtainable only with MRI have been found to be useful in differentiating normal pressure hydrocephalus from atrophy. Overall, MRI is the preferred investigation for dementia once the decision has been made to investigate.

CT can be performed upon patients with contraindications to MRI, such as pacemakers, aneurysm clips or intraocular metallic foreign bodies. Most patients who suffer claustrophobia in an MRI scanner can tolerate the much less confined space of the CT scanner gantry. CT is very sensitive to calcification, which can be completely undetectable on MRI, and spatial resolution of bony structures, including the skull base, is exquisitely demonstrated by CT. Therefore, CT continues to play a very significant role in brain imaging.

1(b)   Magnetic resonance imaging

Patricia Desmond and Brian Tress

The technique of MRI has become an essential tool in the evaluation of neurological disease. Not only is it an important adjunct to CT but in many cases it is the imaging method of choice.

MRI has its roots in the pioneering work of Bloch, Purcell and others in the first half of the century (Bloch, Hansen & Packard, 1946; Purcell, Torry & Pound, 1946). However, more than 40 years elapsed between the first description of the phenomenon of nuclear magnetic resonance (NMR) and the production of the first images of human anatomy by groups at the University of Nottingham in 1976 and 1977. The development and widespread clinical dissemination of these devices occurred in the 1980s.

Basic physics of MRI

Human tissue contains significant amounts of water, proteins, lipids and other macromolecules, which are abundant in hydrogen atoms the nuclei of which are positively charged particles called protons. MRI relies on the fact that protons are magnetically active.

Protons can be thought of as spinning around their own internal axis (Fig. 1.21). One of the fundamental features of electromagnetism is that a moving charge creates its own small magnetic field. In the case of a spinning proton, this self-produced magnetic field is referred to as its magnetic moment.

When patients are placed in a strong magnetic field, the spinning protons inside their bodies can take up one of only two possible orientations. Each proton is either aligned along the direction of or in the opposite direction to the strong magnetic field (Fig. 1.22).

When radiofrequency (rf) pulses of just the right energy (called the Larmor or resonant frequency) are applied, some of the protons aligned with the strong magnetic field will absorb this energy and reverse their direction. The absorbed energy is then emitted as a radiofrequency pulse given off as the protons return to, or 'relax' back to,

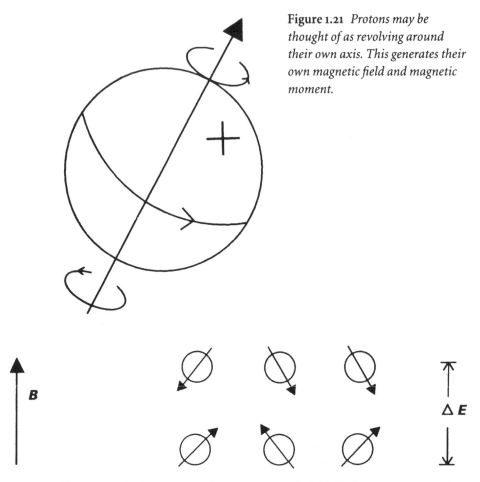

Figure 1.21 *Protons may be thought of as revolving around their own axis. This generates their own magnetic field and magnetic moment.*

Figure 1.22 *In the presence of a strong magnetic field, B, the protons magnetic moments are either aligned with or against the direction of the external field. Each of these states is associated with a different energy.*

their original alignment (and energy). This emitted pulse can be spatially encoded to construct an MR image (Fig. 1.23).

The rate at which the protons relax to their original orientation is determined by two parameters: T_1 (the spin-lattice or longitudinal relaxation) and T_2 (the spin–spin or transverse relaxation) (Fig. 1.24). The observed range of T_1 and T_2 relaxation rates of soft tissues is much greater than the simple variations in tissue density used to provide contrast in plain film X-rays or CT. MRI, therefore, provides substantially improved soft tissue contrast.

In summary, protons have a magnetic moment. An MR image is made by placing a patient inside a strong magnet and pulsing them with a radiowave. The patient's body then emits a radio signal which is received and used to generate the MR image.

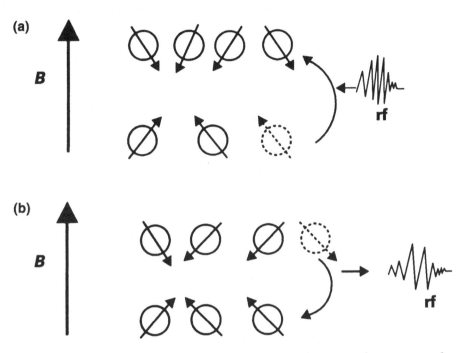

Figure 1.23 *(a) A radiofrequency (rf) pulse at the Larmor frequency may be absorbed by protons in the low-energy state (aligned in the direction of the external field) allowing them to flip to the higher energy state (aligned against the field). (b) As the protons relax back to their initial state, an rf pulse will be emitted. This is the signal detected and used to form the MR image.*

The MRI system

The components of an MRI system are a magnet to produce the field, a radiofrequency system to transmit and receive signals, a gradient system for spatial encoding and a computer system to control the process and to reconstruct the images (Fig. 1.25).

The magnet

The purpose of the magnet is to provide a strong, uniform field to surround the patient. The strength of a magnetic field is measured in units of tesla (T) or gauss (1 tesla equals 10 000 gauss). The magnetic field used for MRI is typically 1.5 T, which is a field strength about 30 000 times greater than the magnetic field of the earth.

Most magnets in clinical use are superconducting magnets. However, not all

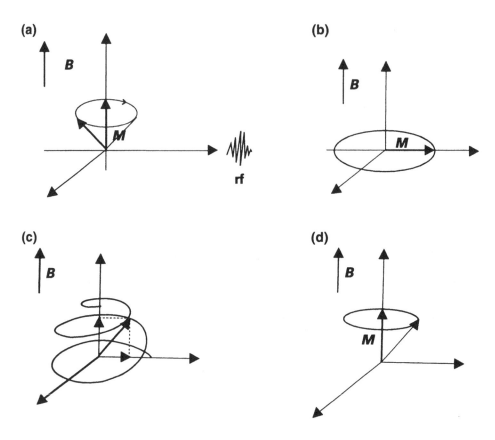

Figure 1.24 *(a) Spinning protons placed in an external magnetic field* B *tend to align with the external field and may be thought of as having a net longitudinal magnetization* M. *(b) After the application of a 90° radiofrequency pulse, the longitudinal magnetisation is tipped into the transverse plane. At this point the longitudinal magnetisation is zero and the transverse magnetisation is maximal and equal to* M. *(c and d) With relaxation, the magnetization vector* M *slowly returns (in a spiral course) to its original position. The loss of transverse magnetization is called transverse relaxation.*

magnetic fields are created using superconductors. The magnet and the shims (shimming coils) may also be made of resistive or permanent magnets or combinations thereof. Resistive magnets require constant direct current power supplies and are not a practical option when very high field strengths are required, as they are inefficient and generate large amounts of heat.

Permanent magnets cannot provide the higher field strengths used in current imaging equipment. Their practical limit is about 0.3 T, beyond which their use is constrained by the required physical size and weight involved.

The most powerful magnetic fields used are generated using coils of superconducting wires that are made from a combination of titanium and niobium. Commercially available clinical systems use field strengths of up to 1.5 T. Field strengths of up to 4.0 T are used on humans only for research. The safety of rapid scanning at high field strength is yet to be determined.

Liquid helium is needed to keep the wires cooled to a temperature of approximately 4 K ($-269\,°C$). At these temperatures, the wires are in a superconducting state, having no

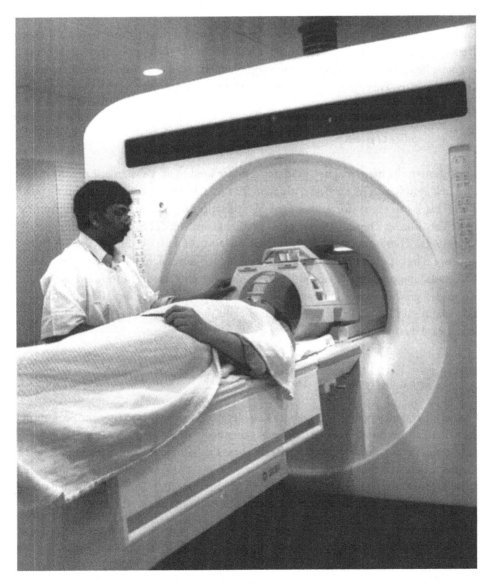

Figure 1.25 *The 1.5 T imaging magnet.*

electrical resistance. In theory, the electrical current, and hence the resultant magnetic field, would need no energy to be maintained. In practice, superconducting magnets require power supplies that are used intermittently to maintain the appropriate current in the supercooled wires. A small amount of liquid helium is also consumed, requiring the supply to be topped-up every four to six weeks. If the coils are allowed to rise above the superconducting temperature, the increased electrical resistance leads to rapid heat production, which will cause the liquid helium to boil off in an uncontrolled manner. This situation is referred to as a 'quench'.

The signal-to-noise ratio is defined as the ratio of the signal intensity detected divided by the intensity of the background noise that is also detected. The signal-to-noise ratio is a major determinant of image quality and is roughly proportional to the strength of the magnetic field. Because it is difficult to obtain a perfectly homogeneous magnetic field, fine adjustments to the main magnetic field are made by mechanical or electrical means. This process is known as shimming the magnet.

Gradient system

In addition to the main magnet, gradient coils are used to vary systematically the magnetic field, producing linear fields, which make slice selection and spatial encoding possible. This is necessary for subsequent identification of the image elements from a particular volume. There are three sets of gradient coils, one for each of the three spatial dimensions. These gradients are switched on and off rapidly during the scanning sequence. The rapid changes in magnetic field induce eddy currents, which in turn tend to degrade image quality. The production of eddy currents, can be minimized by the use of shielded gradient coils. The rapid switching of the gradient fields causes the coils to move slightly and to knock against their anchoring devices, producing the characteristic noise heard during an MR scan.

The radiofrequency system

The radiofrequency system is used both to generate the pulse that excites the protons in the patient's body and to receive the signal generated as these protons relax. The system uses another set of coils for this purpose. In some cases, the same coils are used for both purposes; in others they are specialized for transmission and reception. The signal used to excite the protons is of a very high power (up to 16 000 watts). The signal emitted from the patient is extremely weak (approximately one billionth of a watt). A preamplifier is required to amplify this signal before it can be analyzed for image construction.

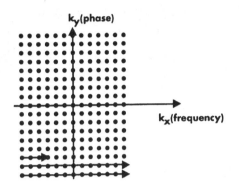

Figure 1.26 *K space is the spatial frequency domain and is related to image space by a Fourier transformation. K space describes the data sampling process. All frequency points are collected at each phase step before proceeding to the next phase step.*

Image formation

The amplified signal from the patient is transferred to the main computer for image formation. An MR image consists of a display of spatially localized signal intensities (voxels), the spatial localization having been provided by the gradient coils. A gradient that selects only a particular slice (in the z axis) is turned on during the radiowave excitation so that only the protons in that slice absorb the energy in the pulse (all other slices are said to be 'off resonance'). Two other gradients (the frequency and the phase-encoding gradients) are used to determine the x and y coordinates of a point in the slice from which the signal is coming.

The computer uses a Fourier transform to analyze the mixture of signals coming from the slice, determining the intensity of the phase and frequency components and thereby generating the appropriate intensity for each x–y coordinate (Fig. 1.26).

Image contrast

Aside from the overall field strength and the density of protons, the strength and contrast of the detected signal depends on timing parameters that are set by the operator. These parameters control the time between successive radiowave pulses (TR), the time between excitation and sampling (TE) and the strength and number of radiofrequency pulses employed. Contrast is also dependent on the two relaxation constants of the tissue being examined (T_1 and T_2). Relaxation occurs in three dimensions but images are presented in two dimensions. T_1 represents relaxation in the longitudinal direction and T_2 relaxation in the transverse direction.

The contrast of particular features varies depending on whether the images are T_1 weighted, T_2 weighted or proton-density weighted (also called spin- density weighted). It is not technically possible to reconstruct a pure T_1 or T_2 image. Weighted images are predominantly based on T_1 or T_2 relaxation but contain some element of the alternate relaxation parameter. Tumors and other tissues with a large amount of freely mobile

(a)
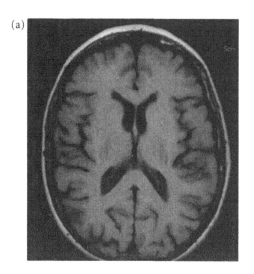

(b)
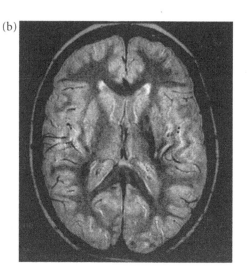

(c)
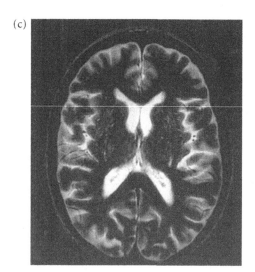

Figure 1.27 *Axial images in a normal 73-year-old female. (a) T₁ axial spin echo image. The CSF is low signal intensity (black) and the white matter is slightly increased in signal intensity compared with the adjacent gray matter. (b) Proton density image. CSF is relatively low signal intensity and the white matter is reduced in signal intensity compared with the gray matter. (c) T₂-weighted image. CSF is high signal intensity (white) and white matter is reduced in signal intensity when compared with the gray matter. T₂-weighted images have more contrast but less anatomical definition than T₁-weighted images.*

water usually appear dark in T_1-weighted images, but bright in proton-density and T_2-weighted images. In general, the T_1-weighted images give a sharper definition of anatomy and the T_2-weighted sequences have more contrast and are more sensitive to the water shifts often associated with pathological states. For most clinical studies, all three types of image are used, with each contributing to the differentiation between normal and abnormal states (Fig. 1.27). More strongly T_1-weighted sequences, called inversion recovery sequences, can be used to further increase contrast when detailed anatomy is an imaging requirement (Fig. 1.28).

Fast imaging techniques

One limitation of standard imaging is the time taken to acquire the information. Usually patients are required to keep still for between three and twelve minutes. In recent times, faster imaging techniques have been developed to ameliorate this situation. These are generically referred to as gradient echo scans (GRE). In conventional imaging (spin echo), a radiofrequency pulse is used to form the echo. In gradient echo imaging the same gradients used for spatial localization are also used to create the echo. This means that slices can now be obtained in seconds rather than minutes. This type of scanning is particularly useful when a three-dimensional data set is to be imaged, rather than a single two-dimensional slice (Fig. 1.29). Obtaining three-dimensional data has the additional advantage of allowing reformatting in any other plane. Even faster imaging will be available in the future when echo planar imaging (EPI) will allow images to be obtained in as little as 45 milliseconds.

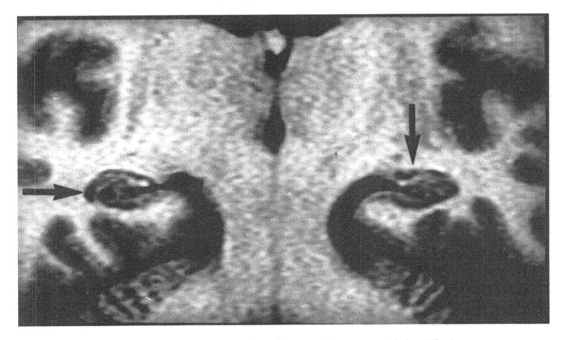

Figure 1.28 *Coronal inversion recovery images of the temporal lobes. The internal structure of the hippocampi (arrows) can be seen. A small cyst of the hippocampal fissure is seen on the right, and the white matter of the alveus running over the superior aspect of the hippocampus on the left is well displayed.*

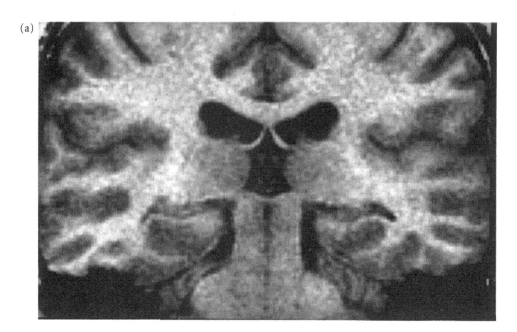

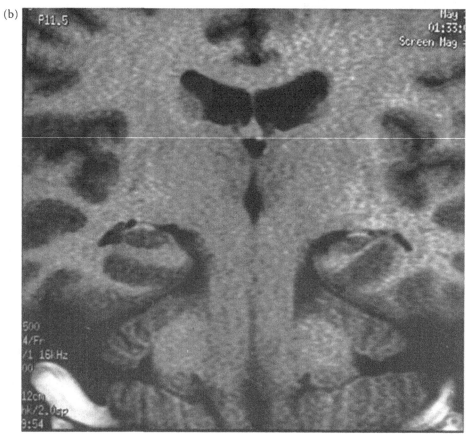

Figure 1.29 *Fast scans. (a) Fast spoiled grass images (FSPGR). A three-dimensional data set with 125 images can be obtained in 12 minutes. These images show comparable detail to the two-dimensional acquisition . (b) Inversion recovery images. With this two-dimensional acquisition, 12 images were obtained in 10 minutes.*

MR volumetrics

With the aid of appropriate computer software, the many thin slices obtained with gradient echo imaging can be used to measure volumes of regions of the brain. Accurate measurements of regions as small as the hippocampus are readily obtainable. These are already of clinical use in the diagnosis of temporal lobe epilepsy and may be of use in the diagnosis of AD (Desmond *et al.*, 1994). It is also possible to measure total brain and CSF volumes, as well as determine the volume of total cerebral gray and white matter. This can be done with an accuracy of approximately 2–3% (Harris *et al.*, 1994). The role of MR volumetrics in the assessment of disease states will be determined by the clinical demand and value of what is still a somewhat time-consuming endeavor.

Contrast

Gadolinium, a rare earth element, is a paramagnetic substance and is the contrast agent used in MR imaging. Gadolinium is toxic in its free state and so must be bound to diethylenetriamine pentaacetic acid (DTPA) to eliminate its toxicity. The biodistribution of gadolinium chelates in the vascular and interstitial compartments is similar to that of iodinated contrast agents. Contrast enhancement is seen on T_1-weighted images. In brain imaging it is used to highlight breaks in the blood brain barrier that are commonly associated with pathological states such as tumors and metastases. One of the major advantages of gadolinium chelates over iodinated contrast is their increased safety margin. Severe reactions are rare (approximately 1 in 350000) (Goldstein *et al.*, 1990).

Safety

There are a few absolute contraindications to MRI. Patients with pacemakers, implanted neurostimulators, cochlear implants, metal in the eye and older ferromagnetic intracranial aneurysm clips should not be placed in an MRI scanner. A patient with a pacemaker is likely to suffer an arrhythmia as a result of currents induced in the pacemaker by changes in the magnetic field that occur during scanning. Similarly, neurostimulators and cochlear implants will also pick up induced currents leading to aberrant stimulation and/or malfunction. A metallic foreign body in the eye can move within the globe in a strong magnetic field and cause irreversible damage to vision. Torque around the base of

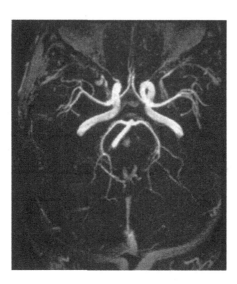

Figure 1.30 *MR angiogram. Circle of Willis in the axial plane.*

an aneurysm clip may open the aneurysmal sac and lead to subarachnoid hemorrhage. One such fatality has been reported. Orthopedic implants do not present a safety problem.

Although there is no convincing evidence to suggest a risk to the fetus, pregnancy is considered a relative contraindication to MRI, especially in the first trimester.

Approximately 5% of patients will experience claustrophobia in the scanner. This can often be allayed by discussion, calming music or, when necessary, anxiolytic drugs.

The safety of very rapid (echo planar) imaging remains under investigation. The increased speed and strength of the gradient fields used in such rapid imaging are capable of inducing currents in peripheral nerves. Muscle twitching and/or pain may be felt. The threshold for cardiac stimulation is at least an order of magnitude higher than that for skeletal muscle and no arrthythmias have been generated. However further studies must be performed to determine the safety of rapid scanning at high field strengths.

Magnetic resonance angiography

Magnetic resonance angiography (MRA) is a technique of obtaining an 'angiogram' in approximately 10 to 12 minutes without even requiring an intravenous injection of contrast medium (Fig. 1.30).

Blood flowing into the imaging plane has increased signal compared with the surrounding tissue. This is often referred to as a 'time of flight' effect. This effect can be maximized by using gradient echo techniques. The images produced have very high signal within the blood vessels and have a uniformly low signal in background structures. These images are called the partitions, or the source images, and form the basis of the MR angiogram. They can be obtained as a two- or three-dimensional data set. The MR angiogram is constructed by using a computer algorithm to select only those elements of maximum signal intensity (MIP) from each of these images. From these a two- or three-dimensional projection of the vessels is formed.

At present MRA lacks the resolution of conventional catheter angiography. However, it is already a useful screening test in the assessment of carotid disease and the detection of asymptomatic intracerebral aneurysms.

Applications of MRI scanning

MRI is the imaging method of choice in a wide variety of neurological disorders. However, the present limited availability of MR scanners means that for the foreseeable future CT will still be used as the initial screening investigation in most centers. The sensitivity of CT to calcification and acute blood products and its excellent bone detail ensures that it will always have a major role to play in neurological imaging.

Applications and clinical potential of MRI

All types of intracranial tumor (primary, metastatic, intraaxial and extraaxial) are best shown on gadolinium-enhanced T_1-weighted images. MRI is superior to CT in detection of the edema, cysts, vascularity, hemorrhage and necrosis associated with the presence of a cerebral tumor (Fig. 1.31). The improved depiction of the tumor and its associated changes often allows a better choice of biopsy site by the treating neurosurgeon. MRI is more sensitive than CT in detecting metastatic tumors (Davis *et al.*, 1991).

Abnormalities within the white matter are better assessed by MRI than by CT. In one clinical series, the specificity of MRI for the diagnosis of multiple sclerosis (MS) in clinically definite MS was as high as 95% (Yetkin *et al.*, 1991) (Fig. 1.32).

Abnormalities within the white matter are a normal finding in an aging population, occurring in over 60% of those aged above 60 years. There is an increased incidence of white matter changes in patients who have a history of hypertension, ischemic heart disease and cerebrovascular disease. No correlation has been demonstrated between the degree of white matter change within the brain and declining cognitive function. Even

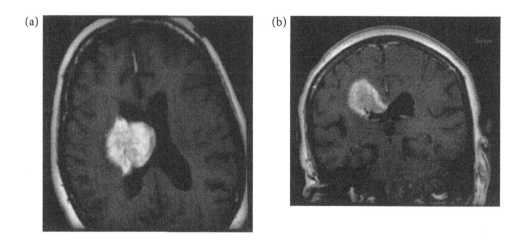

Figure 1.31 *Glioblastoma multiforme. Tumor of the corpus callosum bulges into the right lateral ventricle. The tumor is clearly seen on the postgadolinium axial (a) and coronal (b) images.*

patients with severe white matter changes may have normal cognitive function. However, a patient with a vascular dementia will always show extensive areas of signal abnormality within the cerebral white matter (Fig. 1.33). Therefore the diagnosis of vascular dementia is often impossible on the basis of the scan alone.

Some headway has been made in the imaging diagnosis of AD. Many groups have reported disproportionate atrophy in the amygdala and hippocampus (structures important in the function of memory) in AD patients compared with aged matched controls (e.g. Desmond *et al.*, 1994) (Fig. 1.34).

MRI is the imaging method of choice in the investigation of epilepsy. The most common cause of complex partial seizures is mesial temporal sclerosis. This diagnosis is unable to be made from CT, but MRI is capable of allowing diagnosis of mesial temporal sclerosis (Fig. 1.35) to be made with very high sensitivity and specificity (Jackson *et al.*, 1990). MRI is also able to demonstrate congenital anomalies of brain formation such as pachygyria and gray matter heterotopias, which may be a focus for seizure activity (Fig. 1.36).

MRI is more sensitive than CT in demonstrating acute stroke, and particularly in showing ischemic changes in the brain stem and cerebellum (Fig. 1.37).

Physiological studies such as single photon emission tomography (SPET) or positron emission tomography (PET) provide information about brain function. The development of MR perfusion, functional MR and MR spectroscopy (see below) will provide additional and overlapping information. One of the most important advances for SPET and PET imaging in recent years is the ability to coregister these images with MRI scans.

a)

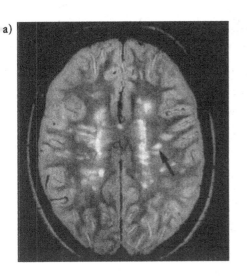

Figure 1.32 *Multiple sclerosis. (a) Proton density image, axial plane: periventricular white matter lesions (arrow) show a lumpy-bumpy configuration, typical of demyelination. (b) Proton density image, sagittal plane. Increased signal intensity at the callosal septal interface (arrow) extending into the corpus callosum is characteristic for demyelination.*

(b)

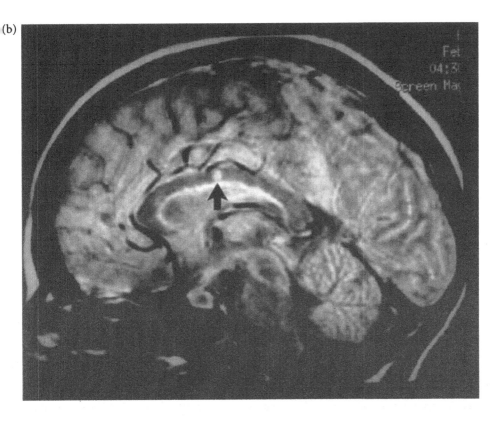

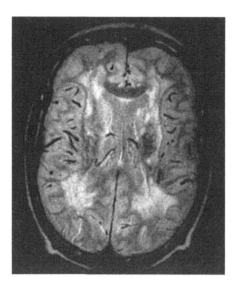

Figure 1.33 *Vascular dementia. Proton density axial images show extensive periventricular and subcortical white matter disease.*

Physiological as well as anatomical information can then be obtained from one combined image.

Future prospects

The advent of faster imaging has been a big factor in the development of new techniques in MR imaging. These include MR diffusion, MR perfusion, MR spectroscopy and functional MRI.

MR diffusion

Molecular self-diffusion is a property of a tissue. It is a measure of molecular mobility, or Brownian (random) motion, within a tissue. Tissues have different diffusion coefficients and this can be used as a source of contrast in diffusion-weighted imaging. Diffusion-weighted imaging has already been shown to be more sensitive than T_2-weighted spin echo imaging in detecting early stroke (Warach, Chien & Li, 1992). Diffusion-weighted imaging may be useful in evaluating the effects of early pharmacological intervention in stroke. It is thought that the initial diffusion image will provide an early quantifiable anatomical marker of ischemic injury.

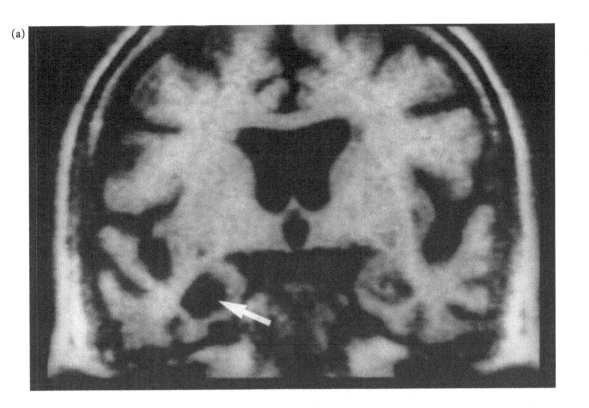

(a)

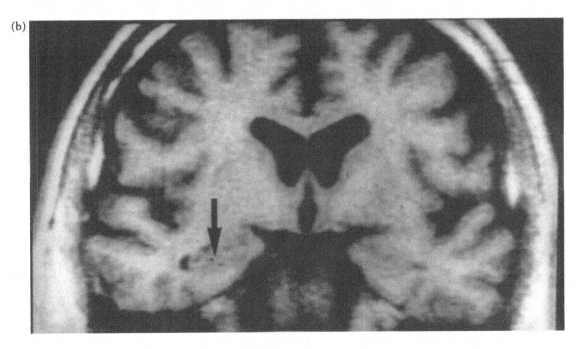

(b)

Figure 1.34 *Coronal inversion recovery images at the level of the interpeduncular fossa in a patient with AD (a) and a normal control (b). There is marked atrophy in the head of the hippocampus in the patient (arrow in (a)), compared with the control (arrow in (b)).*

(a)

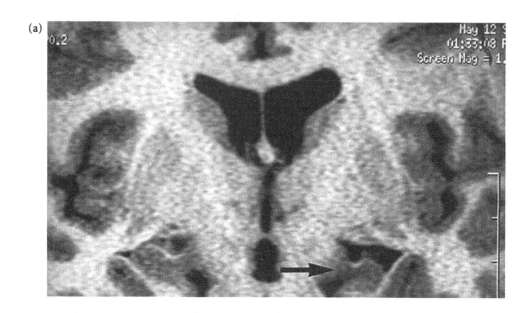

(b)

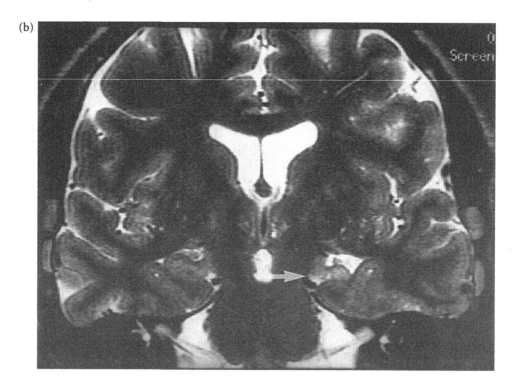

Figure 1.35 *Mesial temporal sclerosis. (a) Inversion recovery coronal image demonstrates marked atrophy of the left hippocampus (arrow). (b) T_2-weighted coronal image shows high signal intensity (arrow) in an atrophic hippocampus.*

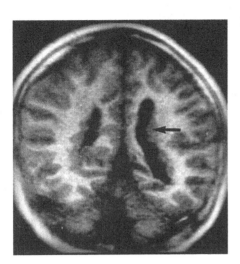

Figure 1.36 *Heterotopic gray matter. Coronal inversion recovery image. Multiple abnormal nodules of gray matter line the lateral ventricles (arrow).*

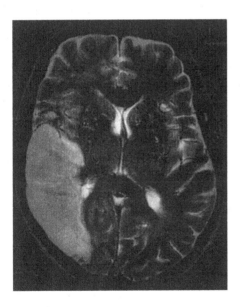

Figure 1.37 *Acute right middle cerebral artery infarct: T_2-weighted axial image. Increased signal is present in the gray and white matter of the lateral segment of the right temporal lobe.*

MR perfusion

MR perfusion imaging relies on fast imaging during the passage of a bolus injection of gadolinium DTPA. The effects of the passage of contrast through the intravascular spaces can be used to give a measure of regional cerebral blood volume. The assessment of perfusion in terms of volume (ml) per weight (100mg) of tissue per minute is not yet obtainable with MR scanning. However, MR perfusion can be used to assess regional cerebral blood volume and these changes closely parallel studies performed with technetium-99m-labeled hexamethylpropyleneamine oxime (HMPAO) SPET.

MR spectroscopy

MR spectroscopy has been used by biochemists for many years to identify constituent chemical elements of a tissue without destruction of the sample. It is only in recent years that an attempt has been made to combine imaging and in vivo spectroscopy. To simplify the spectra generated, the volume sampled must be kept very small, otherwise multiple overlapping spectra will be obtained, and interpretation of the information will be difficult.

At present imaging volumes are of the order of 8–27 cm^3. Early clinical work is promising, with abnormal spectra seen in disease states such as temporal lobe epilepsy, AD and brain infarction (Shonk *et al.*, 1995).

MR imaging of brain activation

One of the most exciting areas of functional MRI is the imaging of brain activation. The working principle is based on the measurable changes in perfusion to the activated region of the brain. This can be performed without the use of intravenous contrast and has been shown to be reliable in detecting the perfusion changes that occur during visual stimulation (Ogawa, Tank & Menon, 1992). Although these techniques are still in their infancy, they promise to become an important aspect of future imaging for neuro-anatomical data and for neurological and psychiatric disorders.

1(c) Single photon and positron emission tomography

Basil Shepstone and Kim Jobst

It is the functional, as opposed to the morphological, capability of nuclear medicine investigations that is their great strength. Initially, the technique involved the injection of suitable gamma-emitting radionuclides into the blood or CSF to produce an image of regional function in the brain (cerebral scintigraphy) or of CSF flow (radionuclide cisternography). Disease was then detected by assessing the degree to which the so-called blood brain barrier could be breached or to what extent the normal channels of CSF flow were altered.

If a solitary gamma-ray detection device, such as a gamma camera, is used to map the radionuclide distribution in one plane at a time, the resulting images are referred to as planar images. Alternatively, if the detector is designed to accumulate images at intervals over 360° around the brain, computer techniques similar to those described in Chapter 1(a) can be used to reconstruct cross-sectional representations of function.

Planar cerebral imaging

Routine cerebral scintigraphy became universally available when appropriate detectors and radionuclides could be combined. The basis of all detection systems is the scintillation unit (Fig. 1.38), containing the all-important sodium iodide crystal and photomultiplier tubes. These constituted the old rectilinear scanners, which preceded the gamma camera, invented by Hal Anger in 1961 (Fig. 1.39). Gamma cameras make use of one large scintillator crystal and a number of photomultiplier tubes arranged so that the spatial relationships of radioactive tracers in the brain can be precisely recorded, stored and displayed in many ways on a screen or as hard copy (Fig. 1.40). Nowadays it is impossible to conceive of a gamma camera system not linked to a computer; this enables so-called regions of interest (ROIs) to be drawn over areas of uptake that can subsequently be aligned with structural maps for anatomical specificity.

These ROIs can also be represented as dynamic activity–time curves, a most useful attribute revealing the functional status of otherwise static anatomical images.

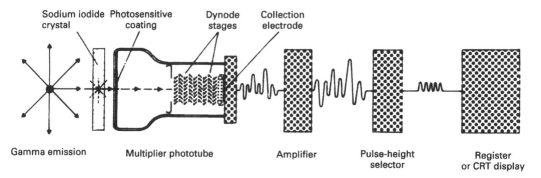

Sodium iodide Photosensitive   Dynode   Collection
crystal   coating   stages   electrode

Gamma emission   Multiplier phototube   Amplifier   Pulse-height   Register
                                                                    selector   or CRT display

Figure 1.38 *The basic scintillation detector. Gamma rays from the patient strike a sensitive sodium iodide crystal, where they are converted into light photons. These, in turn, strike a photosensitive coating and are changed into electrons. The electrons are multiplied by the dynode stages in the photomultiplier until a large number are available to constitute an electrical current. The current is amplified and eventually reaches a television screen. The pulse-height selector filters out pulses produced by the wrong kind of radiation, e.g. cosmic ray activity and unwanted radionuclides administered previously.*

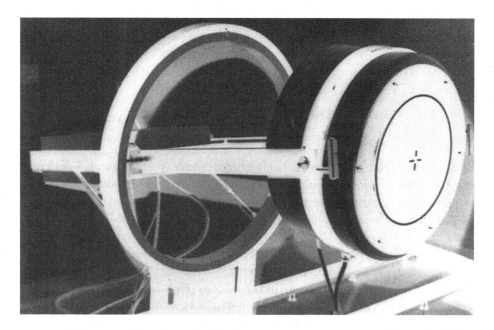

Figure 1.39 *A modern scintillation or gamma camera mounted on a gimball mounting so that the camera can rotate around the patient if necessary to produce cross-sectional images.*

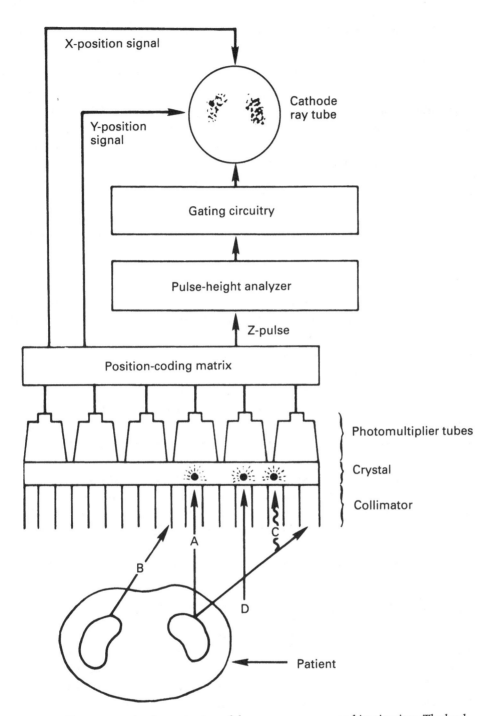

Figure 1.40 *A schematic view of the gamma camera and its circuitry. The lead collimator will only allow parallel rays such as A, C and D to reach the crystal. Rays such as B will be absorbed by the lead. The pulse-height analyzer and gating circuitry will later filter off D (cosmic radiation) and C (scattered radiation) because their energies will not be appropriate. The position-coding matrix circuit will assign the pulse to the correct position on the television screen, which will obviously correspond to the coordinates of the photomultipliers which are activated. The Z-pulse provides intensity.*

The attributes of technetium-99m in the form of the pertechnetate ion, diethylene diaminetetraacetic acid or gluconate made it an ideal tracer for cerebral scintigraphy. Technetium-99m is an easily available radionuclide of nearly pure gamma emission, short half-life and excellent clearance from the body. Therefore, it can safely be administered to the patient in doses capable of producing high count rates and maximum information density.

When pertechnetate is used as a cerebral imaging agent, the normal brain is not visualized because the ion does not cross the normal blood brain barrier. Only if there is a lesion causing the blood brain barrier to 'leak' does uptake occur in the brain itself. The detection of any lesion depends on the uptake of tracer in the surrounding tissue.

The customary procedure in planar brain imaging is to use the injection of tracer to generate what is in effect a cerebral angiogram. Sequential images are recorded at short time intervals, which can later be displayed individually or in so-called 'cine mode'. Otherwise, activity in selected ROIs (e.g. left and right cerebral hemispheres) can be displayed as a function of time. It is then customary to generate an 'equilibrium' or 'blood-pool' image, which is simply a summation of all dynamic images. Finally, late static images are recorded in the antero–posterior, postero–anterior and two lateral projections. Occasionally a view from the top, a vertex projection, is also recorded.

Except for activity in the venous sinuses, such a series of scintigrams will show the normal brain to be relatively clear of activity. However, any lesion involving breakdown of the blood brain barrier will cause a focus of increased uptake. Although this is a sensitive process, it is not specific. Therefore the differential diagnosis of any scintigram in isolation may be wide, making other evidence derived from the clinical history and examination essential to the working diagnosis in many instances. Occasionally the position and/or shape of the uptake may be useful in identifying either diseases or causes of dysfunction, as in the case of strokes or subdural hematomata.

Tumors, strokes, infections and traumatic lesions may all show as foci of increased uptake. An example of a planar cerebral image of a patient with metastases to the brain is shown in Fig. 1.41.

The relatively simple, noninvasive planar cerebral scintigram was, therefore, a sensitive tool for screening. However, it was obvious that it could not compete for anatomical specificity with X-ray CT when it was invented in 1972 (Ambrose & Hounsfield, 1972a,b; Hounsfield 1973). However, the development of X-ray CT was a direct result of pioneering work in nuclear medicine that led to the revolutionary technique of what is now known as emission CT, the adjective 'emission' being used to indicate that the radioactivity is emitted *from* the body, as opposed to transmission CT (conventional CT) where the X-ray beam is transmitted *through* the body. Emission CT should be reduced to the acronym ECT, but because of conflict with another well-known technique, it has instead become known as PET or SPET, standing for positron emission tomography and single photon emission tomography, respectively.

Single photon emission tomography

In 1963, some years before Hounsfield became famous for his invention of X-ray transmission CT, David Kuhl, a medical student at the University of Pennsylvania, and his colleague Dr Edwards hit on the unique idea of obtaining transverse sectional views of the brain (Kuhl & Edwards, 1963). Four small scintillation detectors were arranged to view the patient's head in the anterior, posterior and two lateral directions at the desired level. As they made linear passes across each direction, the radiation events detected were stored on magnetic tape. The detectors were then rotated 15° about the patient's head, still

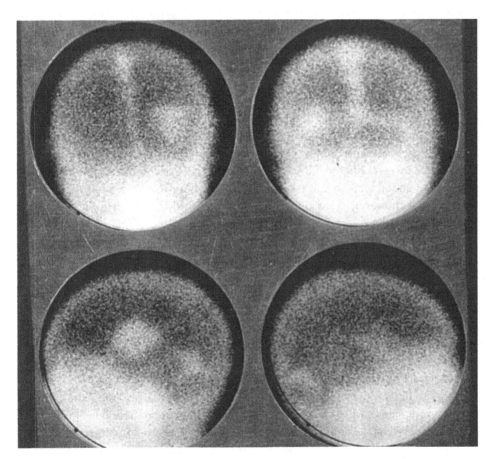

Figure 1.41 *An example of technetium-99m pertechnetate scintigrams showing cerebral metastases from a lung cancer. The radionuclide has penetrated the blood brain barrier into the lesions, depicting them as photon-abundant areas. (Clockwise: anterior, posterior, left lateral and right lateral views. Hardcopy on polaroid film, so areas of high activity are white.)*

in the same plane, and a further series of readings taken. The process was then repeated until the four recorders covered the whole brain. The data were then processed by computer to generate a cross-sectional view of the brain.

It is interesting to note that as early as 1917 the Austrian mathematician Radon showed that a two- or three-dimensional object can be reconstructed from the infinite set of all its projections. These concepts probably were first used to great effect in astronomy and meteorology, where the two-dimensional weather maps reconstructed from satellite readings are well known. There is no mathematical difference between weather satellites recording from earth and detectors recording from a body. The work of Kuhl and Edwards antedated Hounsfield and Cormack's work by some 10 years and it is sad that they were not given a share of the Nobel Prize that accrued to this great achievement in 1979.

Nowadays, the same principle of acquiring such cross-sectional images is still used, but a rotating gamma camera is employed instead of a rectilinear scanner or a static gamma camera, which can only produce planar images.

Planar views will not demonstrate the cross-sectional (or tomographic) distribution of radionuclide in the brain because of the shielding effect of structures lying over and under the plane of interest. For accurate reconstruction of cross-sectional images, count-rate data are acquired at a number of different angles around the head. In order to do this, a gamma camera is used where the camera head is mounted on a swivel bearing so that it can be rotated around the patient, stopping at predetermined angles (e.g. 3° or 5°) to acquire images until the full 360° of rotation have been covered. This is known as the 'step-and-shoot' method and takes about half-an-hour to obtain a full set of data. Some cameras, however, can acquire images continuously rather than by the intermittent step-and-shoot method. Although data are collected over 360°, when they are used to generate the actual images (so-called backprojection) it is usual to average counts in diametrically opposite directions so that only 180 readings are used. Ring detectors are also possible, but their enhanced speed is matched only by their expense.

While tomography improves spatial perception and contrast, spatial resolution is usually no better than with planar imaging and at the surface, at least, is worse. This is because the resolution of an image is largely determined by the distance between the source in the patient and the detector. In tomography, the camera is further from the source than in planar imaging, where there is no revolution of the camera head which can, therefore, be placed much nearer the patient surface.

Using a collimator (a perforated lead plate) with its holes parallel to the plane of rotation, electronic signals will be received through each collimator or hole along the length of the patient (Fig. 1.42). For a given camera angle, these signals are combined to produce line integrals along the patient and the line integrals are, in turn, summated to produce a count profile for each slice. There will be a count profile for each slice at each angle at which the camera is stopped during the 360° rotation.

The eventual image is made up from a large square (a matrix) composed of an array of much smaller squares (pixels). As the overall area of the matrix is constant, the more pixels that are needed, the smaller the pixel size. For example, the pixels in a 256 × 256 matrix will be much smaller than those in a 64×64 matrix. The number of planar projections during the rotation, the time taken for each projection and the pixel/matrix size are referred to as acquisition parameters. The more projections, the longer the time taken for each projection, and the smaller the pixel size, the better the final image. Normally, the pixel size should be half the resolution required. Resolution, besides being dependent on distance, is determined by how the image is acquired and reconstructed.

Image reconstruction can be achieved by either 'iterative' or 'filtered' backprojection techniques.

Figure 1.43 illustrates the principle of iterative methods of reconstruction.

As can be seen in the figure, the principle of the iterative method is that as the number of projections is increased, so the solution will approach reality.

Backprojection refers to the summation techniques of image reconstruction from the projections referred to above. Filtering is a mathematical technique to remove or suppress non-target data or noise to produce a simplified image with clean margins. Recent trends use iterative or repetitive techniques. The basic steps of image reconstruction are as follows:

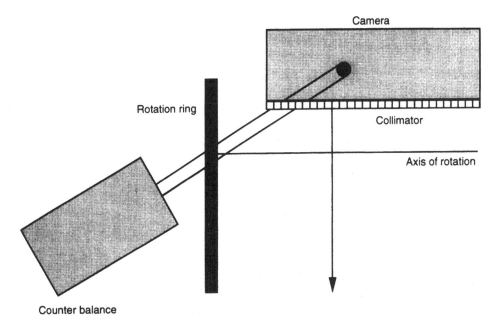

Figure 1.42 *A rotating gamma camera with parallel-hole collimator set up for SPET. The collimator holes (the line-of-sight of which is depicted by the arrow) must be parallel to the ring around which the camera rotates and perpendicular to the long axis of rotation, the latter corresponding to the axis of the supine patient.*

(1) A count profile is determined for each row or pixel
(2) A Fourier transform (see below) is determined for each projection
(3) Each transformed datum is mathematically filtered
(4) The process is then reversed and the inverse Fourier tranform of these filtered data is determined
(5) The filtered data at this particular angle are backprojected
(6) The above steps are repeated for all slices
(7) Slices at different angles are obtained by sampling the data block in the required direction.

The Fourier theorem states that any curve (such as the count–profile curve) can be broken down into a number of sine and cosine waves, each with known amplitude (height) and phase (angle). Each such wave also has a spatial frequency, determined by the reciprocal of its wavelength and expressed in cycles per centimeter or cycles per pixel. In effect this means that a complex profile can be broken down into simple numbers.

Filtering of the data transformed by Fourier analysis involves multiplying each point by a filter value. For ideal data, the filter value increases linearly with the spatial frequency up to the resolution limit of the camera (similar to a ramp and therefore called a ramp filter), but could not exceed the resolution limit of the distance between the holes on the collimator. This method can only be used in the case of high count densities, which would not apply in clinical situations.

As the camera has limited resolution, only noise is obtained beyond the frequency limit and so the filter function must be reduced to zero beyond this frequency. There are several filter functions, which do this in different ways (e.g. Shepp–Logan, Hanning, Hahn, Butterworth filters). The point and rate at which this reduction occurs can be altered and are dependent on the resolution required and the count-rate density in the reconstructed image. The Butterworth filter is perhaps the filter of first choice for clinical studies of the brain because it is mathematically the simplest.

Backprojection requires knowledge of the angle at which the projection was obtained and the centre of the rotation. It involves restoring the data along the direction of the collimator holes, during which the data from the different projections are added and interpolated onto the image matrix. In filtered backprojection, the images must be convolved with a spatial filter that subtracts counts on either side of every 'active pixel'. This reduces the background caused by 'ordinary' backprojection.

Although the data are smoothed within a slice, there is no smoothing between slices. To avoid this, prefiltering is used to smooth the planar projections in two dimensions before reconstruction is started. This can be done with a ramp filter with cut-off such that no high-frequency component remains in the count profiles. The mechanical centre of rotation is difficult to determine, so the electrical centre is used, which is the projection of the mechanical centre on the camera face. Brain images should not be smoothed too much as the fine structure of the brain produces high-frequency constituents that should not be lost.

Attenuation is a big problem in SPET reconstruction. Most systems use reconstruc-

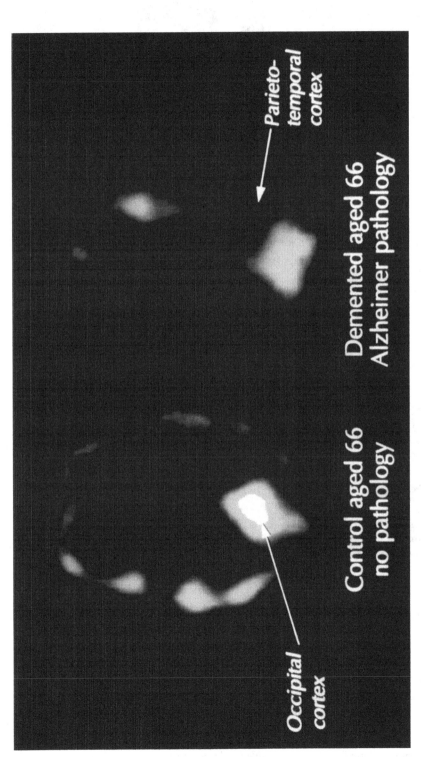

Figure 1.46 SPET images obtained using ^{99m}Tc-labeled HMPAO in a pathologically confirmed normal man (left) and a confirmed case of AD (right), showing the characteristic parietotemporal hypoperfusion of the condition. Such regional blood flow changes may significantly improve clinical diagnostic accuracy (Jobst et al., 1994).

A colour version of this image is available for download from www.cambridge.org/9780521112475.

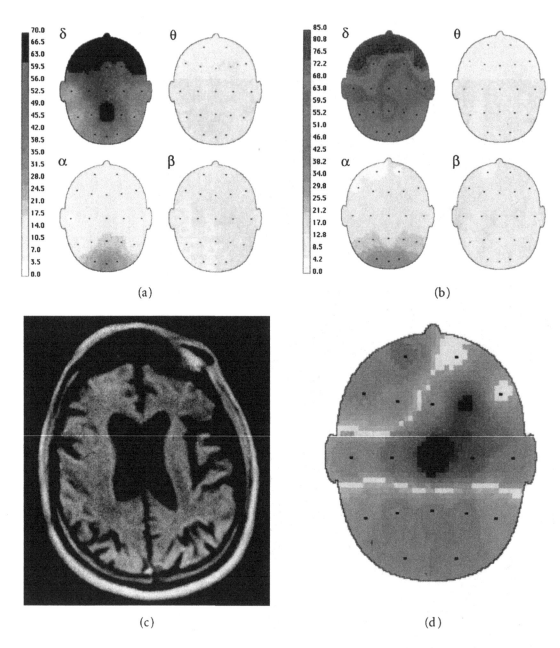

Figure 1.47 *Images of the brain of a 72-year-old male with AD. QEEG brain maps of absolute (a) and relative (b) power, MR image (c) and cordance map (d). QEEG maps are shown as projections onto the scalp from above (patient's right on right of panel); MR image is shown with radiologic convention (patient's right on left of panel). Generalized cerebral atrophy is present, somewhat more marked over the left hemisphere. Low values of cordance are found over the parietal regions bilaterally, the regions classically associated with hypometabolism in AD. Cordance values are greatest over the right frontal region, the area with the least cerebral atrophy.*

A colour version of these images are available for download from www.cambridge.org/9780521112475.

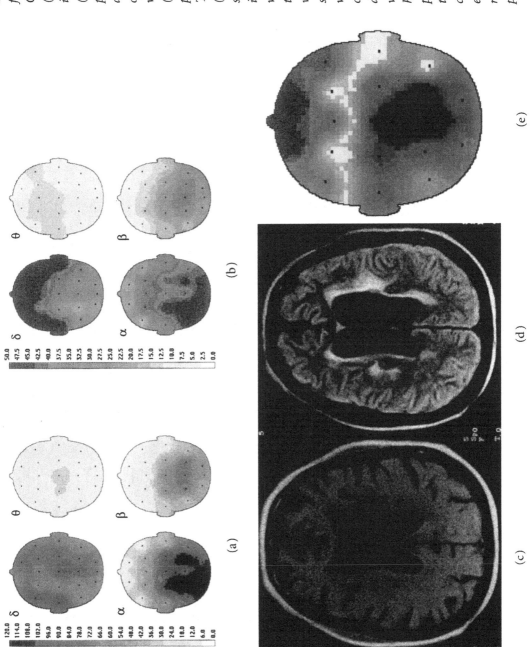

Figure 1.48 A 75-year-old female with vascular dementia: QEEG brain maps of absolute (a) and relative (b) power, MR image (c, d) and cordance map (e). QEEG maps are shown as projections onto the scalp from above (patient's right on right of panel); MR images are shown with radiologic convention (patient's right on left of panel). The MR images show T_1-weighted (c) and T_2-weighted (d) images through the same scan plane. Periventricular hyper-intensities are seen bilaterally, with a small lacunar infarct in the right corona radiata; low values of cordance are seen with a scattered distribution bilaterally, with a subtly greater extension over the right hemisphere. The distribution of lowest cordance values over frontal regions and highest cordance over the right posterior region parallels the topography of the periventricular capping, which appears most extensively anteriorly and has relatively spared the right posterior region.

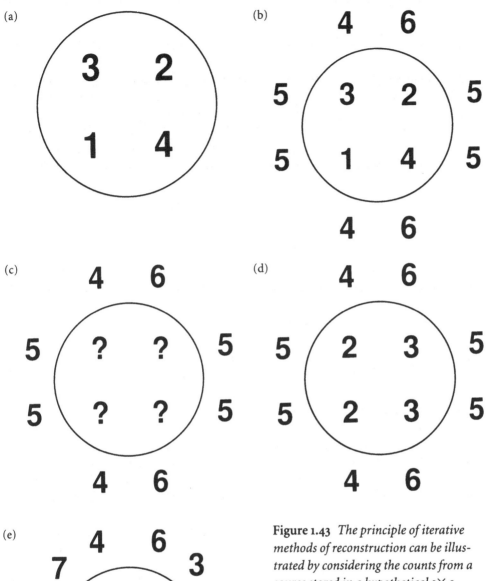

Figure 1.43 *The principle of iterative methods of reconstruction can be illustrated by considering the counts from a source stored in a hypothetical 2× 2 matrix (a). Each number can be interpreted as counts per unit area. The counts on the four orthogonal planar views would then be as shown in (b). The reconstruction process starts with the reverse situation (c), which could be incorrectly reconstructed as (d). However, if the number of planar views is increased to include the diagonals, the number of possible solutions is reduced (e), i.e. as the number of projections increase, so the solution will approach reality.*

tion techniques such as the first-order Cheng correction, which is based on the way in which the body would attenuate a point source. This is adequate for most clinical images, but the Cheng filter really only multiplies the counts in the centre so that they can be visualised. Most projections assume the patient's head to be an elliptical cylinder! Some triple-headed cameras now use the third camera head to acquire a transmission computed image from a cobalt-57 or other radioactive source at the same time as the SPET to use as an attenuation map. Other systems use a computed-transmission image-set, but are less satisfactory as they do not relate to a particular energy.

Quantitative accuracy is dependent on scatter, attenuation, the reconstruction filter, the slice shape and partial volume effects. The partial volume effect is an apparent reduction in the pixel count corresponding to a given radioactive concentration in a small volume relative to the count from the same concentration in a lower volume. It occurs when the object of interest is thinner than the slice thickness or is only partially within the slice.

The biggest problem with quantitative SPET is the spatial filtering to reduce the background. Backprojection produces an arbitrary background that changes with the reconstructed images. The filtering subtracts an arbitrary amount from the image to reduce the background and so the 'absolute' numbers are somewhat arbitrary themselves! (See Fig. 1.44.) True quantification can only be carried out with blood sampling and iterative reconstruction methods, as outlined above.

Therefore in performing SPET it is vital to choose a detector with good energy resolution, planar uniformity and low spatial distortion. These in turn require a high-resolution collimator, the smallest radius of rotation and an appropriate energy-window setting. In reality, scatter and attenuation problems are almost insoluble and it cannot be emphasized too strongly that the same projection data can produce many different images and what is presented to the clinician represents only the 'best guess' of the technologists. However, at the time of writing, progress is being made using xenon-derived correction algorithms and sophisticated coregistration and image-fusion techniques. The tortoise of SPET is rapidly approaching the PET hare!

Positron emission tomography

The location of positron-emitting radionuclides injected into the body are, contrary to expectation, detected by the presence of high-energy gamma rays. These arise when the positrons (which are positively charged electrons) collide with electrons and both are annihilated in an exchange of matter into energy, resulting in two high-energy gamma rays that travel 180° away from each other in opposite directions (Fig. 1.45).

The SPET gamma camera must, therefore, be converted for PET, so that it always has two orthogonally situated detectors, one on each side of the patient, that are

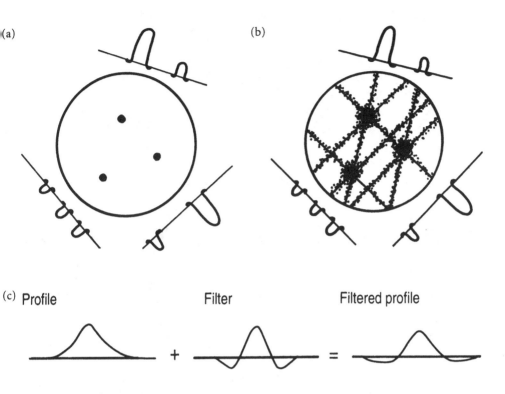

(c) Profile   Filter   Filtered profile

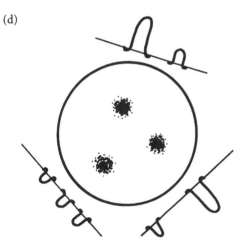

Figure 1.44 *(a) Count profiles relating to a single slice from a hypothetical distribution consisting of three point sources. (b) Backprojection of the count profiles in (a) produces an image of the point sources by summation, but with high background. (c) Mathematical filtering is applied to each point in the profile to cancel out the high background, giving the final image (d).*

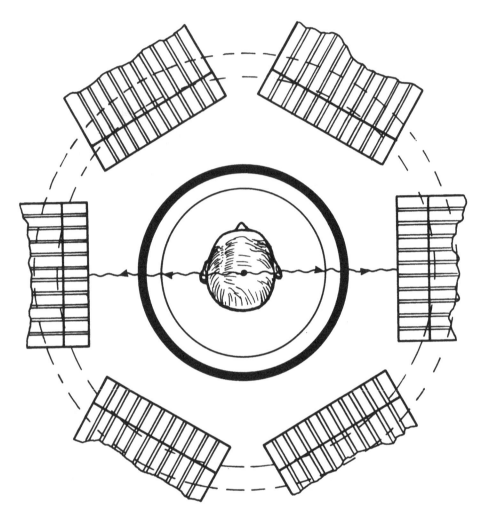

Figure 1.45 *Schematic representation of a PET device. The annihilation gamma rays travel in opposite directions from a joint source within the brain. Using diametrically opposed detectors, the twin gamma rays are selected for coincidence and a cross-sectional image is built up from the coincident scintillations.*

electronically linked so that only coincidental events are recorded. This direct-line geometry obviates the need for selective interference collimators of the kind needed in single photon emission situations, where there is the possibility of interference by gamma rays of different energies, such as background radiation or other unwanted radionuclides injected previously.

The simultaneous reception of a positron event by the two diametrically opposed detectors allows for focus at a given plane in the patient, in contrast to the lack of this facility in a planar gamma camera. It is possible to combine the spatial sensing of the two detectors in such a way that only radioactivity lying on a given plane will be in sharp focus in the final image, and activity from other planes becomes effectively invisible.

Modern positron cameras have a considerable degree of sophistication. Their external appearance is not dissimilar from the now familiar X-ray CT and MRI machines. Internally they now have banks of detectors all carefully aligned so that, in spite of their numbers, they are always in pairs facing each other. For instance, the Neuro-ECAT machine, designed specifically for cerebral studies at the University of California, Los Angeles, has three octagonal detector planes, each with 88 bismuth germanate detectors.

Positron-emitting radionuclides are important because they include a number of key biological elements, such as carbon, oxygen, nitrogen, iron and fluorine, which have no suitable single photon counterpart. However, these radionuclides have overwhelming disadvantages of being cyclotron produced (and therefore very expensive) and having very short half-lives (the half-life of oxygen-15 is only 15 minutes), which means they must be used immediately. By extension, this involves the presence in the hospital of both a cyclotron and a laboratory where these short-lived radionuclides can be incorporated into or converted to an appropriate radiopharmaceutical on-line, as well as being rendered sterile, apyrogenic and generally biologically compatible. The positron camera must also be in the same area.

These requirements involve an extensive investment in space and money, the latter running into millions of US dollars. The result is that only a few selected places have positron facilities. They abound in the USA, and the West German Government considered the technique so important that their major nuclear medicine departments have been provided with positron facilities. The number of PET units worldwide is around 50 at present, with their numbers increasing at about 10% per annum. One or two centers are experimenting with less expensive detectors and longer lived positron emitters.

Radiopharmaceuticals used in PET

Conventional brain scintigraphy has always been a misnomer and should be called 'non-brain imaging', the reason being that the single photon radiopharmaceuticals (technetium-99m pertechnetate, DTPA or gluconate) do not cross the blood brain barrier to penetrate normal brain. Only when the blood brain barrier is damaged do they appear as focal areas of increased uptake in cerebral tissues. The quest has, therefore, been on for some time to produce radiopharmaceuticals capable of investigating the normal brain.

Of all the useful positron-emitting elements cited above, the unexpected fluorine in the form of [^{18}F]-labeled deoxyglucose has proved to be the most useful in cerebral studies. This is now known as the 'FDG method'. After intravenous injection, FDG enters the brain and is phosphorylated by cerebral hexokinase. The metabolic product, FDG-6–PO_4 remains fixed in the brain, where it undergoes only slow dephosphorylation. The change in fluorine-18 activity and glucose concentration with time can be measured by a combination of cerebral scintigraphy and plasma concentration measurements, which enable local cerebral glucose utilization to be determined and represented pictorially in cross-sectional images.

Oxygen-15 is also useful in determining cerebral oxygen utilization and blood volume. The uptake of [^{13}N]ammonia has also been used to estimate blood flow.

Several neutral lipophilic radiolabeled compounds have been developed and it is nowadays customary to divide them into two groups: (i) those whose cerebral distribution is proportional to blood flow and (ii) those where the localization image is dependent on the distribution of receptor binding.

PET investigations have access mainly to receptor-binding radiopharmaceuticals. In particular, these involve the dopamine receptors 3-N-[^{11}C]methyl spiperone, ^{18}F-labeled spiroperidol and haloperidol and the opiate receptor, [^{11}C]carfentanil. For example, serial measurements of the last agent in patients before and after administration of the competitive opiate antagonist nalaxone can differentiate specific from non-specific opiate receptor binding.

Radiopharmaceuticals used in SPET

There is no question that the impetus provided by the success of PET users has stimulated research on more practical gamma-emitting radiopharmaceuticals that cross the intact blood brain barrier and localize in the normal brain tissue. Lesions are being identified by photon-deficient areas in the brain image or changes in the pattern of normal distribution.

Following the distinction between agents depending on CBF and those relying on receptor binding, the former includes the large group of the iodoamphetamines, the cyclic amines and cyclic diaminodithiol, whereas there is still a relative dearth of receptor-binding agents.

Amines are important chemical mediators of brain function and affect transport of brain metabolites, and the rates of syntheses and metabolism. A number of labeled amines that cross the normal blood brain barrier and remain fixed to the brain for sufficient time to permit tomographic imaging have been synthesized in the last few years. Radiolabeled di-beta-(morpholinoethyl)-selenide (MOSE) and di-beta-(piperidinoethyl)-selenide (PIPSE) were early examples of compounds that are neutral and lipid soluble at normal blood pH and so diffuse into cells.

Winchell and his colleagues (Winchell, Baldwin & Lin, 1980) have demonstrated that a large number of amines pass the blood brain barrier, resulting in high brain concentration after intravenous injection. As with PIPSE and MOSE, the penetration of the blood brain barrier results from the free diffusion of the unionized form of the compound. The most promising of these amines has been *N*-isopropyl-*p*-iodoamphetamine (IMP) labeled with iodine-123, which is extracted from brain *proportional to blood flow*. There are three possible mechanisms for tracer localization: pH gradient, metabolism into an impermeable metabolite and receptor binding, but it is not yet certain which, if any, of these three are applicable.

One disadvantage of IMP is that its uptake from sites such as the lung may result in recirculation and redistribution in the brain, altering the image resolution and accuracy of lesion detection. As a result, coupled with what nowadays always seems to be the ultimate aim in synthesizing a new radiopharmaceutical (i.e. to find a technetium-99m-based compound), there has been a search to find a more appropriate agent.

HMPAO labeled with technetium-99m was developed by Amersham International in the UK relatively recently. It differs from ^{123}I-IMP in that the latter requires living brain cells in order to be extracted from the blood, whereas ^{99m}Tc-HMPAO is not brain-cell specific. It is, for instance, being used to detect tumors elsewhere in the body. There may well be a role for both agents because, although they are both dependent on brain blood flow, ^{123}I-IMP also reflects the status of brain cells. SPET CBF imaging using both tracers has shown characteristic perfusion defects in a number of neuropsychiatric diseases and may contribute significantly to differential diagnosis particularly in the dementias (Jobst et al., 1994) (Fig. 1.46 (facing p. 50)).

The exciting prospect for the future is that experience with technetium-99m-labeled CBF agents indicates that it might be possible to image so-called 'recognition-site ligands' if the appropriate tracers can be designed. Iodine-123 remains too expensive to permit the high doses necessary for adequate resolution and which can be achieved with technetium-99m. The lead in this respect has so far been taken by PET, which has been successful in the study of the dopamine receptor system. However, even now [123]I *m*-iodobenzylguanidine has become available for imaging the autonomic nervous system, as well as methyl[123]I iodo-lysergic acid diethylamide (LSD) for serotonin receptors, [123]I *p*-iododexetimide for muscarinic cholinergic receptors and iodine-123 ligands for alpha and beta adrenergic receptors.

The benzodiazepine antagonist iomazenil (Ro 16–0154), an analog of the benzodiazepine ligand flumazenil, has been labeled with iodine-123 and is a useful benzodiazepine radioligand. It has been used in an attempt to localize epiletogenic foci.

The agent ^{123}I iodobenzamide may even equal the ability of the PET agents in imaging dopamine D_2 receptors. Such receptors are known to mediate the antipsychotic and extrapyramidal motor effects of neuroleptics. Measurement of D_2–dopamine receptor occupancy may be used in defining the minimal effective dosage of neuroleptics that gives sufficient occupancy for antipsychotic efficiency with a minimum of side effects.

1(d) Electroencephalography and magnetoencephalography

Andrew Leuchter and Ian Cook

Introduction

The brain is an electrochemical organ. Most of the brain's energy metabolism is devoted to maintaining electrical gradients, which are the basis of resting state potentials and neural transmission. Three neuroimaging techniques create images using these potentials and may be used to examine brain function: electroencephalography (EEG), evoked potentials (EPs), or event-related potentials (ERPs), and magnetoencephalography (MEG).

EEG was introduced to clinical practice in the early 20th century by a German psychiatrist, Hans Berger, who demonstrated changes in the EEG in response to arousal, emotions and activities. Interest in clinical EEG was fueled by Berger's study of the EEGs of institutionalized patients (Berger, 1937), many of whom showed distinct abnormalities, particularly diffuse slowing. Berger also made clear that the EEG has a special role in the assessment of older adults, by reporting that the EEG changed with aging and was abnormal in a high proportion of individuals with dementia.

Much of Berger's work is still relevant today; the EEG remains the single most cost-effective physiologic test to indicate the presence of delirium or dementia in an older adult. The usefulness of conventional EEG has been limited, however, by limited reliability of interpretations and unclear physiologic meaning of results. Over the past several years, the usefulness of EEG has been enhanced through the application of computer-based methods for signal analysis. These methods, classed under the broad rubric of quantitative electroencephalography (QEEG), have rendered EEG measurements more reliable and reproducible and have aided physiologic interpretation of abnormalities. This section will review the basic indications for and findings of QEEG, the scientific basis for the technology and discuss its clinical application.

A second computer-based approach, that of EPs, involves recording following repetitive stimuli and observing the averaged electrical response of the brain to these stimuli. This technique serves to standardize the conditions of recording and permits the study of pathways involved in information processing. EPs have been shown to reveal characteristics of the brain relevant to the processes of aging.

A third approach, quite different from the two previous approaches, is MEG. This is a promising technology for functional imaging that measures magnetic fields generated by electrical sources within the brain. This technology is particularly useful for studying sources deep within the brain and offers superior possibilities for localizing focal abnormalities that produce distinctive signals. MEG has not been widely applied to the study of older patients, but its potential applications will be reviewed.

Clinical applications of conventional EEG

In the elderly, there are three primary clinical situations in which the EEG may provide useful diagnostic information: the assessment of dementia, the assessment and longitudinal follow-up of delirium and evaluation of seizure disorders. First, the EEG may be helpful in distinguishing normal elderly from those with dementia. Examination of the EEG in most normal subjects during aging shows changes beginning in the fifth or sixth decade of life: these include a decrease of 0.5–1.0Hz in the mean frequency of the posterior dominant rhythm (Busse, 1983; Kanowski, 1971; Obrist & Busse, 1965; Roubicek, 1977), increased theta slow-wave activity (Gibbs & Gibbs, 1951; Obrist, 1979) and focal slowing, primarily in the left anterior temporal region. Focal slowing has been reported in 17–59% of healthy elderly subjects (Helmchen, Kanowski & Künkel, 1967; Hughes & Cayaffa, 1977; Katz & Horowitz, 1982; Obrist & Busse, 1965; Otomo & Tsubaki, 1966; Soininen et al., 1982; Torres et al., 1983; Visser et al., 1987), but to be considered normal it should be intermittent and never exceed 25% of the activity in the recording. Similarly, a posterior dominant rhythm in the waking state below 8Hz is never considered normal (Obrist, 1979; Oken & Kaye, 1992). The evolution of beta wave activity in aging is unclear, with some researchers reporting a slight increase (Gibbs, Lorimer & Lennox, 1950; Matousek et al., 1967; Mundy-Castle, 1951; Obrist, 1954) and others a decline after the sixth decade (Busse & Obrist, 1965; Obrist, 1976; Schlagenhauff, 1973; Wang & Busse, 1969).

These findings have both similarities with and differences from those patients with dementia. EEG studies of dementia describe decreases in the frequency and reactivity of the posterior dominant rhythm, as well as an excess of theta and delta wave activity (Andermann & Stoller, 1961; Coben, Danziger & Berg, 1983a; Coben, Danziger & Storandt, 1985; Coben et al., 1990; Dejaiffe et al., 1964; McAdam & Robinson, 1956; Weiner & Schuster, 1956). The posterior dominant rhythm in these patients commonly is below 8Hz, and the theta and delta wave slowing account for a high proportion of the recording, even in patients with equivocal impairment (mini-mental state examination (MMSE) scores ≥24) (Leuchter et al., 1993a). The high prevalence of abnormalities even in the early stages of the illness increases the diagnostic usefulness of the test.

Conventional EEG, however, is of limited diagnostic usefulness in differentiating between different types of dementia. Although focal abnormalities are more common in patients with vascular dementia than those with primary degenerative dementia (74% versus 19% of patients) (Dejaiffe *et al.*, 1964; Harrison *et al.*, 1979; Logar *et al.*, 1987; Roberts, McGeorge & Caird, 1978), they are common in both illnesses. Bilateral paroxysmal activity may be seen in one-quarter of patients with either diagnosis (Dejaiffe *et al.*, 1964; Fortin, 1966; Liddell, 1958). Furthermore, many patients (particularly those with a clinical diagnosis of vascular dementia) will actually have neuropathological changes of both illnesses, and this 'mixed' dementia is particularly difficult to assess (Ettlin *et al.*, 1989).

The EEG also is of limited use for distinguishing between depression and dementia. Many patients who have a primary diagnosis of depression have abnormal EEGs (Leuchter *et al.*, 1993b). An abnormal EEG may identify a subgroup of depressed patients with structural brain disease, or those who are more likely to have memory complaints. Physical illnesses such as hypertension (Visser, 1991), atherosclerosis (Obrist, 1963) and diabetes (Mooradian *et al.*, 1988; Pramming *et al.*, 1988) may cause changes in brain structure and EEG (such as deep white-matter ischemic disease) and brain function (as measured with EEG) (Giaquinto & Nolfe, 1986; Bowen *et al.*, 1990; Obrist *et al.*, 1963; Oken & Kaye, 1992; Visser *et al.*, 1987; Visser, 1991). The clinical significance of these abnormalities is not yet clearly delineated.

A second disorder in which the EEG has a useful diagnostic role is delirium. It was first established by Romano & Engel (1944) that the degree of slowing in the EEG is directly related to the level of confusion in delirious patients. It is, in fact, exceptional to make the diagnosis of delirium in the absence of EEG slowing (Lipowski, 1987; Romano & Engel, 1944). Furthermore, improvements in the EEG reflect improvements in mental status, so that EEG may be used to monitor recovery and the effectiveness of interventions aimed at the underlying causes of delirium (Brenner, 1991; Romano & Engel, 1944). In cases where the mental status examination is equivocal or difficult to perform (such as in a patient on a ventilator or with aphasia), or where the medical interventions being considered are invasive or pose significant risks and decisions rest on whether or not a delirium is resolving, the EEG may be a useful physiologic monitor of delirium. In contrast to patients with dementia, in whom the degree of slowing may be only slightly greater than that seen in normal aging, patients with delirium commonly have much more severe abnormalities (Brenner, 1991; Engel & Romano, 1959; Rabins & Folstein, 1982).

The evaluation of late-onset seizures is not uncommon: the elderly may account for one-quarter of the cases of new-onset epilepsy (Sander *et al.*, 1990), most commonly as a result of stroke, trauma and mass lesions (Ettinger & Shinnar, 1993; Lühdorf, Jensen & Plesner, 1986; Sung & Chu, 1990). The EEG may be used to confirm the presence of epileptiform discharges and to help to establish the type of seizure disorder. It cannot, however, rule out a seizure disorder, since 10 to 47% of patients with late-onset seizure disorders have normal EEGs (Ahuja & Mohanta, 1982; Carney *et al.*, 1969; Hyllested & Pakkenberg, 1963; Lühdorf *et al.*, 1986; Shigemoto, 1981; Woodcock & Cosgrove, 1964). Even when epileptiform abnormalities (i.e. spikes or spike- and-wave complexes) are detected, a diagnosis of a seizure disorder is not certain, since these abnormalities generally are interictal in nature (i.e. not contemporaneous with an actual seizure). In some brain areas (such as occipital cortex), interictal abnormalities may have a low correlation with clinical seizures (Niedermeyer, 1987). In other cases, renal failure or degenerative brain disease such as AD may lead to the development of generalized sharp waves or spike foci that have a low association with clinical seizures. To be certain of the diagnosis, prolonged EEG recording may be necessary to observe changes in the state or behavior of the patient that are linked to electrographic changes (i.e. observe the EEG during a true ictal event). In all cases, seizures are diagnosed on the basis of clinical presentation (Pinkus & Tucker, 1985).

The use of EEG for the evaluation of seizures is dependent upon detection of intermittent or even rare discharges, which may be difficult to discern from EEG background activity. For this purpose, the trained human observer probably is still the best instrument for detecting abnormality. However, the use of EEG for the evaluation of dementia and/or delirium is heavily dependent upon the quantification of activity in different frequency bands (Leuchter & Holschneider, 1994). For this purpose, conventional EEG interpretation is limited in its usefulness. The assessment of 'how much' slowing is contained in the record is difficult even for trained electroencephalographers, who differ on assessments of the same record with disturbing frequency (Woody, 1966; 1968). This is not surprising because (i) there are no well-established guidelines for determining when slow-wave activity is excessive; (ii) it is difficult for the human eye to separate waveforms of different frequencies by visual inspection alone; and (iii) electroencephalographers differ on how much slow-wave activity is acceptable at any given age.

Technique and applications of QEEG

QEEG analysis minimizes and/or eliminates many limitations of conventional EEG, which explains why computer-based techniques are rapidly supplanting conventional EEG. In QEEG, data are digitized at rates of at least 100 samples per channel per second, with rates of 128–256 samples more common. These data are recorded onto magnetic or optical media. The analog waveform is displayed on a high-resolution video display terminal, permitting conventional observation of the recording by the technician, or later visual interpretation by the physician. Later reproduction on paper media is also common.

After digital data are recorded, they commonly are processed through spectral analysis. In this technique, a series of segments (epochs) of EEG data (commonly one to four seconds in length) are processed through Fourier transformation to calculate the energy (power) in the signal that can be accounted for by a series of sinusoidal waveforms of different amplitudes and frequencies. Power commonly is averaged for a series of epochs representing 20–30 seconds of data and may be calculated for frequencies up to half the value of the sampling rate (the Nyquist frequency). Power may be represented as either the intensity of energy in a given band measured in μV^2 (absolute power) or the proportion of energy in a given band measured as a percentage (relative power) (Leuchter & Holschneider, 1994).

Because of the quantitative nature of its measurements, QEEG power measures provide more reliable and reproducible measurements of the energy content of an EEG signal than visual interpretation. The quantitative measures minimize the need for judgments about frequency content, which may not be reliable, thus increasing consistency for measures across individuals or within an individual over time.

QEEG also yields information that could not ordinarily be obtained from the conventional record. One such measure is *coherence*, or synchronization of electrical activity from different regions within an individual (Leuchter *et al.*, 1992). Coherence is analogous to the square of a correlation coefficient between the signals recorded at two locations and is computed from the following formula:

$$C_{xy}(\lambda) = \frac{|S_{xy}(\lambda)|^2}{S_x(\lambda)^* S_y(\lambda)}$$

in which the square of the cross-spectrum is divided by the product of the spectra of the individual channels (Beaumont & Rugg, 1979; Busk & Galbraith, 1975; Leuchter *et al.*, 1992; Thatcher, Krause & Hrybyk, 1986). Coherence indicates whether signals at multiple locations are rising and falling in a time-locked manner in any frequency band and would be difficult or impossible to assess visually except at very low frequencies.

Application of QEEG to older patients has clarified physiologic changes that occur with aging. Studies indicate that, while there is some slowing of the posterior dominant rhythm in the elderly (Busse, 1983; Duffy *et al.*, 1984a; Oken & Kaye, 1992), delta and theta power probably do not increase with normal aging (Duffy *et al.*, 1984a; Katz & Horowitz, 1982; Leuchter *et al.*, 1993b; Matejcek, 1979; Williamson *et al.*, 1990). Recent studies suggest that increased slowing seen on conventional EEG studies probably reflects the health status of the subjects studied (Oken & Kaye, 1992; Rice *et al.*, 1991). The pattern of changes in beta power is more complex, with possible increases through the seventh decade, after which time decreases may be seen (Duffy *et al.*, 1984a; Williamson *et al.*, 1990).

Several studies indicate that QEEG offers at least modest advantages over conventional EEG in detecting a possible dementing illness (Brenner *et al.*, 1986; Duffy *et al.*, 1984b; Nuwer, 1988; Prichep *et al.*, 1983). However, few studies have compared directly conventional EEG with QEEG, and additional research is needed. Several studies have utilized linear combinations of QEEG measures (absolute power, relative power, spectral ratios) to discriminate demented from nondemented subjects. These studies generally have found 85–95% sensitivity and specificity in confirming the presence of a dementing illness (Breslau *et al.*, 1989; Duffy *et al.*, 1984b; Leuchter *et al.*, 1987). Since there appears to be a direct relationship between the amount of QEEG slow-wave power and the level of impairment (Berg *et al.*, 1984; Coben *et al.*, 1983a; Johannesson *et al.*, 1979; Miyasaka *et* al., 1978; Rae-Grant et al., 1987; Leuchter et al., 1993b), most studies have found that QEEG measures are most reliable in identifying patients with at least mild-to-moderate impairment.

QEEG appears to be of greater use for distinguishing depression from dementia than conventional EEG, although which measures are most useful is unclear. The most common finding in depression is increased alpha power, particularly in the frontal regions (Pollock & Schneider, 1989); other findings include increased right temporal slow-wave and bifrontal beta power (Schatzberg et al., 1986). Using a combination of these variables, several investigators have found an overall accuracy in identifying depressed patients of 60–90% (John et al., 1977; 1988; Shagass et al., 1984).

QEEG probably has its clearest clinical application in the examination of patients with delirium. QEEG detects significant changes in the amount of slow-wave power in the course of a delirium. Decreases in slow-wave power appear to precede improvements in mental status (Leuchter & Jacobson, 1991). Quantification of slow-wave power appears to be useful for differentiating delirium from dementia (Jacobson, Leuchter & Walter, 1993a; Koponen et al., 1989) and may be helpful in identifying the onset of delirium as a complication of dementia (Jacobson et al., 1993b). Finally, QEEG power measures are associated with the length both of delirium and of hospitalization (Koponen, 1991; Koponen et al., 1989).

Brain dysfunction that is detectable by EEG appears to result not only from simple destruction of brain tissue but additionally from partial deafferentation of pyramidal cells of the cerebral cortex (Steriade et al., 1990). Two new QEEG methods detect this partial deafferentation with greater precision than previously possible. The first of the measures, called cordance, shows strong associations with brain metabolism (measured by FDG–PET) and perfusion (measured by HMPAO–SPET) in a small series of cases representing a variety of brain diseases (Leuchter et al., 1994a). In a study of 27 patients, most of whom suffered from dementing illnesses, cordance showed significantly stronger correlations with perfusion than traditional QEEG power measures (Leuchter et al., 1994b). Cordance shows promise as a noninvasive method for monitoring brain function; it may provide information similar to PET or SPET scanning at much lower cost, and without the need for expensive equipment or radioisotopes.

A second measure based upon detection of deafferentation is a new algorithm for examining coherence. Coherence, which measures synchronized brain electrical activity, reflects both the structural and functional connections between brain areas (Busk & Galbraith, 1975; Davis & Wada, 1974; O'Connor & Shaw, 1978; Shaw, O'Connor & Ongley, 1977a,b; Tucker, Roth & Bair, 1986). Coherence previously had been thought to be mediated by either corticocortical or corticosubcortical fibers; a new, neuroanatomically based paradigm recently has been proposed in which coherence is measured along the surface projections of known fiber tracts (i.e. projections of the visual pathways). In validation of this method, Leuchter and colleagues (1994c) recently showed that coherence measured along surface projections in the frontal or visual association pathways was sensitive to the presence of periventricular white matter lesions (detected on MRI). This association between deep white matter lesions and decreased coherence was seen in subjects with dementia as well as in normal controls and suggests that coherence may detect 'disconnection' between brain areas caused by structural damage.

Coherence also appears to be useful in differentiating between the two most common forms of dementia, vascular dementia (sometimes called multiinfarct dementia or MID) and dementia caused by AD. Neuropathologic data show that these illnesses affect different types of brain connection, with AD selectively causing degeneration of long corticocortical fibers, and multiinfarct dementia causing diffuse damage to corticosubcortical white matter networks. Leuchter and colleagues (1992; 1994d) have shown that a combination of different surface projection measures (coherence ratio) detects high proportions of subjects with AD or multiinfarct dementia and may predict long-term outcomes in dementia.

As examples of the use of these measures in assessing brain dysfunction in dementia, Fig. 1.47 (facing p. 50) presents the absolute and relative power brain maps of a 72-year-old male with moderate dementia owing to AD, along with a representative MRI slice of his brain and the cordance maps. The absolute and relative power maps (Fig. 1.47a,b) indicate an excess of energy in the slow-wave bands but are not etiologically specific for this patient's encephalopathic process. The MR image (Fig. 1.47c) shows the prominence of cerebral sulci and enlargement of the ventricles, indicative of central cerebral atrophy; the atrophic changes are more marked in his left hemisphere. The cordance map (Fig. 1.47d) shows the presence of high cordance (red regions) over the central primary motor and sensory cortical regions and over the right hemisphere; there are lower values of cordance seen over the parietal regions bilaterally and over the left temporal and frontal regions as well. The high values of cordance seen here are associated with the areas of greatest perfusion and metabolism and correlate topographically with the extent of this patient's cerebral atrophy. This patient's coherence ratio value was 0.53, in the range associated with AD.

Fig. 1.48 (facing p. 50) shows similar images for a 75-year-old female with vascular dementia. Her absolute and relative power maps show an excess of slow-wave energy, with a subtle asymmetry suggesting that brain function is better preserved over the left hemisphere, but without a clear indication of the etiology of the dementia. Her MR image reveals deep white matter ischemic changes in the periventricular region. Her cordance map shows high values of cordance over the parietal regions and well-preserved cordance over much of the central and temporal regions as well, with multifocal loss of concordance over the frontal regions, more prominent over the right hemisphere. Her coherence ratio was in the vascular dementia range, with a value of -0.42.

Technique and applications of EPs

EPs are also a second measure that could not be assessed without computer assistance. In these paradigms, electrical activity is recorded while the subjects are exposed to repetitive visual (i.e. flashes of light or patterns), auditory (i.e. clicks or tones) or other stimuli (i.e. electrical stimulation of the skin). A computer averages the response to the time-locked, repeated stimuli, thus enhancing the signal evoked by the stimuli while averaging out other brain activity unrelated to the stimuli. The resulting display is a voltage wave form of the average response potentials. These potentials appear as a series of positive and negative waveforms occurring at specific time intervals following a stimulus and are labeled according to their polarities (P for positive, N for negative) and latencies from time of the stimulus (in milliseconds).

The EPs of greatest usefulness for the examination of elderly patients are those with medium to long latencies, termed 'endogenous' or 'cognitive' potentials. These potentials probably represent processing of stimuli in higher centers (including primary or association cortex) and reflect processes of attention and intention, as well as the effects of age.

It was first established by Goodin and colleagues (1978a) that some of these long-latency EPs are prolonged in the elderly. The first paradigm studied was the response to an anticipated 'rare' auditory stimulus. This positive waveform, which occurred approximately 300 milliseconds following stimulation in young adults (P300), occurred with a longer latency in the elderly. P300 latency appears to increase by 0.9 to 1.8 milliseconds each year (Hillyard & Picton, 1987; Polich, 1991) and is independent of changes in motor reaction time. There is disagreement regarding the rate of increase with age, with some investigators reporting a linear increase (Pfefferbaum et al., 1984a; Picton et al., 1984; Polich, Howard & Starr, 1985; Squires et al., 1980; Syndulko et al., 1982) and others a curvilinear increase (Brown, March & La Rue, 1983; Mullis et al., 1985). Similar observations have been made using different auditory evoked potentials (AEPs), visual evoked potentials (VEPs), and somatosensory evoked potentials (SSEPs) (Beck, Swanson & Dustman, 1980; Brown et al., 1983; Picton et al., 1984; Syndulko et al., 1982). There is no consistent effect reported for the amplitude of these potentials during aging (Beck et al., 1980; Brown et al., 1983; Goodin et al., 1978a; Pfefferbaum et al., 1980; Picton et al., 1984; 1986; Snyder & Hillyard, 1976).

Several investigators have attempted to use short-latency EPs for the diagnosis of dementia (Coben et al., 1983b; Harkins, 1981; Visser et al., 1976). Prolonged-flash VEP latency and increased amplitude (Coben et al., 1983b; Visser et al., 1976; Wright, Harding & Orwin, 1984), as well as some changes in brain-stem AEPs (Harkins, 1981) and SSEPs (Huisman et al., 1985) have been reported in patients with dementia. However, the differences in the exogenous potentials between demented subjects and normal controls are too small or inconsistent to permit definitive classification.

Most of the research on the late components of EPs in dementia has been focused on the P300 peak. It has been established that P300 latency is prolonged in dementia. Goodin, Squires & Starr (1978b) first reported an abnormally large increase in the P300 latency in a group of patients with dementias of different etiologies; they also noted that the increase in latency correlated with severity of dementia as assessed by the MMSE. Although these findings have been confirmed by several laboratories, prevalence of reported 'abnormal' latency varies from 13% to 83%, with most studies reporting that 70–80% of demented patients have prolonged P300 latency (Brown, Marsh & La Rue

1982; 1983; Gordon *et al.*, 1986; Patterson, Michalewski & Starr, 1988; Squires *et al.*, 1980; Syndulko *et al.*, 1982) (see Fig. 1.48*b*). P300 latency is of questionable value for the detection of dementia, since both sensitivity (Leppler & Greenberg, 1984; Pfefferbaum *et al.*, 1984b; Polich *et al.*, 1986; Syndulko *et al.*, 1984) and specificity (Calloway *et al.*, 1985; Gordon *et al.*, 1986; Hansch *et al.*, 1982; Lukas *et al.*, 1990; Pfefferbaum *et al.*, 1979; Rosenberg, Nudelman & Starr, 1985; St Clair, Blackwood & Christine, 1985) are limited.

EPs also have been utilized with limited success in the assessment of delirium. Some but not all studies have shown abnormalities of the short-latency AEPs in hepatic and renal encephalopathy (Chu & Yang, 1987; Pierelli *et al.*, 1985; Rossini *et al.*, 1984; Trzepacz, Sclabassi & Van Thiel, 1989; Yang, Chu & Liaw, 1986). Both VEPs and SSEPs show more consistent abnormalities in these syndromes (Casellas *et al.*, 1985; Kuba *et al.*, 1983; Levy & Bolton, 1986; Levy, Bolton & Losowsky, 1990; Pierelli *et al.*, 1985; Rossini *et al.*, 1981; Trzepacz *et al.*, 1989; Yen & Liaw, 1990; Zeneroli *et al.*, 1984). P300 potentials may show increased latency as well, although it may be problematic to obtain patient cooperation for this paradigm (Sandford & Saul, 1988). Despite the limitations of EPs in delirium, a recent review suggested that VEPs may be the most sensitive neurophysiologic measure for detecting subclinical hepatic encephalopathy (van der Rijt & Schalm, 1992).

Technique and applications of MEG

An entirely different approach to the recording of brain electromagnetic activity is the basis for MEG. All electrical sources generate magnetic fields. Electrical sources within the brain have been modeled as electrical dipoles consisting of assemblies of neurons oriented in a tangential (i.e. parallel to the skull) or radial (i.e. perpendicular to the skull) direction (Pizella & Romani, 1990). MEG utilizes a device called a superconducting quantum interference device (SQUID) magnetometer to detect these magnetic fields within the brain. This is a supercooled detection coil that is extremely sensitive to low-intensity magnetic fields generated by dipoles within the brain (Fagaly, 1990). The fields generated by the brain are of extremely low strength (approximately 10^{-8} gauss), but sensitivity of the detectors in the range to 10^{-10} gauss is now practically possible.

MEG has several advantages over EEG. The SQUID need not be in contact with the scalp and it is insensitive to the effects of muscle tension and activity. In addition, as opposed to the EEG signal which is 'blurred' and filtered by the skull, MEG is relatively unaffected by these interposed structures. Finally, in contrast to EEG, MEG detects sources deep within the brain. Recent advances in SQUID technology have allowed relatively precise localization of these dipole sources (Rose & Ducla-Soares, 1990).

MEG also has several disadvantages. First, because of the weak signal being studied, there may be significant problems with artifact from other electrical fields in the environment. Theoretically, the gradiometer technique permits identification and rejection of signals from nearby electrical equipment and other sources. This technique relies upon the fact that signals fall off with the cube of distance from the source; a distant and powerful field, therefore, would appear very similar to each member of a pair of sensing coils, while a nearby weak field would show considerable difference between the coils. In practice, signal-to-noise problems pose a challenge for MEG, and magnetic shielding is useful for eliminating environmental noise sources (Weinberg, 1991) though it is often costly. Second, although MEG is sensitive to deep sources within the brain, recent results show that it is relatively insensitive to dipoles oriented near the surface. Therefore, it is more suited to detection of sources lying within a sulcus and may not detect signals from sources on the surface of a gyrus. EEG is sensitive to both types of dipole, and in this sense MEG and EEG are complementary techniques, with MEG providing information about dipole orientation that is not readily accessible from EEG.

At present, the sole widespread clinical application of MEG is to epilepsy, where its power in dipole localization is useful for localizing seizure foci (Coben *et al.*, 1990; Fenwick, 1990). Few data are available to determine what MEG reveals about changes in the brain with aging.

Conclusion

At present, although QEEG is finding wide and increasing clinical application, the technique remains an adjunct to conventional EEG (APA Task Force on Quantitative Electrophysiological Assessment, 1991). There are several reasons why it has this secondary position. First, interpretation of paper tracings remains the 'gold standard' for detection of epileptiform abnormalities. Second, although QEEG provides reliable and reproducible measurements of the slow-wave power in a recording, there is little agreement on how much slowing is excessive, or on the use of normative databases to determine how much slowing is excessive. Third, there is concern about problems with artifacts that may unpredictably influence results.

QEEG and EEG seem to be evolving as complementary techniques. For the foreseeable future, EEG probably will remain the primary test for detection of epileptiform abnormalities. QEEG probably will supercede conventional EEG for most other applications in the elderly. As studies continue to prove the reliability of QEEG for detecting brain disease as well as the reliability of current standards for rejecting artifact, QEEG will find greater degrees of clinical acceptance. The application probably will be greatest in the elderly, where quantification of slow-wave power is particularly valuable.

QEEG occupies a unique niche among the functional imaging technologies. While PET and SPET provide more direct information about metabolism or perfusion of brain tissue, these techniques are costly and invasive and are not well suited to repeated measurements. QEEG complements these techniques. It is noninvasive and does not require costly equipment. Furthermore, QEEG provides information about the function of fiber systems within the brain and is a more direct measure of cortical deafferentation. In the future in some select situations, QEEG using the cordance method may be the preferred method for assessing perfusion and metabolism. Similarly, coherence measurements are useful for detection of dysfunction in tracts linking brain areas and may be useful for detection of the effects of white matter lesions.

For similar reasons, QEEG has a variety of uses in the research setting. This is particularly true for the assessment of drug effects, monitoring the course of illness or the screening of novel treatments, where serial and frequent study is particularly important. The combination of anatomic (MRI and CT) with physiologic measures of brain function (SPET, PET and QEEG) holds great promise for the future, in terms both of detecting and of understanding the pathophysiology of brain disease.

MEG remains a promising technology for the identification of electrical sources within the brain, but it remains relatively costly and its advantages for the study of the elderly are unclear. At present, applications for the elderly remain largely in the research realm.

The reliability as well as the efficiency of computer-based methods make the emergence of QEEG into widespread clinical use an inevitability. Just as computers have reduced the physician time demands and increased the reliability of ECG interpretation, QEEG will become a mainstay of EEG interpretation. As research continues to demonstrate the applicability of new algorithms to clinical situations, QEEG will become a widespread method for imaging the brain.

References

Ahuja, G.K. & Mohanta, A. (1982). Late onset epilepsy. *Acta Neurologica Scandinavica*, 66, 216–226.

Ambrose, J. & Hounsfield, G. (1972a). Computerised transverse axial tomography. *British Journal of Radiology*, 46, 148–149.

Ambrose, J. & Hounsfield, G. (1972b). Computerised transverse axial scanning (tomography). Part 2: clinical applications. *British Journal of Radiology*, 46, 1023–47.

American Psychiatric Association Task Force on Quantitative Electrophysiological Assessment (1991). Quantitative electroencephalography: a report on the present state of computerized EEG techniques. *American Journal of Psychiatry*, 148, 961–964.

Anderman, K. & Stoller, A. (1961). EEG patterns in hospitalized and non-hospitalized aged. *Electroencephalography and Clinical Neurophysiology*, 13, 319.

Beaumont, J.G. & Rugg, M.D. (1979). The specificity of intrahemispheric EEG alpha coherence asymmetry related to psychological task. *Biological Psychology*, 9, 237–248.

Beck, E.C., Swanson, C. & Dustman, R.E. (1980). Long latency components of the visually evoked potential in man: effects of aging. *Experimental Aging Research*, 6, 523–545.

Berg, L., Danziger, W.L., Storandt, M. *et al.* (1984). Predictive features in mild senile dementia of the Alzheimer type. *Neurology*, 34, 563–569.

Berger, H. (1937). On the electroencephalogram of man: twelfth report. *Archiv für Psychiatrie und Nervenkrankheiten*, 106, 165–187.

Bloch, F., Hansen, W.L. & Packard, M.E. (1946). Nuclear Induction. *Physical Review*, 69, 127.

Bowen, B., Barker, W., Lowenstein, D., Sheldon, J. & Duara, R. (1990). MR signal abnormalities in memory disorder and dementia. *American Journal of Neuroradiology*, 11, 283–290.

Brenner, R.P. (1991). Utility of electroencephalography in delirium: past views and current practice. *International Psychogeriatrics*, 3, 211–229.

Brenner, R.P., Ulrich, R.F., Spiker, D.G. *et al.* (1986). Computerized EEG spectral analysis in elderly normal, demented and depressed subjects. *Electroencephalography and Clinical Neurophysiology*, 64, 483–492.

Breslau, J., Starr, A. Sicotte, N., Higa, J. & Buchsbaum, M.S. (1989). Topographic EEG changes with normal aging and SDAT. *Electroencephalography and Clinical Neurophysiology*, 72, 281–289.

Brown, W.S., Marsh, J.T. & La Rue, A. (1982). Event-related potentials in psychiatry: differentiating depression and dementia in the elderly. *Bulletin of the Los Angeles Neurological Societies*, 47, 91–107.

Brown, W.S., Marsh, J.T. & La Rue, A. (1983). Expotential electrophysiological aging: P300 latency. *Electroencephalography and Clinical Neurophysiology*, 55, 277–285.

Busk, J. & Galbraith, G. (1975). EEG correlates of visual-motor practice in man. *Electroencephalography and Clinical Neurophysiology*, 38, 415–422.

Busse, E.W. (1983). Electroencephalography. In *Alzheimer's Disease: The Standard Reference*, ed. B. Reisberg, pp. 231–236. New York: The Free Press.

Busse, E. & Obrist, W. (1965). Pre-senescent electroencephalographic changes in normal subjects. *Journal of Gerontology*, 20, 315–320.

Calloway, E., Halliday, R., Naylor, H. & Schechter, G. (1985). Effects of oral scopolamine on human stimulus evaluation. *Psychopharmacology*, 85, 133–138.

Carney, L.R., Hudgins, R.L., Espinosa, R.E. & Klass, D.W. (1969). Seizures beginning after the age of 60. *Archives of Internal Medicine*, 124, 707–709.

Casellas, F., Sagalés, T., Calzada, M.D., Accarino, A., Vargas, V. & Guarner, L. (1985). Visual evoked potentials in hepatic encephalopathy. *Lancet*, i, 394–395.

Chu, N.-S. & Yang, S.-S. (1987). Brainstem auditory evoked potentials in different types of hepatic disease. *Electroencephalography and Clinical Neurophysiology*, 67, 337–339.

Coben, L.A., Chi, D., Synder, A.Z. & Storandt, M. (1990). Replication of a study of frequency analysis of the resting awake EEG in mild and probable Alzheimer's disease. *Electroencephalography and Clinical Neurophysiology*, 75, 148–154.

Coben, L.A., Danziger, W.L. & Berg, L. (1983a). Frequency analysis of the resting awake EEG in mild senile dementia of Alzheimer type. *Electroencephalography and Clinical Neurophysiology*, 55, 372–380.

Coben, L.A., Danziger, W.L. & Hughes, C.P. (1983b). Visual evoked potentials in mild senile dementia of the Alzheimer's type. *Electroencephalography and Clinical Neurophysiology*, 55, 121–130.

Coben, L.A., Danziger, W. & Storandt, M. (1985). A longitudinal EEG study of mild senile dementia of Alzheimer type: changes at 1 year and at 2.5 years. *Electroencephalography and Clinical Neurophysiology*, 61, 101–112.

Dahlbeck, S.W., McCluney, K.W., Yeakley, J.W. *et al.* (1991). The interuncal distance: a new MR measurement for the hippocampal atrophy of Alzheimer disease. *American Journal of Neuroradiology*, 12, 932–932.

Davis, P.C., Hudgins, P.A., Peterman, S.B. & Hoffman, J C. (1991). Diagnosis of cerebral metastases: double dose delayed CT vs contrast enhanced MR imaging. *American Journal of Neuroradiology*, 12, 293–300.

Davis, S.M., Tress, B.M., Hopper, J.L., Kaye, A.H. & Rossiter, S.C. (1987). Dynamic CT brain scanning in the haemodynamic evaluation of cerebral arterial occlusive disease. *Neuroradiology*, 29, 259–265.

Davis, A. & Wada, J. (1974). Hemispheric asymmetry: frequency analysis of visual and auditory evoked responses to non-verbal stimuli. *Electroencephalography and Clinical Neurophysiology*, 37, 1–9.

Dejaiffe, G., Constantinidis, J., Rey-Bellet, J. & Tissot, R. (1964). Corrélations électrocliniques dans les démences de l'age avancé. *Acta Neurologica Belgica*, 64, 677–707.

Desmond, P.M., O'Brien, J.T., Tress, B.M. *et al.* (1994). Volumetric and visual assessment of the mesial temporal structures in Alzheimer's disease. *Australian and New Zealand Journal of Medicine*, 24, 547–553.

Duffy, F.H., Albert, M.S. & McAnulty, G. (1984a). Brain electrical activity in patients with presenile and senile dementia of the Alzheimer type. *Annals of Neurology*, 16, 439–448.

Duffy, F.H., Albert, M.S., McAnulty, G. & Garvey, J. (1984b). Age-related differences in brain electrical activity in healthy subjects. *Annals of Neurology*, 16, 430–438.

Engel, G. & Romano, J. (1959). Delirium, a syndrome of cerebral insufficiency. *Journal of Chronic Diseases*, 9, 260–277.

Ettinger, A.B. & Shinnar, S. (1993). New-onset seizures in an elderly hospitalized population. *Neurology*, 43, 489–492.

Ettlin, T.M., Staehelin, H., Kischka, U. *et al.* (1989). Computed tomography, electroencephalography, and clinical features in the differential diagnosis of senile dementia. *Archives of Neurology*, 46, 1217–1220.

Fagaly, R.L. (1990). Neuromagnetic instrumentation. *Advances in Neurology*, 54, 11–32.

Fenwick, P.B. (1990). Behavioural treatment of epilepsy. *Postgraduate Medical Journal*, 66, 336–338.

Fortin, A. (1966). La signification clinique du tracé EEG de la maladie de Alzheimer. *Acta Neurologica Belgica*, 66, 106–115.

Giaquinto, S. & Nolfe, G. (1986). The electrocephalogram in the normal elderly: a contribution to the interpretation of aging and dementia. *Electroencephalography and Clinical Neurophysiology*, 63, 540–546.

Gibbs, F.A. & Gibbs, E.L. (1951). Changes with age awake. In *Atlas of Electroencephalography*, ed. F.A. Gibbs & E L. Gibbs, pp. 82–88. Reading, MA: Addison-Wesley.

Gibbs, E., Lorimer, F. & Lennox W. (1950). Clinical correlates of exceedingly fast activity in the electroencephalogram. *Diseases of the Nervous System*, 11, 323–326.

Goldstein, H.A., Kashanian, F.K., Blumetti, R.F., Holyoak, W.L., Hugo, F.P. & Blumfield D.M. (1990). Safety assessment of gadolinium dimeglumine in U.S. clinical trials. *Radiology*, 174, 17–23.

Goodin D., Squires, K., Henderson, B. & Starr, A. (1978a). Age-related variations in evoked potentials to auditory stimuli in normal human subjects. *Electroencephalography and Clinical Neurophysiology*, 44, 447–458.

Goodin, D.S., Squires, K.C. & Starr, A. (1978b). Long latency event-related components of the auditory evoked potential in dementia. *Brain*, 101, 635–648.

Gordon, E., Kraiuhin, C., Harris, A., Meares, R. & Howson, A. (1986). The differential diagnosis of dementia using P300 latency. *Biological Psychiatry*, 21, 1123–1132.

Hansch, E.C., Syndulko, K., Cohen, S.N., Goldberg, Z.I., Potvin, A.R. & Tourtelotte, W.W. (1982). Cognition in Parkinson disease: an event-related potential perspective. *Annals of Neurology*, 11, 599–607.

Harkins, S.W. (1981). Effects of presenile dementia of the Alzheimer's type on brainstem transmission time. *International Journal of Neuroscience*, 15, 165–170.

Harris, G.J., Barta, P.E., Peng, L.W. et al. (1994). MR volume segmentation of gray and white matter using manual thresholding: dependence on image brightness. *American Journal of Neuroradiology*, 15, 225–230.

Harrison, M.J., Thomas, D.J., Du-Boulay, G.M. & Marshall, J. (1979). Multi-infarct dementia. *Journal of the Neurological Sciences*, 40, 97–103.

Helmchen, H., Kanowski, S. & Künkel, H. (1967). Die Altersabhängigkeit der Lokalisation von EEG-Herden. *Schweitzer Archiv für Neurologie und Psychiatrie*, 209, 474–483.

Hillyard, S.A. & Picton, T.W. (1987). Electrophysiology of cognition. In *Handbook of Physiology*, 5th edn, ed. V.B. Mountcastle, F. Plum & S.R. Geiger, pp. 519–584. Bethesda, MD: American Physiology Society.

Hopper, J.L., Davis, S.M., Tress, B.M., Kaye, A.H., Rossiter, S.C. & Derrick, P.L. (1987). Analysis of dynamic computed tomography scan brain images. *Investigative Radiology*, 22, 651–657.

Hounsfield, G N. (1973). Computerised transverse axial scanning (tomography). Part 1. Description of the System. *British Journal of Radiology*, 46, 1016–1022.

Hughes, J.R. & Cayaffa, J.J. (1977). The EEG in patients at different ages without organic cerebral disease. *Electroencephalography and Clinical Neurophysiology*, 42, 776–784.

Huisman, U.W., Posthuma, J., Visser, S.L., Jonker, C. & de Rijke, W. (1985). The influence of attention on visual evoked potentials in normal adults and dementia. *Clinical Neurology and Neurosurgery*, 87, 11–16.

Hyllested, K. & Pakkenberg, H. (1963). Prognosis of epilepsy of late onset. *Neurology*, 13, 651–654.

Jackson, G.D., Berkovic, S.F., Tress, B.M., Kalnins, R.M., Fabinyi G.C. & Bladin, P.F. (1990). Hippocampal sclerosis can be reliably detected by magnetic resonance imaging. *Neurology*, 40, 1869–1875.

Jacobson, S., Leuchter, A. & Walter, D. (1993a). Conventional and quantitative EEG in the diagnosis of delirium among the elderly. *Journal of Neurology, Neurosurgery and Psychiatry*, 56, 153–158.

Jacobson, S., Leuchter, A.F., Walter, D. & Weiner, H. (1993b). Serial quantitative EEG among elderly subjects with delirium. *Biological Psychiatry*, 34, 135–140.

Jobst, K.A., Hindley, N.J., King, E. & Smith, A. D. (1994). The diagnosis of Alzheimer's disease: a question of image? *Journal of Clinical Psychiatry*, 55 (Suppl. 11), 22–31.

Jobst, K. A., Smith, A.D., Szatmari, M. et al. (1992). Detection in life of Alzheimer's disease using a simple method of measurement of medial temporal lobe atrophy by computed tomography. *Lancet*, 340, 1179–1183.

Johannesson, G., Hagberg, B. Gustafson, I. & Ingvar, D.H. (1979). EEG and cognitive impairment in presenile dementia. *Acta Neurologica Scandinavica*, 59, 225–240.

John, E.R., Karmel, B.Z., Corning, W.C. et al. (1977). Neurometics: numerical taxonomy identifies different profiles of brain functions within groups of behaviorally similar people. *Science*, 196, 1393–1410.

John, E.R., Prichep, L.S., Fridman, J. & Easton, P. (1988). Neurometics: computer-assisted differential diagnosis of brain dysfunctions. *Science*, 239, 162–169.

Johnson, D.W., Stringer, W.A., Marks, M.P., Yonas, H., Good, W.F. & Gur, D. (1991). Stable xenon CT cerebral blood flow imaging: rationale for and role in clinical decision making. *American Journal of Neuroradiology*, 12, 201–213.

Kanowski, S. (1971). EEG und Alterpsychiatrie. *Nervenarzt*, 42, 347–355.

Katz, R.I. & Horowitz, G.R. (1982). Electroencephalogram in the septuagenarian: studies in a normal geriatric population. *Journal of the American Geriatrics Society*, 30, 273–275.

Koponen, H. (1991). Delirium in the elderly: a brief overview. *International Psychogeriatrics*, 3, 177–179.

Koponen, H., Partanen, J., Paakkonen, A., Mattila, E. & Riekkinen, P.J. (1989). EEG spectral analysis in delirium. *Journal of Neurology, Neurosurgery and Psychiatry*, 52, 980–985.

Kuba, M., Peregrin, J., Vit, F., Hanusová, I. & Erben, J. (1983). Pattern- reversal visual evoked potentials in patients with chronic renal insufficiency. *Electroencephalography and Clinical Neurophysiology*, 56, 438–442.

Kuhl, D.E. & Edwards, R.O. (1963). Image separation radioisotope scanning. *Radiology*, 80, 653–661.

Leppler, J.G. & Greenberg, H.J. (1984). The P3 potential and its clinical usefulness in the objective classification of dementia. *Cortex*, 20, 427–433.

Leuchter, A.F., Cook, I.A., Lufkin, R.B. *et al.* (1994a). Cordance: a new method for assessment of cerebral perfusion and metabolism using quantitative electroencephalography. *Neuroimage*, 1, 208–219.

Leuchter, A.F., Cook, I.A., Mena, I. *et al.* (1994b). Assessment of cerebral perfusion and metabolism using quantitative EEG cordance. *Psychiatry Research: Neuroimaging*, 55, 141–152.

Leuchter, A.F., Cook, I.A., Newton, T.F. *et al.* (1993a). Regional differences in brain electrical activity in dementia: use of spectral power and spectral ratio measures. *Electroencephalography and Clinical Neurophysiology*, 87, 385–393.

Leuchter, A.F., Daly, K., Rosenberg-Thompson, S. & Abrams, M. (1993b). The prevalence of electroencephalographic abnormalities among patients with possible organic mental syndromes. *Journal of the American Geriatrics Society*, 41, 605–611.

Leuchter, A.F., Dunkin, J.J., Lufkin, R.B., Anzai, Y., Newton, T.F. & Cook, I.A. (1994c). The effect of white-matter disease on functional connections in the aging brain. *Journal of Neurology, Neurosurgery and Psychiatry*, 57, 1347–1354.

Leuchter, A.F. & Holschneider, D. (1994). Quantitative electroencephalography: neurophysiological alterations in normal aging and geriatric neuropsychiatric disorders. In *Textbook of Geriatric Neuropsychiatry*, ed. E. Coffey & J. Cummings, pp. 215–240. Washington, DC: American Psychiatric Press.

Leuchter, A.F. & Jacobson, S. (1991). Quantitative measurement of brain electrical activity in delirium. *International Psychogeriatrics*, 3, 231–247.

Leuchter, A.F., Newton, T.F., Cook, I.A., Walter, D.O., Rosenberg-Thompson, S. & Lachenbruch, P. (1992). Changes in brain functional connectivity in Alzheimer-type and multiinfarct dementia. *Brain*, 115, 1543–1561.

Leuchter, A.F., Simon, S.L., Daly, K.A. *et al.* (1994d). Quantitative EEG correlates of outcome in elderly psychiatric patients. I. Cross-sectional and longitudinal assessment of patients with dementia. *American Journal of Geriatric Psychiatry*, 2, 200–209.

Leuchter, A.F., Spar, J., Walter, D. & Weiner, H. (1987). Electroencephalographic spectra and coherence in the diagnosis of Alzheimer's-type and multiinfarct dementia. *Archives of General Psychiatry*, 44, 993–998.

Levy, L.J. & Bolton, R.P. (1986). Visual evoked potentials in hepatic encephalopathy. *Journal of Hepatology*, 3, 7P.

Levy, L.J., Bolton, R.P. & Losowsky, M.S. (1990). The visual evoked potential in clinical hepatic encephalopathy in acute and chronic liver disease. *Hepatogastroenterology*, Suppl. II, 37, 66–73.

Liddell, D.W. (1958). Investigations of EEG findings in presenile dementia. *Journal of Neurology, Neurosurgery and Psychiatry*, 21, 173–176.

Lipowski, Z. (1987). Delirium (acute confusional states). *Journal of the American Medical Association*, 258, 1789–1792.

Liston, E. (1979). Clinical findings in presenile dementia. *Journal of Nervous and Mental Disease*, 167, 337–342.

Logar, C., Grabmair, W., Schneider, G. & Lechner, H. (1987). EEG Veränderungen bei seniler Demenz vom Alzheimer Typ. *Zeitschrift für Elektroenzephalographie, Elektromyographie und Verwandte Gebiete*, 18, 214–216.

Lühdorf, K., Jensen, L.K. & Plesner, A.M. (1986). Etiology of seizures in the elderly. *Epilepsia*, 27, 458–463.

Lukas, S.E., Mandelson, S.H., Kourii, E., Boldric, M. & Amass, L. (1990). Ethanol-induced alteration in EEG alpha activity and apparent source of the auditory P300 evoked response potential. *Alcohol*, 7, 471–477.

McAdam, W. & Robinson, R.A. (1956). Senile intellectual deterioration and the electroencephalogram: a quantitative correlation. *Journal of Mental Science*, 102, 819–825.

Matejcek, M. (1979). Pharmaco-encephalography: the value of quantified EEG in psychopharmacology. *Pharmakopsychiatrie Neuro-Psychopharmakologie*, 12, 126–136.

Matousek, M., Volavka, J., Roubicek, J. & Roth, Z. (1967). EEG frequency analysis related to age in normal adults. *Electroencephalography and Clinical Neurophysiology*, 23, 162–167.

Miyasaka, M., Nakano, T., Ohmori, K., Ohtaka, T. & Mori, K. (1978). The mental deterioration in the aged and the computerized EEG analysis. *Folia Psychiatrica et Neurologica Japonica*, 32, 95–108.

Mooradian, A.D., Perryman, K., Fitten, J., Kavonian, G.D. & Morley, J.E. (1988). Cortical function in elderly non-insulin dependent diabetic patients. *Behavioral and Electrophysiologic Studies*, 148, 2369–2372.

Mullis, R.J., Holcomb, P.J., Diner, B.C. & Dykman, R.A. (1985). The effects of aging on the P3 component of the visual event-related potential. *Electroencephalography and Clinical Neurophysiology*, 62, 141–149.

Mundy-Castle, A.C. (1951). Theta and beta rhythm in the electroencephalograms of normal adult. *Electroencephalography and Clinical Neurophysiology*, 3, 477–486.

Niedermeyer, E. (1987). Epileptic seizure disorders. In *Electroencephalography: Basic Principles, Clinical Applications and Related Fields*, ed. E. Niedermeyer & F. Lopes da Silva, pp. 405–510. Baltimore, MD: Urban and Schwarzenberg.

Nuwer, M.R. (1988). Quantitative EEG: II. Frequency analysis and topographic mapping in clinical settings. *Journal of Clinical Neurophysiology*, 5, 45–85.

Nuwer, M.R., Jordan, S.E. & Ahn, S.S. (1987). Evaluation of stroke using EEG frequency analysis and topographic mapping. *Neurology*, 37, 1153–1159.

O'Brien, J.T., Desmond, P., Ames, D., Schweitzer, I., Tuckwell, V. & Tress B. (1994). The differentiation of depression from dementia by temporal lobe magnetic resonance imaging. *Psychological Medicine*, 24, 633–640.

Obrist, W. (1954). The electroencephalogram of normal aged adults. *Electroencephalography and Clinical Neurophysiology*, 6, 235–244.

Obrist, W.D. (1963). The electroencephalogram of healthy aged males. In *Human Aging: A Biological and Behavioral Study*, ed. J. E. Birren, R. N. Butler, S. W. Greenhouse, L. Sokoloff & M. R. Yarrow, pp. 79–93. Washington DC: US Government Printing Office.

Obrist, W.D. (1976). Problems of aging. In *Handbook of Electroencephalography and Clinical Neurophysiology*, ed. A. Remond, pp. 275–292. Amsterdam: Elsevier.

Obrist, W.D. (1979). Electroencephalographic changes in normal aging and dementia. In *Brain Function in Old Age, Bayer Symposium VII*, ed. F. Moffmeister & C. Müller, pp. 102–111. Berlin: Springer-Verlag.

Obrist, W.D. & Busse, E.W. (1965). The electroencephalogram in old age. In *Applications of Electroencephalography in Psychiatry*, ed. W. P. Wilson, pp. 185–205. Durham, NC: Duke University Press.

Obrist, W.D., Sokoloff, L., Lassen, N.A., Lane, M.H., Butler, R.N. & Feinberg, I. (1963). Relation of EEG to cerebral blood flow and metabolism in old age. *Electroencephalography and Clinical Neurophysiology*, 15, 610–619.

O'Connor, K. & Shaw, J. (1978). Field dependence, laterality and the EEG. *Biological Psychology*, 6, 93–109.

O'Connor, K.P., Shaw, J.C. & Ongley, C.O. (1979). The EEG and differential diagnosis in psychogeriatrics. *British Journal of Psychiatry*, 135, 156–162.

Ogawa, S., Tank, D.W. & Menon, R. (1992). Intrinsic signal change accompanying sensory stimulation: functional brain mapping with magnetic resonance imaging. *Proceedings of the National Academy of Sciences, USA*, 89, 5981–5955.

Oken, B.S. & Kaye, J.A. (1992). Electrophysiologic function in the healthy, extremely old. *Neurology*, 42, 519–526.

Otomo, E. & Tsubaki, T. (1966). Electroencephalography in subjects sixty years and over. *Electroencephalography and Clinical Neurophysiology*, 20, 77–82.

Patterson, J.V., Michalewski, H.J. & Starr, A. (1988). Latency variability of the components of auditory event-related potentials to infrequent stimuli in aging, Alzheimer type dementia, and depression. *Electroencephalography and Clinical Neurophysiology*, 71, 450–460.

Pfefferbaum, A., Ford, J.M., Roth, W.T. & Kopell, B.S. (1980). Age-related changes in auditory event-related potentials. *Electroencephalography and Clinical Neurophysiology*, 49, 266–276.

Pfefferbaum, A., Ford, J.M. Wenegrat, B.G., Roth, W.T. & Kopell, B.S. (1984a). Clinical application of P3 component of event-related potentials. I. Normal aging.

Electroencephalography and Clinical Neurophysiology, 59, 85–103.

Pfefferbaum, A., Horvath, T.B., Roth, W.T. & Kopell, B.S. (1979). Event-related potential changes in chronic alcoholics. *Electroencephalography and Clinical Neurophysiology*, 47, 637–647.

Pfefferbaum, A., Wenegrat, B.G., Ford, J.M. et al. (1984b). Clinical applications of the P3 component of event-related potentials II: dementia. *Electroencephalography and Clinical Neurophysiology*, 59, 104–124.

Picton, T.W., Cherri, A.M., Champagne, S.C., Stuss, D.T. & Nelson, R.F. (1986). The effects of age and task difficulty on the late positive component of the auditory evoked potential. *Electroencephalography and Clinical Neurophysiology*, 38, 132–133.

Picton, T.W., Stuss, D.T., Champagne, S.C. & Nelson, R.F. (1984). The effects of age on human event-related potentials. *Psychophysiology*, 21, 312–325.

Pierelli, F., Pozzessere, G., Sanarelli, L., Valle, E., Rizzo, P.A. & Morocutti, C. (1985). Electrophysiological study in patients with chronic hepatic insufficiency. *Acta Neurologica Belgica*, 85, 284–291.

Pinkus, J. & Tucker, G. (1985). *Behavioural Neurology*. New York: Oxford University Press.

Pizella, V. & Romani, G.L. (1990). Principles of magnetoencephalography. *Advances in Neurology*, 54, 1–9.

Polich, P. (1991). P300 in the evaluation of aging and dementia. In *Event-Related Brain Research*, ed. C.H.M. Brunia, G. Mulder & M.N. Verbaten, pp. 304–323. New York: Elsevier.

Polich, J., Ehlers, C.L., Otis, S., Mandell, A.J. & Bloom, F.E. (1986). P3 latency reflects the degree of cognitive decline in dementing illness. *Electroencephalography and Clinical Neurophysiology*, 63, 138–144.

Polich, J., Howard, L. & Starr, A. (1985). Aging effects on the P300 component of the event-related potential from auditory stimuli: peak definition, variation, and measurement. *Journal of Gerontology*, 40, 721–726.

Pollock, V.E. & Schneider, L.S. (1989). Topographic electroencephalographic alpha in recovered depressed elderly. *Journal of Abnormal Psychology*, 3, 268–273.

Pramming, S., Thorsteinsson, B., Stigsby, B. & Binder, C. (1988). Glycaemic threshold for changes in electroencephalograms during hypoglycaemia in patients with insulin dependent diabetes. *British Medical Journal*, 296, 665–667.

Prichep, L., Mont, F.G., John, E.R. & Ferris, S.H. (1983). Neurometric electroencephalographic characteristics of dementia. In *Alzheimer's Disease: The Standard Reference*, ed. B. Reisberg, pp. 252–257. New York: Macmillan.

Purcell, E.M., Torry, H.C. & Pound, C.V. (1946). Resonance absorption by nuclear magnetic moments in a solid. *Physical Review*, 69, 37.

Rabins, P. & Folstein, M.F. (1982). Delirium and dementia: diagnostic criteria and fatality rates. British *Journal of Psychiatry*, 140, 149–153.

Rae-Grant, A., Blume, W., Lau, C., Hachinski, V.C., Fisman, M. & Merskey, H. (1987). The electroencephalogram in Alzheimer-type dementia. *Archives of Neurology*, 44, 50–54.

Rice, D., Buchsbaum, M., Hardy, D. & Burgwald, L. (1991). Focal left temporal slow EEG activity is related to a verbal recent memory deficit in a non-demented elder population. *Journal of Gerontology*, 4, 144–151.

Roberts, M., McGeorge, A.P. & Caird, F.I. (1978). Electroencephalography and computerized tomography in vascular and nonvascular dementia in old age. *Journal of Neurology, Neurosurgery and Psychiatry*, 41, 903–906.

Romano, J., & Engel, G. (1944). Electroencephalographic data. *Archives of Neurology and Psychiatry*, 51, 356–377.

Rose, D.F. & Ducla-Soares, E. (1990). Comparison of electroencephalography and magnetoencephalography. *Advances in Neurology*, 54, 33–37.

Rosenberg, C., Nudelman, K. & Starr, A. (1985). Cognitive evoked potentials (P300) in early Huntington's disease. *Archives of Neurology*, 42, 984–987.

Rossini, P.M., diStefano, E., Febbo, A., DiPaolo, B. & Basciani, M. (1984). Brainstem auditory evoked responses in patients with chronic renal failure. *Electroencephalography and Clinical Neurophysiology*, 57, 507–514.

Rossini, P.M., Pirchio, M., Treviso, M., Gambi, D., DiPaolo, B. & Albertazi, A. (1981). Checkerboard reversal pattern and flash VEPs in dialyzed and nondialyzed subjects. *Electroencephalography and Clinical Neurophysiology*, 52, 435–444.

Roubicek, J. (1977). The electroencephalogram in the middle-aged and elderly. *Journal of the American Geriatrics Society*, 25, 145–152.

Sage, M.R. & Wilson, A.J. (1994). Special report. The blood-brain-barrier: an important concept in neuroimaging. *American Journal of Neuroradiology*, 1, 601–622.

Sander, J.W.A.S., Hart, Y.M., Johnson, A.L. & Shorvon, S.D. (1990). National general practice study of epilepsy: newly diagnosed epileptic seizures in a general population. *Lancet*, 336, 1267–1271.

Sandford, N.L. & Saul, R E. (1988). Assessment of hepatic encephalopathy with visual evoked potentials compared with conventional methods. *Hepatology*, 8, 1094–1098.

Schatzberg, A.F., Elliot, G.R., Lerbinger, J.E., Marcel, B. & Duffy, F.H. (1986). Topographic mapping in depressed patients. In *Topographic Mapping of Brain Electrical Activity*, ed. F.H. Duffy, pp. 389–391. Boston, MA: Butterworths.

Schlagenhauff, R.E. (1973). Electroencephalogram in gerontology. *Clinical Electroencephalography*, 4, 153–163.

Shagass, C., Romer, R.A., Straumanis, J.J. & Josiassen, R.C. (1984). Psychiatric diagnostic discriminations with combinations of quantitative EEG variables. *British Journal of Psychiatry*, 144, 581–592.

Shaw, J., O'Connor, K. & Ongley, C. (1977a). The EEG as a measure of cerebral functional organization. *British Journal of Psychiatry*, 130, 260–264.

Shaw, J., O'Connor, K. & Ongley, C. (1977b). EEG coherence as a measure of cerebral functional organization. In *Architectonics of the Cerebral Cortex*, ed. M. A. B. Brazier & H. Petsche, pp. 245–255. New York: Raven Press.

Shigemoto, T. (1981). Epilepsy in middle age or advanced age. *Folia Psychiatrica et Neurologica Japonica*, 35, 287–293.

Shonk, T.K., Moats, R.A., Gifford, P. *et al.* (1995). Probable Alzheimer disease: diagnosis with proton MR spectroscopy. *Radiology*, 195, 65–72.

Snyder, E. & Hillyard, S.A. (1976). Long-latency evoked potentials to irrelevant, deviant stimuli. *Behavioral Biology*, 16, 319–331.

Soininen, H., Partanen, V.J., Helkala, E.L. & Riekkinen, P.J. (1982). EEG findings in senile dementia and normal aging. *Acta Neurologica Scandinavica*, 65, 59–70.

Squires, K.C., Chippendale, T.J., Wrege, K.S., Goodin, D.S. & Starr, A. (1980). Electrophysiological assessment of mental function in aging and dementia. In *Aging in the 1980s*, ed. L.W. Poon, pp. 125–134. Washington, DC: American Psychological Association.

St Clair, D., Blackwood, D. & Christine, J.E. (1985). P3 and other long latency auditory evoked potentials in presenile dementia Alzheimer type and alcoholic Korsakoff syndrome. *British Journal of Psychiatry*, 147, 702–706.

Steriade, M. Gloor, P., Llinas, R., Llinás, R.R., Lopes da Silva, F.H. & Mesulam, M.-M. (1990). Basic mechanisms of cerebral rhythmic activities. *Electroencephalography and Clinical Neurophysiology*, 76, 481–508.

Sung, C.-Y & Chu, N.-S. (1990). Epileptic seizures in elderly people: aetiology and seizure type. *Age and Ageing*, 19, 25–30.

Syndulko, K., Cohen, S.N., Pettler-Jennings, P., Shah, J., Friedman, A., Potvin, A.R. & Tourtelotte, W.W. (1984). P300 and neurocognitive function in neurologic patients. In *Evoked Potentials. II. The Second International Evoked Potentials Symposium*, ed. R.H. Nodar & C. Barber, pp. 441–445. Boston, MA: Butterworth.

Syndulko, K., Hansch, M.A., Cohen, S.N. *et al.* (1982). Long-latency event-related potentials in normal aging and dementia. In *Clinical Applications of Evoked Potentials in Neurology*, ed. J. Courjon, F. Maugiere & M. Revol, pp. 279–285. New York: Raven Press.

Thatcher, R.W., Krause, P.J. & Hrybyk, M. (1986). Cortico-cortical associations and EEG coherence: a two-compartmental model. *Electroencephalography and Clinical Neurophysiology*, 64, 123–143.

Torres, F., Faoro, A., Loewenson, R. & Johnson, E. (1983). The electroencephalogram of elderly subjects revisited. *Electroencephalography and Clinical Neurophysiology*, 56, 391–398.

Tress, B.M., Davis, S.M., Lavan, J., Kaye, A.H. & Hopper J.L. (1986). Incremental dynamic computed tomography: a practical method of imaging the carotid bifurcation. *American Journal of Neuroradiology*, 7, 49–54.

Trzepacz, P.T., Sclabassi, R.J. & Van Thiel, D.H. (1989). Delirium: a subcortical phenomenon? *Journal of*

Neuropsychiatry and Clinical Neurosciences, 1, 283–290.

Tucker, D., Roth, D. & Bair, T. (1986). Functional connections among cortical regions: topography of EEG coherence. *Electroencephalography and Clinical Neurophysiology*, 63, 242–250.

Van der Rijt, C.C.D. & Schalm, S.W. (1992). Quantitative EEG analysis and evoked potentials to measure (latent) hepatic encephalopahy. *Journal of Hepatology*, 14, 141–142.

Visser, S.L. (1991). The electroencephalogram and evoked potentials in normal aging and dementia. In *Event-related Brain Research*, ed. C.H.M. Brunia, G. Mulder & M.N. Verbaten, pp. 289–303. New York: Elsevier.

Visser, S.L., Hooijer, C., Jonker, C., van Tilburg, W. & de Rijke, W. (1987). Anterior temporal focal abnormalities in EEG in normal aged subjects: correlations with psychopathological and CT brain scan findings. *Electroencephalography and Clinical Neurophysiology*, 66, 1–7.

Visser, S.L., Stan, F.C., van Tilburg, W., DenVelde, W., Blom, J.L. & de Rijke, W. (1976). Visual evoked response in senile and presenile dementia. *Electroencephalography and Clinical Neurophysiology*, 40, 385–392.

Wang, H. & Busse, E. (1969). EEG of healthy old persons – a longitudinal study. I. Dominant background activity and occipital rhythm. *Journal of Gerontology*, 24, 419–426.

Warach, S., Chien, D. & Li, W. (1992). Rapid diffusion imaging of acute cerebral infarction. *Neurology*, 42, 1717–1723.

Weinberg, H. (1991). Review of MEG studies. In *Introduction to Brain Topography*, ed. P.K.H. Wong, pp. 113–143. New York: Plenum Press.

Weiner, H. & Schuster, D.B. (1956). The electroencephalogram in dementia – some preliminary observations and correlations. *Electroencephalograhy and Clinical Neurophysiology*, 8, 479–488.

Williamson, P.C., Merskey, H., Morrison, S. *et al.* (1990). Quantitative electroencephalographic correlates of cognitive decline in normal elderly subjects. *Archives of Neurology*, 47, 1185–1188.

Winchell, H.S., Baldwin, R.M. & Lin T.H. (1980). Development of I–123-labelled amines for brain studies: localization of I–123 indophenyl alkyl amines in rat brain. *Journal of Nuclear Medicine*, 21, 940–246.

Woodcock, S. & Cosgrove, J.B.R. (1964). Epilepsy after the age of 50. *Neurology*, 14, 34–40.

Woody, R.H. (1966). Intra-judge reliability in clinical EEG. *Journal of Clinical Psychology*, 22, 150.

Woody, R.H. (1968). Inter-judge reliability in clinical EEG. *Journal of Clinical Psychology*, 24, 251–256.

Wright, C.E., Harding, G.F. A. & Orwin, A. (1984). Presenile dementia – the use of the flash and pattern VEP in diagnosis. *Electroencephalography and Clinical Neurophysiology*, 57, 405–415.

Yang, S.-S., Chu, N.-S. & Liaw, Y.F. (1986). Brainstem auditory evoked potentials in hepatic encephalopathy. *Hepatology*, 6, 1352–1355.

Yen, C.L. & Liaw, Y.F. (1990). Somatosensory evoked potentials and number connection test in the detection of subclinical hepatic encephalopathy. *Hepatogastroenterology*, 37, 332–334.

Yetkin, F.Z., Haughton, V.M., Papke, R.A., Fischer, M.E. & Rao, R.M. (1991). Multiple sclerosis: specificity of MR for diagnosis. *Radiology*, 178, 447–451.

Zeneroli, M.L., Pinelli, G., Gollini, G. *et al.* (1984). Visual evoked potential: a diagnostic tool for the assessment of hepatic encephalopathy. *Gut*, 25, 291–299.

Part 2
Neuroimaging in specific psychiatric disorders of late life

2 The normal elderly

Hillel Grossman, Gordon Harris, Sandra Jacobson
and Marshal Folstein

Introduction

Aging is a complex process both dreaded and honored, celebrated for its achievements and mourned for its deficits. The quest of ages has been to understand aging with the hope of forestalling, reversing or even abolishing this process. Contemporary scientific investigations into aging can be seen as further endeavors along this path. There has been much focus in contemporary science on the brain as the locus of key aspects of the aging process; the wisdom, insight, clarity of the old as well as the forgetfulness, dulling and slowing of senescence.

Neuroimaging is a powerful tool for the exploration of the brain and has in many ways supplanted the neuropathological investigation of autopsy-derived specimens as the gold standard for the study of the brain. Autopsy studies have always been limited by the difficulties in gathering large numbers of brains, a selection bias usually involving previously ill subjects and artifacts related to agonal events as well as the fixation of the brain. Neuroimaging allows the study of large populations *in vivo*. As well, subjects can be studied repeatedly, allowing for prospective studies. However, the newness of these technologies remains evident in the ambiguities that surround interpretation of many so-called abnormalities. There is no fully comprehensive or standardized normative baseline across the age spectrum for comparative interpretation of any neuroimaging-derived data. Questions abound about neuroimaging findings and what they represent in terms of neuropathology and certainly in terms of brain function.

This chapter will explore the uses of structural and functional neuroimaging techniques in the study of normal aging. For each technique there will be a review of findings by brain region and then an exploration of the antecedents (risk factors) for the abnormality as well as the consequences or clinical significance.

Interpreting neuroimaging research

Before approaching this literature it is necessary to point out some of the specific difficulties in comparing neuroimaging studies. Studies tend to differ in selection of subjects, imaging technique and imaging and statistical analysis.

Selection of subjects

The primary difficulty in selecting subjects for a study of aging lies in the basic question: what is aging and who are the aged? Many early imaging studies of aging relied upon demented or ill populations and extrapolated to the healthy elderly. However, it is far from clear that correlations found in demented or ill subjects will hold true for normal aging. This speaks directly to a conceptual problem of whether normal aging differs from dementia by degree or whether the demented are a categorically separate entity. In reviewing imaging studies, one finds that prior studies are often criticized for having populations characterized as 'normal' that are too diseased (e.g. including subjects who have cerebrovascular risk factors such as hypertension, diabetes or even small strokes) or are selected from a 'hypernormal' sample of the elderly who are entirely disease free, high functioning and perhaps not representative of the majority of the elderly population. The ideal study recognizes the heterogeneity of the elderly population and controls carefully for this sort of variability. Rowe & Kahn (1987) advocate the terms *usual* and *successful* as a means of describing and classifying some of this heterogeneity in normal aging. Drayer (1988) and others have suggested that neuroimaging may be a key to understanding the risk factors or contributors to usual or successful aging.

Imaging technique

CT and MRI are the two techniques used for the study of brain structure in modern neuroimaging. They are so different that the literature from each must be dealt with separately and cannot be compared directly. Details of these techniques will be found in Chapters 1(a) and 1(b). MRI is more accurate than CT in detecting lesions and in delineating their extent, far more sensitive than CT in detecting white matter abnormalities and has been validated more closely with autopsy than CT. There are several technical factors that are important in analyzing an MRI study.

Magnet size
The strength of the magnet can vary tenfold from 0.2 (low field) to 1.5 or 2.0 T (high field). Stronger magnets generally provide much clearer resolution.

Aquisition parameters

MR images can be obtained in a variety of planes and slicing parameters. The ideal study utilizes very thin slices with no gaps in between slices. Many studies, however, have used thick slices with gaps in between them such that a mathematical interpolation is necessary to estimate the data that exist within the gap or within the thickness of the slice. This is particularly disadvantageous when looking at small structures such as the hippocampus or basal ganglia, which can be lost in the gap or thickness.

Image analysis

The clinical use of neuroimaging varies greatly from its research use. In clinical operations, it is only necessary for an experienced interpreter of images to look at a scan and provide a qualitative reading. For example, a clinical film reader would attest that the film at hand demonstrates a degree of atrophy disproportionate to what is expected for a subject in that age group. Such a qualitative approach is inadequate in research studies, especially in aging when abnormalities are not necessarily detectable by the naked eye and when the object of study itself is normal variation.

Quantification has taken many different approaches. The most primitive are visual rating scales using which an experienced reader provides a reading usually of the degree of atrophy or a count of the number of white matter hyperintensities (WMHI). The next tier involves planimetric measurements either directly from a radiographic film or conducted on a computer console. Ventricle–brain ratios and brain–caudate ratios are examples of this. Volumetric techniques involve some method of counting pixels or three-dimensional voxels of information in an automated or semiautomated fashion. This represents the most objective and sensitive technique for detecting variations and is particularly beneficial in studies of aging in which it is presumed that the variations are subtle and not always obvious to more gross measurements.

Statistical analysis

Statistical analysis of neuroimaging data can be complex. Of greatest importance is the institution of appropriate controls for factors other than aging that might contribute to variability in brain size or function. Such factors include sex, education and head size. The most common means of controlling for these variables are by multivariate analysis. Head size can be controlled for by using the intracranial volume obtained from the imaging data and taking the structure of interest as a proportion of the total intracranial volume. Obviously, there is no change over the course of adulthood in head size or total intracranial volume, though the proportion of tissue versus CSF can and certainly does change across the lifespan. Another important analysis in studying small structures is the need to control for total brain volume. For example, if a study detects atrophy in the caudate nucleus it would still be necessary to demonstrate that this is not simply a reflection of generalized atrophy but rather is specific to the caudate.

Brain changes with aging

Brain size and atrophy

Brain development involves many processes of growth and regress through the life course. Brain size increases dramatically after birth through the first decade of life primarily as a result of gray matter processes such as cell proliferation, arborization and synaptogenesis. The overall growth in the second decade is much more gradual owing to the parallel processes of neuronal pruning and growth, especially axonal myelination. From the third decade through the fifth or sixth decade there is stability in brain size. Subsequently, there is a gradual decline that seems to accelerate with each passing decade. The decrease in brain size is evident neuropathologically as decreased brain weight at autopsy, with CT as increased ventricular size, and with MRI as loss of brain tissue and volume. There is a great deal of variability in the extent of brain atrophy and this variability increases with age.

Neuropathology

On autopsy, the decrease in brain size is evident by lower brain weights, a decrease in gray and white matter and a decreased number of neurons. This has been noted particularly in the superior frontal and superior temple gyri, precentral gyrus, hippocampus, thalamus, amygdala and inferior olive, and Purkinje and dentate of the cerebellum. There is an increase in both central and sulcal CSF, most prominent in the frontal and parietal regions. There is also an increase in the pericerebellar subarachnoid space (Drayer, 1988). On microscopic studies, there is a progressive accumulation of lipofuscin, melanin and ceroid within the neurons. One can also see neuritic plaques, neurofibrillary tangles and granulovacuolar degeneration similar to that seen in Alzheimer's pathology, though less in number. As noted, the problems with autopsy data include difficulty of access to subjects, so that most studies have small numbers as well as a huge sampling bias (some studies are of subjects who have died in hospital of nonneurological causes) and probably are not representative of aging or the elderly. Autopsy subjects obtained in this fashion rarely have good premorbid characterization of cognitive function or risk factors. In addition, there are artifacts inherent in the autopsy process as described previously. Functional data are not obtainable from a neuropathological specimen.

CT

Decrease in brain size in CT studies is manifest by larger ventricles and cortical sulci. This has been seen consistently in aging studies, with the atrophy beginning in the fifth decade and increasing in prominence in the sixth and seventh decades. There is, however, a marked heterogeneity, such that 30–50% of those studied will have ventricles and sulci that fall within the range of young adults (Drayer, 1988). CT studies have relied primarily upon visual rating scales or planimetric measurements and have, therefore, been limited by the strength of the naked eye.

MRI of total brain and CSF

Atrophy is manifest on MRI by enlarged ventricles and sulci, similar to observations by CT. However, MRI studies are better able to detect and quantify subtle contrast and the lack of bony artifact. All studies that analyzed total brain volume have found a decrease with aging. Similarly, all studies have noted an increase in both cortical and ventricular or central CSF. Some have noted a disproportionate increase in cortical CSF relative to the ventricles. The increase in CSF develops earlier and to a greater extent in men than in women. Studies that looked for specific regionalization of brain atrophy noted the frontal lobe to be preferentially affected. Coffey *et al.* (1992) observed that the frontal lobe tended to atrophy at a rate of 0.55% over the course of each year, in contrast to the temporal lobe, which decreased at a rate of 0.23% per year. Others (DeCarli *et al.*, 1994) also found a disproportionate loss of frontal lobe tissue relative even to other parts of the brain that had demonstrated atrophy. Jernigan, Press & Hesselink (1990) found a loss of volume in all peripheral cortical areas and some mesial cortical regions including posterior insula, hippocampus and parahippocampus. A few studies report differences in laterality, though Coffey *et al.* (1992) noted that there was no difference in the rate of atrophy between hemispheres.

Tissue characteristics

MRI allows the distinction of tissue compartments, gray matter, white matter and CSF based on their intrinsic characteristics (hydrogen ion concentration and alignment). Recent volume studies have found no detectable differences in the volume of white matter between old and young subjects (e.g. Jernigan *et al.*, 1991). This clearly contrasts with the progressive decline in gray matter and increase in CSF associated with aging. What emerges is that the different tissue compartments follow distinct developmental courses across a lifetime. Miller, Alston & Corsellis (1980) in a much cited pathological study described a nonlinear decrease in the gray-to-white matter ratio. They noted that in the third decade of life the ratio was 1.3; it decreased to 1.1 in the sixth decade of life but then increased again to 1.2 in the eighth decade. Harris *et al.* (1994) in a large MRI study replicated the findings of Miller and colleagues on autopsy and noted ratios of 1.24 in the third decade of life, 1.15 in the fifth decade of life and 1.4 in the eighth decade of life. These authors suggested that white matter atrophy exceeds gray matter atrophy in later life and hypothesized that in late life neuronal cell loss leads to a loss of both nerve cells in the gray matter as well as myelinated fibers in the white matter. Myelinated fibers are much larger than the nerve cells and this is reflected by the greater loss of white matter and gray matter in later life than in earlier life. Jernigan *et al.* (1991), however, suggest that the volume of white matter remains constant but that its quality, as reflected by T_2 values, changes with age. Abnormalities in white matter characteristics in aging have attracted much attention and merit a separate discussion below.

Specific structures

Hippocampus

Coffey *et al.* (1992) found in their sampling of 76 adults ranging in age from 30–91 that the hippocampal–amygdaloid complex decreases at a rate of 0.30% per year. Jernigan *et al.* (1991) similarly noted a linear decrease in volume of a mesial cortical gray region comprising the posterior insula, hippocampus and parahippocampal gyrus.

Basal ganglia

Subcortical gray matter volume decreases with age, with the greatest loss in the caudate. Caudate and lenticular nucleus volumes are significantly smaller in the elderly even when controlling for generalized atrophy. Jernigan *et al.* (1991) found no significant loss in the lentiform nuclei. This inconsistency is a good example of the influence of imaging technique on the data. Jernigan *et al.* (1991) used a T_2-weighted image; this is highly sensitive to iron (see below), which might interfere with the volume measurement of iron-laden structures like the globus pallidus. The thalamus showed no significant decline with age in all studies.

Diencephalon

Only one study delineated the diencephalon specifically (Jernigan *et al.*, 1991) and found selective loss of an anterior diencephalon region of interest, including anterior hypothalamic, septal and basal forebrain nuclei.

Cerebellum

Neuropathological studies have demonstrated a decrease in cerebellar size and neuronal density with aging in the cerebellar hemispheres and the vermis. Raz *et al.* (1992) demonstrated a strong correlation between age and decreasing area in the cerebellar vermis in a study of 60 subjects ranging in age from 18 to 78. They found the reduction in size limited to the dorsomedial vermis. These regions develop later and have more cortical connections than the ventral vermis. They speculate that the dorsomedial vermis might be more vulnerable to the effects of aging owing to downstream effects of cortical neuronal loss, distance from blood supply and a phylogenetic axiom: 'last to come (in evolution) – first to go (in senium)'. Escalona *et al.* (1991) found no correlation between age and cerebellar volume in 37 subjects, though this study did not control for variation in brain or skull size and did not study the vermis separate from the other cerebellar hemispheres. Mikulis *et al.* (1992) retrospectively reviewed the scans of 221 subjects obtained for clinical purposes and suggested a pattern of change in the positioning of the cerebellar tonsils. In childhood, the tonsils gradually ascend through the foramen magnum as a result of growth of the brain stem and cerebellum. In early and mid-adulthood, the position of the tonsils relative to the foramen magnum remains stable. In late life, neuronal loss leads to a further ascent of the tonsils.

Pituitary

Doraiswamy *et al.* (1992) in a series of studies involving 70 subjects found that pituitary height and cross-sectional area decreased with age between ages 20 and 65. This was most obvious in women but also discernible as a trend in men. The clinical significance of the decrease in pituitary size in later life is unknown.

Gender

Most studies have combined data for men and women together, but there are significant gender effects in aging (Cowell *et al.*, 1994; Gur *et al.*, 1991). As noted above, the increase in CSF volume is much steeper in men than in women. Similarly, men had a disproportionate amount of atrophy in the left hemisphere while females tend to be symmetrical in their degree of atrophy. In addition, the finding in several studies of an increase in cortical atrophy compared with central atrophy is much more pronounced in men than in women. Cowell *et al.* (1994) maintain that sexual dimorphism continues with aging and that it is regionalized and lateralized. They note that the disproportionate frontal lobe atrophy is much more pronounced in men than in women. In addition, men have much more pronounced loss in the right frontal lobe and in the left temporal lobe. They suggest that there is a protective influence of hormones in these regions and that in women the posterior regions of the brain might be more susceptible to the influences of aging.

White matter hyperintensities

WMHI merit their own discussion. The study of WMHI demonstrates both the promise of neuroimaging, particularly MRI, in the detection of subtle brain abnormalities and the newness of these technologies. There is much ambiguity surrounding the interpretation of many of these detected 'abnormalities' and their significance. There has grown a substantial literature since the early 1980s regarding these hyperintensities both in normal aging and in disease processes. WMHI have been held out as the key to distinguishing usual from successful aging (Drayer, 1988; Rowe & Kahn, 1987) and as the elusive 'organic' histopatholology previously sought after but not detected in the idiopathic psychiatric disorders such as schizophrenia and major affective disorders.

At the turn of the century, Binswanger described a rare variant of arteriosclerotic dementia characterized by severe atrophy of white matter and relative sparing of the cerebral cortex. Binswanger referred to his cases as having '*encephalities subcorticalis chronica progressiva*'. Subsequently this has been referred to as subcortical arteriosclerotic encephalopathy or, simply, Binswanger's disease. The clinical syndrome associated with this pathology is characterized by a subacute syndrome including syncope, gait disturbance, hyperreflexia, dementia and elements of pseudobulbar palsy including dysphagia, dysarthria and emotional incontinence (Cummings & Benson, 1983). The etiology was presumed for many years to be vascular, related to atherosclerotic involvement of deep penetrating medullary arteries and/or a watershed effect involving deep white matter.

Binswanger's disease or vascular-related degeneration of white matter was considered rare until the advent of contemporary neuroimaging in the 1970s. Several CT scan studies noted white matter abnormalities occurring with some frequency. On CT, these abnormalities appeared as hypodensities and were referred to as 'rims' or 'caps' when seen in the periventricular areas and as 'unidentified bright objects' when seen in the deep white matter.

With the advent of MRI and enhanced ability to visualize white matter, such lesions were noted with even greater frequency as hyperintensities on proton density and T_2-weighted images. These signal hyperintensities are found in the periventricular regions, deep white matter and subcortical gray matter. While some early reports suggested a reconsideration of the frequency of Binswanger's disease, it soon became clear that the clinical significance of these hyperintensities and whether they reflected disease were unresolved questions. There are several outstanding questions that remain 10 years after the appearance of the first studies of WMHI:

(1) Do WMHI represent disease?
(2) If they do not represent actual disease do they presage or predict disease?
(3) Are WMHI a feature of normal aging?

To answer all the above briefly: WMHI do not on their own represent disease. There is a more complex answer that depends upon the size of the hyperintensity, its location and, most importantly, its histopathology, as will be discussed in detail below. However, the most common WMHI certainly cannot be considered as manifestations of disease in the absence of clinical symptoms. It is not known if so-called benign WMHI predict the development of disease. Few prospective studies have been conducted and those undertaken have been of limited duration (up to 12 months). Some further basic questions regarding WMHI are:

(1) Are there more WMHI with aging?
(2) Where are they located?
(3) Of what clinical importance are they? Namely, how does location, size or histopathology impact upon clinical function.

The neuropathology literature regarding WMHI will be reviewed first, followed by the neuroimaging literature.

Neuropathology

Neuropathological studies have noted focal abnormalities in cerebral white matter occurring most commonly in (descending order): periventricular areas; deep optic radiations, basal ganglia and centrum semiovale. A broad spectrum of histology has been found to accompany these white matter abnormalities. The basic question is whether the WMHI represent damaged tissue or simply an excess of CSF, which can occur in a variety of physiological circumstances. White matter abnormalities on autopsy have been found to be:

(1) *Etat crible* or arteriolar ectasia; there is enlargement of the perivascular space creating an 'extensive network of tunnels filled with perivascular fluid' (Awad *et al.*, 1986)
(2) Myelin pallor
(3) Lacunar infarction
(4) Gliosis
(5) Vascular malformations.

These represent the abnormalities seen in white matter on neuropathology. Several studies have looked at the neuropathology of WMHI seen on MRI. They have pointed out a distinction in the pathology of periventricular and nonperiventricular abnormalities. Periventricular abnormalities are associated with nonischemic processes. For example, defects in the ependymal lining, or gliosis, and fibrosis of small vessels in the subcallosal fasciculus. Nonperiventricular hyperintensities have a more heterogeneous appearance, including dilated perivascular spaces, small infarctions or no detectable abnormality. Periventricular hyperintensities tend to be thin and symmetrical. Those that have an irregular border, that are deep, extending or confluent are more likely to represent demyelination, spongiosis and frequently frank infarction. The limitations of autopsy studies are extensive: the inclusion of patients with disease, lack of premorbid characterization of the subjects, artifacts of death and fixation and no comprehensive analysis of white matter in that only selections are examined microscopically. The selections usually do not include deep white matter or basal ganglia, frequent sites for MRI-detected abnormalities.

Neuroimaging
Neuroimaging provides access to healthy elderly subjects and examines the entire brain comprehensively. Most CT scan studies utilized visual rating scales to quantify the white matter abnormalities. A minority of studies utilized planimetric measurements (such as ventricle to brain ratios) and even fewer studies utilized volumetric techniques. WMHI are detectable on CT but generally must be quite large in order to be seen. Presumably, this is why CT studies have demonstrated stronger correlations between WMHI and other evidence of aging; only large lesions are being entered into the correlation. For example, Kobari, Stirling Meyer & Ichijo (1990) studied 37 subjects who were 'cognitively normal' and noted that white matter abnormalities (referred to as leukoaraiosis) were present in 22%. They noted that the severity and presence of WMHI correlated with the degree of cerebral atrophy, age and cerebral perfusion (by xenon-enhanced CT).

MRI is far superior to CT in the detection and delineation of WMHI. Virtually all studies of WMHI have noted an increase in the presence of the hyperintensities with age. Of note, the vast majority of these studies have been cross-sectional, sampling a broad age range with an increased preponderance of hyperintensities noted in the oldest age groups. Breteler *et al.* (1994), in a true community sample, noted WMHI in 27% of their group in the age range 65 to 84 years. The frequency and severity of hyperintensities increased with age such that while only 11% demonstrated hyperintensities in the 65–69 year age group this increased to 59% in the 80–84 year-old group. Christiansen *et al.* (1994) in a study of 142 volunteers noted that 20% of those in the group aged 21–30 years had WMHI and this figure increased to 100% for the group aged 61–80 years. Both Christiansen *et al.* and Breteler *et al.* utilized high-field (1.5 T) scanners, though the former study used thinner slices without any interslice gap.

Hyperintensities can vary in location, though most studies looked at periventricular intensities only. Coffey *et al.* (1992) in a study of 76 volunteers ranging from 30 to 91 years of age found that 64% of their sample had WMHI in the deep white matter. Only 12% had hyperintensities in the periventricular white matter and 21% had hyperintensities in the pons. The risk for subcortical hyperintensities increased with age only in the deep white matter and pons but not in the basal ganglia or periventricular white matter. The odds of showing hyperintensities increased by 5 to 9% per year depending on the brain region. In virtually all studies that rated the severity of WMHI, most subjects had lesions of only mild severity, though severity tended to increase with advancing age.

Regarding the questions whether WMHI are 'normal' or are suggestive of disease, there have been several approaches. Many have looked to see if hyperintensities correlate with other measures of aging or disease such as brain atrophy or cognitive impairment. Again there is a mixed story. Kobari *et al.* in a 1990 CT study noted that the severity of atrophy was the best predictor of the presence of white matter abnormality, though age and decreased CBF to the subcortical area were also significantly predictive. Christiansen *et al.* (1994), in a high-field study, found no correlation between WMHI and a decrease in brain volume nor with an increase in ventricular volume. Breteler *et al.* (1994), however, in another high-field study noted that the severity of WMHI correlated directly with ventricular–brain ratio even after controlling for age and sex. DeCarli *et al.* (1994) using a 0.5 T magnet and 7 mm slices noted that WMHI volume is an independent predictor of decreased brain volume and increased CSF, though this effect was mostly in larger (greater than 0.5% of total intracranial volume) hyperintensities.

Neuropsychological correlates of WMHI

WMHI correlations with cognition is a complex story with numerous conflicting studies. As noted above, conflicting studies can be a result of several factors.

(1) Subject populations differed between studies in sample size, age range, gender ratios as well as exclusion criteria. Many studies rigidly excluded subjects with any cerebral vascular risk factors and others excluded only those with frank infarction. Some studies excluded subjects with cerebral vascular disease but included subjects with medical disease. Again there has been no standardization in the selection of subject populations.

(2) Many studies differed in magnet size, and slice size, as well as parameters of the actual image. For example, some studies looked at hyperintensities on T_2-weighted images and others looked at proton density-weighted images. As discussed previously, magnet and slice size can determine whether small hyperintensities will be visualized or not and the imaging parameters can dictate whether a blood vessel will be considered an abnormal area of white matter.

(3) Quantification of hyperintensities utilizes rating scales depending upon a visual impression of an expert rater. Only three studies have utilized volumetric technique in the analysis of white matter (Breteler et al., 1994; DeCarli et al., 1994; Jernigan et al., 1990). Volumetric technique has been demonstrated to be more sensitive than the naked eye in detecting small hyperintensities as well as providing a more subtle measure of the severity than rating scales, which are usually a 0 to 3 scale.

(4) Studies have ranged from using simple screening instruments to full-scale neuropsychological batteries. Even within the large batteries, however, some have been more regionally focused to elicit frontal or subcortical dysfunction, again making it difficult to compare negative and positive studies.

Most of the earlier studies of WMHI looking at cognitive correlates of WMHI found no correlation between the presence of hyperintensities and presence or severity of dementia; however, many of these studies were limited in technical parameters that affected the detection of WMHI or in the neuropsychological battery used. Most of the studies utilized a general screening instrument such as the (MMSE) (Folstein, Folstein & McHugh, 1975). Tupler et al. (1992) utilized a broader neuropsychological battery and a high-resolution magnet and found a strong correlation between a measure of attention, mental speed, as well as a measure of visual recognition. However, when age and educational level were included in their statistical model, they were found to account entirely for the correlation. As noted above, WMHI must achieve a larger size before they are detected on CT. This suggests a threshold effect for the development of cognitive impairment. This is precisely what two recent studies have argued. Boone et al. (1993) in a study of recruited subjects between the ages of 45 and 83 noted impairments in digit span and Wisconsin card sort in a subset with subjects with WMHI that were greater than 10 cm^2 in total. Schmidt et al. (1993) in a study of 150 subjects (mean age 60 years) found that most subjects with WMHI tended to be older and performed worse on timed tasks of complemental processing. However, the cognitive measures did not correlate with actual area measurements of WMHI. Schmidt interpreted this correlation between cognitive performance and the presence but not severity of WMHI as emphasizing the importance of the histopathology of a particular lesion over its size. This is in contrast to Boone et al. (1993) and DeCarli et al. (1994) who emphasized the importance of the size of the lesion. DeCarli et al. (1994) in a recent study utilizing a 0.5 T magnet noted that WMHI volumes were a significant independent predictor on several neuropsychological variables including general IQ, visual memory, digit symbol, and trails A and B. DeCarli et al. (1994) found that the correlation was continuous across the severity spectrum of WMHI; however, in subjects with very large quantities of WMHI (greater than 0.5% the total intracranial volume) WMHI volumes correlated with neuropsychological deficits as well as with systolic blood pressure, metabolic perfusion, total cranial volume and total CSF. This suggests again that there is a threshold effect for size that is robustly correlated with several parameters of disease. Cognitive function may be more vulnerable than measures of perfusion or brain volume. It is noteworthy that the studies that have detected positive correlations have generally been recent studies utilizing large numbers of community-recruited volunteers and have found correlations particularly in frontal/subcortical functions. Studies that have utilized the Trails tests (Breteler et al., 1994; DeCarli et al., 1994; Schmidt et al., 1993) have all found positive correlations. In contrast, studies that have utilized broad screening measures, tests of language, memory or visuospatial function, have generally demonstrated no correlation with WMHI and deficits in these areas. This suggests that there might be a particular profile for the cognitive impairment that occurs as a result of white matter deterioration or dysfunction: impairments in attention, 'executive function' and mental speed. DeCarli et al. (1994) point out that the long association superior-longitudinal fasciculi pass immediately adjacent to the lateral ventricles, the most common site for WMHI. Damage to the fasciculi might explain the frontal pattern of cognitive impairment that can be detected with WMHI. Breteler et al. (1994) similarly suggest a 'disconnection syndrome' as a means of accounting for frontal lobe type deficits at sites of injury distal to the actual frontal lobes.

WMHI correlations with atrophy. These have been examined in at least four studies. Kobari et al. (1990) in a CT study reported that atrophy was the strongest predictor of the presence of WMHI, followed by age and then by regional cerebral blood flow (rCBF). Christiansen et al. (1994), however, found no correlation between WMHI and the loss of brain volume or increased ventricular volume. DeCarli et al. (1994) found that WMHI are an independent predictor of loss of brain volume and increase in CSF, though this effect was primarily seen in the minority of subjects with very large quantities of WMHI (greater than 0.5% of the total intracranial volume). Breteler et al. (1994) found the severity of WMHI correlating directly with ventricle-to-brain ratio even after controlling for age and sex.

WMHI correlations with cerebrovascular risk factors. The majority of studies found no correlation between WMHI and cerobrovascular risk factors such as history of stroke, hypertension, diabetes or cardiac disease, nor with laboratory values including serum glucose, serum triglycerides, serum cholesterol, cardiolipin antibodies, coagulation factors or Doppler evidence of stenosis. The lack of correlation is evident in studies that look at the presence or absence of WMHI as well as in studies that look continuously at the number of risk factors and the actual size or frequency of WMHI. Some studies (Breteler et al., 1994; DeCarli et al., 1994) have noted that an increased history of stroke, myocardial infarction and, raised systolic blood pressure related to the prevalence and severity of WMHI. DeCarli et al. (1994) reported this correlation only in those subjects who had very large quantities of WMHI.

Summary

WMHI increase with aging, starting about the sixth decade of life. They are most often detected in periventricular regions but can also be seen in the deep white matter as well as deep gray matter. They do not in themselves represent frank disease, though their clinical significance depends upon the size of the hyperintensity, its location and the neuropathology. Periventricular hyperintensities are more likely to represent benign processes and have minimal, if any, effect on cognition; lesions that are situated at a distance from the ventricles are more likely to represent infarction and to impact upon cognition. There is a particular cognitive profile associated with WMHI that includes deficits of a frontal/subcortical pattern and that is not readily detected with general cognitive screens. There are very limited data regarding prognosis of WMHI, but available data suggest that they do not predict or presage the development a more fulminant disease process. WMHI are representative of both the benefits and pitfalls of rapidly expanding technology. The initial surprise at detecting hyperintensities frequently in normal subjects led to an erroneous assumption that this represented a disease or pre-disease state related to cerebral vascular disease. This was not borne out by multiple studies. Research in the field since the mid-1980s has brought forth a more nuanced explanation of WMHI, which recognises multiple etiologies, pathobiologies and clinical effects.

Functional brain changes

Emission tomography

As people age, the brain suffers neuronal loss and atrophy. Neuropathology studies in healthy, normal elderly subjects have reported neuronal loss primarily in frontal, parietal and temporal lobes (Brody, 1955; Tomlinson, Blessed & Roth, 1968). The ratio of gray matter to white matter changes during aging in a nonlinear fashion, a result observed in both neuropathology (Miller *et al.*, 1980) and *in vivo* MRI studies (Harris *et al.*, 1994). Cerebral atrophy can be quantified in the living human brain by measuring the percentage of CSF on MR images. During normal aging, the CSF percentage increases significantly (Harris *et al.*, 1991b; Jernigan *et al.*, 1990). Although cerebral age-related changes are substantial, the decay is gradual when compared with the devastating effects of senile dementing illnesses such as AD.

Functional neuroimaging techniques such as PET and SPET allow the observation of cerebral glucose metabolic rate, blood flow or receptor concentration in the living human brain. These techniques have been used to study the effects of aging on global cerebral function, and on specific cerebral regions. Age-related changes in neurotransmitter/neuroreceptor systems have also been studied with emission tomography and radioligands that bind to specific receptor systems. Although not all studies have reported concordant results, some findings appear robust and are consistent with the neurophysiology of the aging process.

A number of studies have sought to determine whether general cerebral physiological measures decline with increasing age in normal healthy subjects. These studies have presented contradictory results. Some studies reported significant decline in global cerebral glucose metabolism or blood flow with aging (Kuhl et al., 1982; Levine, Hanson & Nickles, 1994; Takada et al., 1992) but several other research groups did not find such age-related effects (de Leon et al., 1983; 1984; 1987; Duara et al., 1983; 1984; Schlageter et al., 1987; Waldemar et al., 1991). Several groups have suggested that these global effects must be evaluated with corrections for cerebral atrophy, and a number of different atrophy correction techniques have been presented (Chawluk et al., 1987; 1990; Clark et al., 1987; Gottschalk & Hoffer, 1988; Herscovitch et al., 1986; Schlageter et al., 1987; Videen et al., 1988). One research team reported a significant effect of age on global glucose metabolism, which declined with age. However, after correcting for global atrophy, which was correlated with age and inversely correlated with metabolism, the age effects on metabolism were no longer significant (Yoshii et al., 1988). Another research group reported no age effects on global metabolism in healthy males, either with or without correcting for global atrophy (Schlageter et al., 1987). Although the observations of global aging effects on cerebral function are discrepant and further clarification is needed, the presence or absence of global cerebral changes with age are less interesting and informative than reports of localized functional changes.

Decreases in cerebral function associated with the aging process are not uniform throughout the brain. Several studies have reported that these changes were most notable in the three 'association centers' described by Flechsig (1896): regions of the human cerebral cortex devoted to cross-modal sensory association (Villiger, 1931). These regions are currently described as the heteromodal association cortex (Mesulam, 1985). This cortical system coordinates behavioral cognitive and sensory–motor activities and is highly integrated and reciprocally connected. These telencephalic brain regions are the most recently evolved and are the slowest to complete maturation: heteromodal association cortex neurons do not complete myelination or pruning until late adolescence (Benes, 1989). These regions are also susceptible to the neuropathological effects of several degenerative or developmental neurologic or psychiatric illnesses, such as AD (Harris et al., 1991a; Pearlson et al., 1992) and schizophrenia (Schlaepfer et al., 1994).

While the literature is unclear regarding global cerebral functional decline with aging, there is more consistency in results indicating localized regional decline in the heteromodal association cortex of the frontal, temporal and parietal lobes. Some articles describe decline in all three of these regions (Martin et al., 1991; Pantano et al., 1984; Yoshii et al., 1988), although another report observed these decreases only in the left hemisphere (Takada et al., 1992). Not all research teams reported differences in all three of these regions. Several groups observed age-related decline primarily in frontal cortical regions (de Leon et al., 1987; Kuhl et al., 1982; Salmon et al., 1991; Waldemar et al., 1991), while parietal changes were noted in another study (Burns & Tyrrell, 1992). Therefore, these heteromodal association cortex regions, which are relatively new in evolutionary terms and which mature and myelinate in late adolescence, are susceptible to multiple types of neuropathology and are also most affected during the normal aging process.

Functional decline in heteromodal association cortices may help explain the memory impairment that is common in normal aging. In one PET study, researchers observed rCBF changes associated with memory encoding and retrieval tasks (Grady et al., 1995). The CBF responses of a group of young normal volunteers were compared with those of an elderly normal subject group. While the young subjects had increased rCBF during the memory encoding task in left prefrontal and temporal cortex and in hippocampus, the elderly subjects did not have blood flow increases in these regions. During the memory retrieval task, both groups had right prefrontal increases, and the young subjects also had increased right parietal perfusion. Therefore, age-related memory impairments may be associated with decreased regional activation during memory encoding.

In addition to changes in cerebral metabolism and blood flow, PET and SPET are able to observe *in vivo* neuroreceptor physiology. Radioactively labeled compounds have been developed that bind to neuroreceptors, allowing creation of functional neuroimages of their distribution. Researchers have observed the neuroreceptor concentration (B_{max}) or binding rate constants (binding potential, uptake rate constant, or dissociation rate constant) of radioligands to neuroreceptors to study dopamine receptors (D_2, D_1), 5–HT$_2$ (S_2) serotonin receptors, muscarinic cholinergic receptors (M_1, M_2) and H$_1$ histamine receptors.

The greatest number of age-related neuroreceptor studies have been directed at the nigrostriatal dopaminergic system. Studies using the D_2 dopamine receptor radioligand [^{11}C]raclopride (Antonini et al., 1993; Rinne et al., 1993) or N-[^{11}C]methylspiperone (NMSP) (Iyo & Yamasaki, 1993; Wong et al., 1984) have shown a decline in nigrostriatal D_2 dopamine receptor concentration and binding rate constants with advancing age. Additionally, decline in D1 dopamine receptors has been observed using the radioligand ^{11}C-SCH23390 (Iyo & Yamasaki, 1993; Suhara et al., 1991). Several studies have been performed to measure D_2 receptor uptake binding rate constants or receptor number using PET and ^{18}F-labeled L-dopa. Several research groups observed an age-related decline in the uptake and binding of the labeled L-dopa (Cordes et al., 1994; Martin et al., 1989), although other groups did not duplicate this observation (Eidelberg et al., 1993; Sawle et al., 1990). Generally, however, these studies indicate an age-related loss of nigrostriatal dopaminergic neurons.

In addition to studies of the dopaminergic system, several PET reports have focused on changes in other neuroreceptor systems with advancing age. These studies have indicated that many neuroreceptor systems decline with aging. Serotonin 5–HT$_2$ receptors were found to decrease with age (Iyo & Yamasaki, 1993; Wong et al., 1984). Other research groups observed decline in the functioning of muscarinic cholinergic M_1 and M_2 receptors (Dewey et al., 1990; Suhara et al., 1993) and histamine H$_1$ receptors (Yanai et al., 1992). All these studies suggest a gradual decline with aging in multiple neuroreceptor systems.

In conclusion, the brain suffers a diminution of several aspects of its functioning during the aging process. There is no clear evidence of a global decline in cerebral metabolism or blood flow during aging, as studies in this area have been inconsistent, and the effects of atrophy during aging on these global measures may complicate this issue. However, in studies of regional brain function, the results have been more consistent. There appears to be a concentration of age-related functional decline in regions devoted to heteromodal association, located in the frontal, temporal and parietal cortex. These regions are involved in advanced cognitive functioning and reach myelinated maturation relatively late in life (late adolescence). In addition, these regions are susceptible to neuropathology in several disparate disorders and appear to be particularly affected by the aging process. Several neuroreceptor systems, including the dopaminergic, serotonergic, muscarinic cholinergic and histaminergic systems, demonstrate deterioration in PET receptor radioligand studies, indicating a decline in numbers of receptors and a reduction in binding rate constants. Thus, PET and SPET studies have been informative in the depiction of the *in vivo* processes of aging in the human brain.

In addition to PET and SPET, there are new imaging modalities that may contribute additional information in future studies. The advent of echo-planar MRI has led to the development of two new functional imaging modalities; the blood oxygenation level-dependent (BOLD) technique, and the dynamic susceptibility contrast (DSC) MRI method. The BOLD method enables the observation of changes in rCBF without the use of any contrast injection (Ogawa *et al.*, 1993). With BOLD imaging, scans are acquired every one to three seconds over a period of minutes, and rCBF changes can be observed during repeated and varied cognitive activation tasks. Since there is no external contrast agent, subjects can have multiple noninvasive scans. The BOLD method does not provide a baseline functional image. DSC MRI generates images of rCBV that are similar to PET and SPET blood flow images by using a bolus injection of an MRI contrast agent, which alters the local MRI signal, during echo-planar acquisition (Belliveau *et al.*, 1990). This technique has several important advantages over nuclear medicine imaging: DSC MRI uses no ionizing radiation, it can produce images of higher in-plane spatial resolution (1–2 mm) than PET or SPET, it is faster, requiring only about two minutes for acquisition, and it can be less expensive, since both functional and structural scanning are done in a single imaging session, while PET and SPET are frequently done as a complement to structural MR or CT imaging. It also requires less scheduling and inconvenience to the patient. To compare DSC MR with nuclear medicine imaging, functional images produced by DSC and MRI were measured in a group of patients with AD and in matched elderly control subjects (Harris *et al.*, 1996). The regional deficits were almost identical to those observed in similar subject groups using SPET with similar image quantitative analysis methods (Harris *et al.*, 1991a; Pearlson *et al.*, 1992), lending further validation to the utility of DSC MRI as an alternative functional imaging modality to radionuclide tomographic imaging.

EEG and magnetic activity mapping

EEG or brain electrical activity mapping and MEG mapping are functional imaging methods marked by superior temporal resolution (on the order of milliseconds) in comparison with other modalities (see Chapter 1(d)). This characteristic makes these methods particularly useful in determining the time course of various cognitive, sensory and motor functions. Both modalities can image evoked as well as spontaneous brain activity, with MEG being slightly better than EEG mapping in terms of spatial resolution.

EEG mapping was introduced in the 1980s to a community of electro-encephalographers with a well-established tradition of conventional EEG methods and has not been widely used clinically, in part because it never obviated the need to perform conventional waveform analysis. The impetus for development of MEG came at about the same time but was provided by physicists and engineers who were looking for applications for the newly developed SQUID. MEG development has been characterized by a more quantitative approach and motivated by a strong interest in characterizing signal sources. At this time, MEG remains a research tool, albeit of considerable promise.

EEG mapping

In EEG mapping, electrical signals (EEG or evoked potentials) are captured by traditional means but are recorded digitally and processed electronically (with values between electrodes obtained by interpolation). These data are used to produce topographic maps of different quantitative EEG functions, such as absolute and relative spectral power, amplitude, coherence and mean frequency. These maps are presented in color or gray scale on a computer screen, and the images can be printed out directly using a laser or color printer. With some systems, images can be cartooned to show real-time changes in electrocerebral activity, for example, with task or with psychotropic drug administration.

In comparison with traditional EEG methods of display and interpretation, quantitative analysis with topographic mapping of EEG is superior in several ways. Computer analysis of EEG is more sensitive than visual inspection to low-voltage slowing as well as to subtle asymmetries and focalities. In addition, maps as output provide a means of summarizing complex EEG information topographically, approximating more closely the way in which the clinician actually thinks about brain function. Finally, electrical activity maps can be coregistered with maps of metabolism or blood flow or even structure, providing a more complete picture of normal and abnormal brain function.

As noted above, however, EEG mapping is not yet in widespread clinical use. Mapping methods have been validated in various ways (including correlation with traditional EEG) and still are undergoing development. As with other imaging modalities, a critical issue confronting users of EEG mapping is that of normative data. Commercially available mapping systems offer the capability of performing a statistical comparison of patient data with that of a proprietary database; these databases, however, are of variable quality, depending of course on the care taken to recruit, apply exclusionary criteria and adequately study these 'normal' subjects. In practice, most EEG laboratories doing quantitative analysis now have their own normative databases, established using known standards.

As with other functional neuroimaging methods, the question of reliability has been raised for EEG mapping. Pollock and colleagues addressed this issue in a study of 50 patients age 56–76 years who underwent EEG study at two points in time with a 4.5 month test interval; they found high reliabilities for most EEG amplitude measures over this interval (Pollock, Schneider & Lyness, 1991). Finally, the issue of standardization of state has been raised with reference to EEG mapping. It is known that alpha and beta wave activity are sensitive to eyes-open versus eyes-closed condition and to task; it is critically important, therefore, that comparisons be made between like conditions either for serial studies or for comparisons between laboratories.

EEG findings in the normal elderly were once believed to include decreased frequency of the posterior dominant (alpha) rhythm, increased theta and delta slowing, decreased beta activity and focal temporal abnormalities (Breslau *et al.*, 1989; Torres *et al.*, 1983). In most of those studies, these abnormal EEG findings were attributed to aging *per se*. More recent studies aided by quantitative analysis and topographic mapping suggest that these findings are not seen in *healthy* elderly patients (Duffy, McAnulty & Albert, 1993; Maurer & Kierks, 1992). In fact, a study of 202 healthy patients distributed across five decades (age 30–80 years) demonstrated a trend towards *decreased* slow and increased fast activity with age (Duffy *et al.*, 1993). In another study of 52 subjects aged 20–91 years, aging was associated with decreased theta and delta wave slowing, and decreased activity in all bands (Hartikainen *et al.*, 1992). Cognitive performance in normal elderly subjects has been found to correlate with beta activity in frontal areas (Williamson *et al.*, 1990). In one of the few studies reporting evoked potential findings in the normal elderly, Maurer & Kierks (1992) found that P300 evoked potentials showed increased latency and decreased amplitude with aging, but maintenance of normal topography, with a parieto-temporooccipital maximum.

Using spectral ratios (e.g. power in 18–22Hz versus 2–6Hz bands), Leuchter and colleagues (1987) were able to distinguish normals from patients with AD on the basis of spectral content in the left temporal region. Quantitative EEG analysis offers yet another means of evaluating the EEG: spectral coherence, which is the correlation in spectral content between two electrode positions. Coherence is a reflection of anatomy as well as functional connections between brain regions. Decreased coherence is associated with normal aging (Duffy *et al.*, 1995).

As these studies show, quantitative analysis and topographic mapping of EEG data have the potential to extend the diagnostic capabilities of EEG. Topographic maps are more sensitive than conventional EEG to subtle asymmetries and to low-voltage activity. In addition, maps make EEG data easier to interpret and facilitate comparisons with images from other modalities such as MRI and SPET. Finally, maps can be cartooned to show brain activity over time (with task etc.). Future developments in neural network modeling (Anderer *et al.*, 1994; Veselis, Reinsel & Wronski, 1993) and dipolar source modeling promise to make EEG mapping an important tool for understanding normal aging and for distinguishing different types of pathology.

MEG

Details of MEG rationale and technique were given in Chapter 1(d). To date, MEG studies have looked at alpha rhythms, sleep spindles, ictal and interictal activity, and auditory-, visual- and somatosensory-evoked responses, among other parameters. Good correlation has been found between EEG and MEG alpha rhythms (Sato, Balish & Muratore, 1991).

A controversy arose subsequent to publication in 1990 of the results of a study in which investigators created test sources in the brain by directing current to depth electrodes implanted in epileptic patients (Cohen, Cuffin & Yunokunchi, 1990). Magnetic and electrical fields produced by these artificial dipoles were measured; sources were ascertained by an 8 mm average error for MEG and 10 mm average error for EEG. The authors concluded that MEG is not superior to EEG in localization. The study was criticized on several grounds, (Hari et al., 1991; Williamson, 1991) and a consensus statement was issued in 1991 by the European Concerted Action on Biomagnetism Group (COMAC-BME) suggesting that EEG and MEG should be considered complementary techniques (Anogianakis et al., 1992).

MEG has been used to map the sensorimotor cortex and to identify the central sulcus (Gallen et al., 1995; Orrison et al., 1992; Sobel et al., 1993), to map the retina onto the visual cortex (Ahlfors, Ilmoniemi & Hamalainen, 1992), to determine tonotopic organization of auditory cortex (Pantev et al., 1988; Romani, Williamson & Kaufman, 1982; Tiitinen, 1993) and to illustrate specificity of different brain areas to phonetic features (Kuriki, Okita & Hirata, 1995). Auditory stimuli elicit early components that originate in the brain stem, then a sequence of rhythmic evoked response components (at 15–20 milliseconds) that have been localized to the thalamocortical projection (Ribary, 1991) and supratemporal auditory cortex (Pantev et al. 1991). The temporal sequence of activation in human auditory primary and association cortices has been studied using MEG (Lu & Kaufman, 1992). MEG also has been used to demonstrate plasticity of cortical sensory areas (Elbert et al., 1994; Mogilner et al., 1993).

MEG and MRI were used in tandem to localize the somatosensory and auditory cortices in seven healthy persons 30–80 years of age studied with a 37–channel biomagnetometer (Sobel et al., 1993). Data were acquired over the contralateral hemisphere after tactile stimulation of the thumb and the second and fifth digits of each hand, and of the lower lip. Data also were acquired in response to a series of monaural tone bursts. Source modeling procedures enabled these investigators to localize activated neuronal populations. The authors suggest that these methods could be used to relate brain function to structure in preoperative planning (for tumors, for example) and in the work-up and treatment of epilepsy, among other disorders.

It is apparent even from these few reports that MEG is an exceptionally powerful research tool, likely to reveal important information about cognitive, sensory and motor function. The clinical utility of MEG, however, has yet to be demonstrated. Investigators are working on many fronts to extend the practical application of this modality. Studies are underway to develop more precise models of the head based on actual skull shape, to create more realistic models of spike foci and to develop larger, multiarray systems of data acquisition. It is predicted that MEG methods might replace the WADA test for cerebral dominance and obviate the need for placement of depth electrodes in epilepsy studies. The real value of MEG will likely only be realized when EEG and MEG efforts are integrated.

References

Ahlfors, S.P., Ilmoniemi, R.J. & Hamalainen, M.S. (1992). Estimates of visually evoked cortical currents. *Electroencephalography and Clinical Neurophysiology*, 82, 225–236.

Anderer, P., Saletu, B., Kloppel, B *et al.* (1994). Discrimination between demented patients and normals based on topographic EEG slow wave activity: comparison between *z* statistics, discriminant analysis and artificial neural network classifiers. *Electroencephalography and Clinical Neurophysiology*, 91, 108–117.

Anogianakis, G., Badier, J.M. Barrett, G. *et al.* (1992). A consensus statement on relative merits of EEG and MEG. *Electroencephalography and Clinical Neurophysiology*, 82, 317–319.

Antonini, A., Leenders, K.L., Resit, H., Thomann, R., Beer, H.F. & Locher, J. (1993). Effect of age on D_2 dopamine receptors in normal human brain measured by positron emission tomography and ^{11}C-raclopride. *Archives of Neurology*, 50, 474–480.

Awad, I.A., Johnson, P.C., Spetzler, R.E. & Hodak, J.A. (1986). Incidental subcortical lesions identified on magnetic resonance imaging in the elderly, II, postmortem pathological correlations. *Stroke*, 17, 1090–1097.

Belliveau, J.W., Rosen, B.R., Kantor, H.L. *et al.* (1990). Functional imaging by susceptibility-contrast NMR. *Magnetic Resonance Medicine*, 14, 538–546.

Benes, F.M. (1989). Myelination of cortical-hippocampal relays during adolescence. *Schizophrenia Bulletin*, 15, 585–593.

Boone, K.B., Ghaffarian, S., Lesser, I.M., Hill-Gutierrez, E. & Berman, N.G. (1993). Wisconsin Card Sorting Test performance in healthy, older adults: relationship to age, sex, education, and IQ. *Journal of Clinical Psychology*, 49, 54–60.

Breteler, M.M.B., van Swieten, J.C., Bots, M.L. *et al.* (1994). Cerebral white matter lesions, vascular risk factors and cognitive function in a population-based study: the Rotterdam study. *Neurology*, 44, 1246–1252.

Breslau, J., Starr, A., Sicotte, N. *et al.* (1989). Topographic EEG changes with normal aging and SDAT. *Electroencephalography and Clinical Neurophysiology*, 72, 281–289.

Brody, H. (1955). Organization of the cerebral cortex. III. A study of aging in the human cerebral cortex. *Journal of Comparative Neurology*, 102, 511–556.

Burns, A. & Tyrrell, P. (1992). Association of age with regional cerebral oxygen utilization: a positron emission tomography study. *Age and Ageing*, 21, 316–320.

Chawluk, J.B., Alavi, A., Dann, R. *et al.* (1987). Positron emission tomography in aging and dementia: effect of cerebral atrophy. *Journal of Nuclear Medicine*, 28, 431–437.

Chawluk, J.B., Dann, R., Alavi, A. *et al.* (1990). The effect of focal cerebral atrophy in positron emission tomographic studies of aging and dementia. *International Journal of Radiation Applications and Instrumentation, Part B, Nuclear Medicine and Biology*, 17, 797–804.

Christiansen, P., Larsson, H.B., Thomsen, C., Wieslander, S.B. & Henriksen, O. (1994). Age dependent white matter lesions and brain volume changes in healthy volunteers. *Acta Radiologica*, 35, 117–122.

Clark, C., Hayden, M., Hollenberg, S., Li, D. & Stoessl, A.J. (1987). Controlling for cerebral atrophy in positron emission tomography data. *Journal of Cerebral Blood Flow and Metabolism*, 7, 510–512.

Coffey, C.E., Wilkinson, W.E., Parashos, I.A. *et al.* (1992). Quantitative anatomy of the aging human brain: a cross-sectional study using magnetic resonance imaging. *Neurology*, 42, 527–536.

Cohen, D., Cuffin, B.N. & Yunokunchi, K. (1990). MEG versus EEG localization test using implanted sources in the human brain. *Annals of Neurology*, 28, 811–817.

Cordes, M., Snow, B.J., Cooper, S. *et al.* (1994). Age-dependent decline of nigrostriatal dopaminergic function: a positron emission tomographic study of grandparents and their grandchildren. *Annals of Neurology*, 36, 667–670.

Cowell, P.E., Turetsky, B.I., Gur, R.C., Grossman, R.I., Shtasel, D.L. & Gur R.E. (1994). Sex differences in aging of the human frontal and temporal lobes. *Journal of Neuroscience*, 14, 4748–4755.

Cummings, J.L. & Benson, D.F. (1983). Dementia in vascular and infectious disorder. In *Dementia, a Clinical Approach*, ed. J.L. Cummings & D.F. Benson, pp. 125–167, Boston, MA: Butterworth.

DeCarli, C., Murphy, D.G., Gillette, J.A. *et al.* (1994). Lack of age-related differences in temporal lobe volume of very healthy adults. *American Journal of Neuroradiology*, 15, 689–696.

de Leon, M.J., Ferris, S.H., George, A.E. *et al.* (1983). Computed tomography and positron emission transaxial tomography evaluations of normal aging and Alzheimer's disease. *Journal of Cerebral Blood Flow Metabolism*, 3, 391–394.

de Leon, M.J., George, A.E., Ferris, S.H. *et al.* (1984). Positron emission tomography and computed tomography assessments of the aging human brain. *Journal of Computer Assisted Tomography*, 8, 88–94.

de Leon, M.J., George, A.E., Tomanelli, J. *et al.* (1987). Positron emission tomography studies of normal aging: a replication of PET III and 18–FDG using PET VI and 11–CDG. *Neurobiology of Aging*, 8, 319–323.

Dewey, S.L., Volkow, N.D., Logan, J. *et al.* (1990). Age-related decreases in muscarinic cholinergic receptor binding in the human brain measured with positron emission tomography (PET). *Journal of Neuroscience Research*, 17, 569–575.

Doraiswamy, P.M., Potts, J.M., Axelson, D.A. *et al.* (1992) MR assessment of pituitary gland morphology in healthy volunteers: age- and gender-related differences. *American Journal of Neuroradiology*, 13, 1295–1299.

Drayer, B.P. (1988). Imaging of the aging brain, part I. Normal Findings. *Radiology*, 166, 785–796.

Duara, R., Grady, C., Haxby, J. *et al.* (1984). Human brain glucose utilization and cognitive function in relation to age. *Annals of Neurology*, 16, 702–713.

Duara, R., Margolin, R.A., Robertson-Tchabo, E.A. *et al.* (1983). Cerebral glucose utilization, as measured with positron emission tomography in 21 resting healthy men between the ages of 21 and 83 years. *Brain*, 106, 761–775.

Duffy, F.H., Jones, K.J., McAnulty, G.B. *et al.* (1995). Spectral coherence in normal adults: unrestricted principal components analysis; relation of factors to age, gender and neuropsycologic data. *Clinical Electroencephalography*, 26, 30–46.

Duffy, F.H., McAnulty, G.B. & Albert, M.S. (1993). The pattern of age-related differences in electrophysiological acitivity of healthy males and females. *Neurobiology of Aging*, 14, 73–84.

Eidelberg, D., Takikawa, S., Dhawan, V. *et al.* (1993). Striatal ^{18}F-dopa uptake: absence of an ageing effect (see comments). *Journal of Cerebral Blood Flow and Metabolism*, 13, 881–888.

Elbert, T., Flor, H., Birbaumer, N. *et al.* (1994). Extensive reorganization of the somatosensory cortex in adult humans after nervous system injury. *NeuroReport*, 5, 2593–2597.

Escalona, P.R., McDonald, W.M., Doraiswamy, P.M. *et al.* (1991), In vivo stereological assessment of human cerebellar volume: effects of gender and age. *American Journal of Neuroradiology*, 12, 927–929.

Flechsig, P. (1896). *Die Lokalisation der Geistigen Vorgänge Insbesondere der Sinnesempfindungen des Menschen.* Leipzig: Verlag von Veit.

Folstein, M.F., Folstein, S.E. & McHugh, P.R. (1975). 'Mini-mental state', a practical method of grading the cognitive state of patients for the clinician. *Journal of Psychiatric Research*, 12, 189–198.

Gallen, C.C., Schwartz, B.J., Bucholz, R.D. *et al.* (1995). Presurgical localization of functional cortex using magnetic source imaging. *Journal of Neurosurgery*, 82, 988–994.

Gottschalk, A. & Hoffer, P.B. (1988). Positron emission tomography in aging and dementia: effect of cerebral atrophy. *Investigative Radiology*, 23, 879–880.

Grady, C.L., McIntosh, A.R., Horwitz,B. *et al.* (1995). Age-related reductions in human recognition memory due to impaired encoding. *Science*, 269, 218–221.

Gur, R.C., Mozley, P.D., Resnick, S.M. *et al.* (1991). Gender differences in age effect on brain atrophy measured by magnetic resonance imaging. *Proceedings of the National Academy of Sciences,USA*, 88, 2845–2849.

Hari, R., Hamalainen, M., Ilmoniemi, R. *et al.* (1991). MEG versus EEG localization test. *Annals of Neurology*, 30, 222–223.

Harris, G.J., Lewis, R.F., Satlin, A. *et al.* (1996). Dynamic susceptibility constrast magnetic resonance imaging of regional cerebral blood volume in Alzheimer's disease. *American Journal of Psychiatry*, in press.

Harris, G.J., Links, J.M., Pearlson, G.D. & Camargo, E.E. (1991a). Cortical circumferential profile of SPECT cerebral perfusion in Alzheimer's disease. *Psychiatry Research*, 40, 167–180.

Harris, G.J., Rhew, E.H., Noga, T. & Pearlson, G.D. (1991b). User-friendly method for rapid brain and CSF volume calculation using transaxial MRI images. *Psychiatry Research Neuroimaging*, 40, 61–68.

Harris, G.J., Schaepfer, T.E., Peng, L.W., Federman, E.B. & Pearlson, G.D. (1994). Magnetic resonance imaging evaluation of the effects of ageing on grey–white ratio in the human brain. *Neuropathology and Applied Neurobiology*, 20, 290–293.

Hartikainen, P., Soininen, H., Partanen, J. *et al.* (1992). Aging and spectral analysis of EEG in normal subjects: a link to memory and CSF AChE. *Acta Neurologica Scandinavica*, 86, 148–155.

Herscovitch, P., Auchus, A.P., Gado, M., Cho, D. & Raichle, M.E. (1986). Correction of positron emission tomography data for cerebral atrophy. *Journal of Cerebral Blood Flow and Metabolism*, 6, 120–124.

Iyo, M. & Yamasaki, T. (1993). The detection of age-related decrease of dopamine D_1, D_2 and serotonin $5-HT_2$ receptors in living human brain. *Progress in Neuro Psychopharmacology and Biological Psychiatry*, 17, 415–421.

Jernigan, T.L., Archibald, S.L., Berhow, M.T. *et al.* (1991). Cerebral structure on MRI, part I: localization of age-related changes. *Biological Psychiatry*, 29, 55–67.

Jernigan, T.L., Press, G.A. & Hesselink, J.R. (1990). Methods for measuring brain morphologic features on magnetic resonance images: validation and normal aging. *Archives of Neurology*, 47, 27–32.

Kobari, M., Stirling Meyer, J. & Ichijo, M. (1990). Leuko-araiosis, cerebral atrophy and cerebral perfusion in normal aging. *Archives of Neurology*, 47, 161–165.

Kuhl, D.E., Metter, E.J., Riege, W.H. & Phelps, M.E. (1982). Effects of human aging on patterns of local cerebral glucose utilization determined by the [18F]fluorodeoxyglucose method. *Journal of Cerebral Blood Flow and Metabolism*, 2, 163–171.

Kuriki, S., Okita, Y. & Hirata, Y. (1995). Source analysis of magnetic field responses from the human auditory cortex elicited by short speech sounds. *Experimental Brain Research*, 77, 127–134.

Leuchter, A.F., Spar, J.E., Walter, D.O. *et al.* (1987). Electroencephalographic spectra and coherence in the diagnosis of Alzheimer's-type and multiinfarct dementia. *Archives of General Psychiatry*, 44, 993–998.

Levine, R.L., Hanson, J.M. & Nickles, R.J. (1994). Cerebral vasocapacitance in human aging. *Journal of Neuroimaging*, 4, 130–136.

Lu, Z.L. & Kaufman, L. (1992). Human auditory primary and association cortex have differing lifetimes for activation traces. *Brain Research*, 572, 236–241.

Martin, A.J., Friston, K.J., Colebatch, J.G. & Frackowiak, R.S. (1991). Decrease in regional cerebral blood flow with normal aging. *Journal of Cerebral Blood Flow and Metabolism*, 11, 684–689.

Martin, W.R., Palmer, M.R., Patlak, C.S. & Calne, D.B. (1989). Nigrostriatal function in humans studied with positron emission tomography. *Annals of Neurology*, 26, 535–542.

Maurer, K. & Kierks, T. (1992). Functional imaging procedures in dementias: mapping of EEG and evoked potentials. *Acta Neurologica Scandinavica*, Suppl. 139, 40–46.

Mesulam, M.M. (1985). *Principles of Behavioral Neurology*. Philadelphia, PA: F.A. Davis.

Mikulis, D.M., Diaz, O., Egglin, T.K. & Sanchez, R. (1992). Variance of the position of the cerebellar tonsils with age: preliminary report. *Radiology*, 183, 725–728.

Miller, A.K.H., Alston, R.L. & Corsellis, J.A.N. (1980). Variation with age in the volumes of grey and white matter in the cerebral hemispheres of man: measurements with an image analyser. *Neuropathology and Applied Neurobiology*, 6, 119–132.

Mogilner, A., Gorssman, J.A., Ribary, U. et al. (1993). Somatosensory cortex plasticity in adult humans revealed by magnetoencephalography. *Proceedings of the National Academy of Sciences, USA*, 90, 3593–3597.

Ogawa, S., Menon, R.S., Tank, D.W., et al. (1993). Functional brain mapping by blood oxygenation level-dependent contrast magnetic resonance imaging. *Biophysical Journal*, 64, 803–812.

Orrison, W.W., Rose, D.F., Hart, B.L. et al. (1992). Noninvasive preoperative cortical localization by magnetic source imaging. *American Journal of Neuroradiology*, 13, 1124–1128.

Pantano, P., Baron, J.C., Lebrun-Grandié, P., Duquesnoy, N., Bousser, M.G. & Comar, D. (1984). Regional cerebral blood flow and oxygen consumption in human aging. *Stroke*, 15, 635–641.

Pantev, C., Hoke, M., Lehertz, K. et al. (1988). Tonotopic organization of the human auditory cortex revaled by transient auditory evoked magnetic fields. *Electroencephalography and Clinical Neurophysiology*, 69, 160–170.

Pantev, C., Makeig, S., Hoke, M. et al. (1991). Human auditory evoked gamma-band magnetic fields. *Proceedings of the National Academy of Sciences, USA*, 88, 8996–9000.

Pearlson, G.D., Harris,G.J., Powers, R.E., et al. (1992). Quantitative changes in mesial temporal volume, regional cerebral blood flow, and cognition in Alzheimer's disease. *Archives of General Psychiatry*, 49, 402–408.

Pollock, V.E., Schneider, L.S. & Lyness, S.A. (1991). Reliability of topographic quantitative EEG amplitude in healthy late-middle-aged and elderly subjects. *Electroencephalography and Clinical Neurophysiology*, 79, 20–26.

Raz, N., Torres, I.J., Spencer, W.D., White, K. & Acker, J.D. (1992). Age-related regional differences in cerebellar vermis observed in vivo. *Archives of Neurology*, 49, 412–416.

Ribary, U. (1991). Magnetic field tomography of coherent thalamocortical 40-Hz oscillations in humans. *Proceedings of the National Academy of Sciences, USA*, 88, 11 037–11 041.

Rinne, J.O., Hietala, J., Ruotsalainen, U. et al. (1993). Decrease in human striatal dopamine D_2 receptor density with age: a PET study with [^{11}C]raclopride. *Journal of Cerebral Blood Flow and Metabolism*, 13, 310–314.

Romani, G.L., Williamson, S.J. & Kaufman, L. (1982). Tonotopic organization of the human auditory cortex. *Science*, 216, 1339–1340.

Rowe, J.W. & Kahn, R.L. (1987). Human aging: usual and successful. *Science*, 237, 143–149.

Salmon, E., Maquet, P., Sadzot, B., Degueldre, C., Lemaire, C. & Franck, G. (1991). Decrease of frontal metabolism demonstrated by positron emission tomography in a population of healthy elderly volunteers. *Acta Neurologica Belgica*, 91, 288–195.

Sato, S., Balish, M. & Muratore, R. (1991). Principles of magnetoencephalography. *Journal of Clinical Neurophysiology*, 8, 144–156.

Sawle, G.V., Colebatch, J.G., Shah, A., Brooks, D.J., Marsden, C.D. & Frackowiak, R.S. (1990). Striatal function in normal aging: implications for Parkinson's disease. *Annals of Neurology*, 28, 799–804.

Schlaepfer, T.W., Harris, G.J., Tien, A.Y. et al. (1994). Pattern of decreased regional cortical gray matter volume in schizophrenia using magnetic resonance imaging. *American Journal of Psychiatry*, 151, 842–848.

Schlageter, N.L., Horwitz, B., Creasey, H. et al. (1987). Relation of measured brain glucose utilisation and cerebral atrophy in man. *Journal of Neurology, Neurosurgery and Psychiatry*, 50, 779–785.

Schmidt, R., Fazekas, F., Offenbacher, H. et al. (1993). Neuropsychologic correlates of MRI white matter hyperintensities: a study of 150 normal volunteers. *Neurology*, 43, 2490–2494.

Sobel, D.F., Gallen, C.C., Schwartz, B.J. et al. (1993). Locating the central sulcus: comparison of MR anatomic and magnetoencephalographic functional methods. *American Journal of Neuroradiology*, 14, 915–925.

Suhara, T., Fukuda, H., Inoue, O. et al. (1991). Age-related changes in human D_1 dopamine receptors measured by positron emission tomography. *Psychopharmacology*, 103, 41–45.

Suhara, T., Inoue, O., Kobayashi, K., Suzuki, K. & Tateno, Y.

(1993). Age-related changes in human muscarinic acetylcholine receptors measured by positron emission tomography. *Neuroscience Letters*, 149, 225–228.

Takada, H., Nagata, K., Hirata, Y. *et al.* (1992). Age-related decline of cerebral oxygen metabolism in normal population detected with positron emission tomography. *Neurological Research*, 14, 128–131.

Tiitinen, H. (1993). Tonotopic auditory cortex and the magnetoencephalographic (MEG) equivalent of the mismatch negativity. *Psychophysiology*, 30, 537–540.

Tomlinson, B.E., Blessed, G. & Roth, M. (1968). Observations on the brains of nondemented old people. *Journal of Neurological Science*, 7, 331–356.

Torres, F., Faoro, A., Loewenson, R. *et al.* (1983). The electroencephalogram of elderly subjects revisited. *Electroencephalography and Clinical Neurophysiology*, 56, 391–398.

Tupler, L.A., Coffey, C.E., Logue, P.E., Djang, W.T. & Fagan, S.M. (1992). Neuropsychological importance of subcortical white matter hyperintensity. *Archives of Neurology*, 49, 1248–1252.

Veselis, R.A., Reinsel, R. & Wronski, M. (1993). Analytical methods to differentiate similar electroencephalographic spectra: neural network and discriminant analysis. *Journal of Clinical Monitoring*, 9, 257–267.

Videen, T.O., Perlmutter, J.S., Mintun, M.A. & Raichle, M.E. (1988). Regional correction of positron emission tomography data for the effects of cerebral atrophy. *Journal of Cerebral Blood Flow and Metabolism*, 8, 662–670.

Villiger, E. (1931). *Brain and Spinal Cord*. Philadelphia, PA: J.B. Lippincott.

Waldemar, G., Hasselbalch, S.G., Anderson, A.R. *et al.* (1991). 99mTc-d,1-HMPAO and SPECT of the brain in normal aging. *Journal of Cerebral Blood Flow and Metabolism*, 11, 508–521.

Williamson, P.C., Merskey, H., Morrison, S. *et al.* (1990). Quantitative electroencephalographic correlates of cognitive decline in normal elderly subjects. *Archives of Neurology*, 47, 1185–1188.

Williamson, S.J. (1991). MEG versus EEG localization test. *Annals of Neurology*, 30, 222.

Wong, D.F., Wagner, H.N., Dannals, R.F. *et al.* (1984). Effects of age on dopamine and serotonin receptors measured by positron tomography in the living human brain. *Science*, 226, 1393–1396.

Yanai, K., Watanabe,T., Meguro, K. *et al.* (1992). Age-dependent decrease in histamine H_1 receptor in human brains revealed by PET. *NeuroReport*, 3, 433–436.

Yoshii, F., Barker, W.W., Chang, J.Y. *et al.* (1988). Sensitivity of cerebral glucose metabolism to age, gender, brain volume, brain atrophy, and cerebrovascular risk factors. *Journal of Cerebral Blood Flow and Metabolism*, 8, 654–661.

3 Alzheimer's disease

Hans Förstl and Alistair Burns

Introduction

Alzheimer's disease (AD) is characterized clinically by the presence of a dementia syndrome and by the absence of other specific causes of dementia (Burns & Förstl, 1994; McKhann et al., 1984). Diagnostic criteria have been developed with the aim of predicting accurately who will have the pathological hallmarks of AD at postmortem. One of the most widely quoted set of guidelines is those of the National Institute for Neurological and Communicative Disorders and Stroke and the Alzheimer's Disease and Associated Disorders Association (NINCDS/ADRDA, McKhann et al., 1984), which are divided into 'definite' (autopsy confirmed), 'probable' and 'possible' criteria. The clinical suspicion of AD can only be verified by neuropathological examination of brain tissue. Similar to the clinician, the neuropathologist has to rely on inclusion and exclusion criteria, quantify the histopathological hallmarks and rule out other diseases that may significantly contribute to the clinical syndrome. Clinical and neuropathological criteria are essentially arbitrary but validation of each against the other is a legitimate attempt to achieve validity. Discrimination of AD from normal aging and other forms of dementia is the ultimate aim of such studies.

Normal neuroradiological and electrophysiological findings or nonspecific changes are compatible with a diagnosis of probable AD, whereas evidence of severe vascular changes, space-occupying lesions or Creutzfeldt–Jakob disease is not. The primary goal of such investigations in demented patients is the detection of treatable associated or accompanying illnesses. In view of the difficulty in examining the brain *in vivo* (largely because of the protective nature of the skull), brain imaging represents a unique opportunity to view the structure and function of the brain in AD.

This chapter will summarize:

- The typical structural and functional findings in AD,
- The discrimination between AD and normal aging based on neuroimaging results
- The correlations between radiological and clinical findings.

Morphological changes: cranial CT and MRI

Age-related brain changes have been reviewed in Chapter 2. Some degree of ventricular and sulcal enlargement, WMHI and more discrete vascular changes can be observed in a significant proportion of elderly individuals free from dementia. It has been demonstrated that there are larger volumetric differences between younger AD patients and age-matched controls than between elderly patients and controls, which can be explained by age-related changes (Sullivan *et al.*, 1993). The proportion of subjects with completely normal brain scans decreases with age. However, the presence of moderate to severe changes, for example of brain atrophy, raises the suspicion that there may be an underlying disease process, perhaps AD, which is still 'subclinical'. A distinction has, therefore, been suggested between '*successful*' aging with neither cognitive deficits nor brain changes and '*normal*' aging, accompanied by debatable neuroimaging findings but without clinical dysfunction (Coffey *et al.*, 1992; Drayer, 1988).

The discrimination between AD and normal aging is limited by two prinicipal methodological problems: first, the variance of neuroradiological findings within the nondemented elderly population and within the group of patients with clinically diagnosed AD; second, the fact that the clinical diagnosis can only be verified neuropathologically in 80–90% of the patients, mostly in moderate or severe stages of illness (Burns, 1991; Förstl & Fischer, 1994). A complete discrimination between patients and controls would, therefore, be unlikely. The neuropathological confirmation rate is strikingly similar to discrimination achieved by cranial CT (Table 3.1).

The reported data refer to estimates of brain atrophy, by visual ratings or by a variety of standardized measurements. The interrater agreement for visual ratings of ventricular size, but not for sulcal or fissure enlargement, global brain atrophy and white matter alterations, was acceptable in a large multicenter study (Davis *et al.*, 1992). Reliability can be improved and more efficient cut-off values can be developed if linear or computer-assisted planimetric or volumetric measurements are introduced (Burns, 1991; Kido *et al.*, 1989). The results of these methods are, however, closely correlated with each other, and this may partly explain the similarity of this discriminative efficiency between the studies listed in Table 3.1. Several authors have observed that the efficiency of standardized CT scan analysis in distinguishing normal aging from AD approaches the efficiency of neuropsychological testing. A combination of both methods has been reported to improve correct identification of AD (Eslinger *et al.*, 1984; Spano *et al.*, 1992). There is evidence that increasing sophistication of CT analysis does improve discrimination between AD and normal aging. Visual ratings having the poorest discriminatory ability with computerized ratings of scans on patients studied longitudinally revealing better discrimination (Burns, 1991; Förstl *et al.*, 1996b).

The clinical diagnosis of AD can be difficult in the early stages of illness. There are a limited number of reports on the discrimination of early AD and normal aging; examples are listed in Table 3.2. Ichimaya *et al.* (1986) reported a perfect distinction between six patients with mild AD and normal controls using volumetric CT scan analysis. Erkinjuntti

Table 3.1 *Discrimination between groups of nondemented controls and matched samples of patients with AD using cranial CT*

Reference	AD				Controls				Clinical criteria	Measurement	Discrimination (%)
	n	Male:female ratio	Mean age ±SD (years)	Age range (years)	n	Male:female ratio	Mean age ±SD (years)	Age range (years)			
Albert et al. (1984)	10	10:10	58	53–64	8	6:2	58	53–64	Specified	Linear	83
Arai et al. (1983)	18		61±7		14		55±8		Specified	Planimetric	94
Burns et al. (1991)	138	31:107	80±6	64–93	36				NINCDS-ADRDA	Planimetric	81
Damasio et al. (1983)	46	15:31	74±6	60–90	46	12:34	74±6	61–90	Roth criteria	Planimetric	84
Eslinger et al.(1984)	26	12:14	75±6	64–88	26	7:19	75±6	64–88	DSM-IIIR	Linear	73
Ettlin et al. (1989)	15	3:12	NS	83±15	MID/mixed[a]		NS		Neuro-pathology	Visual rating	80
Förstl et al. (1991)	60	14:46	75	66–82	30	7:23	75	66–84	NINCDS-ADRDA	Planimetric	78
George et al. (1990)	20	10:10	NS	60–85	34	16:18	NS	56–87	Specified	Ventricles, linear hippocampus, visual	74, 80
Jacoby & Levy (1980)	40	11:29	NS	60–99	50	10:40	NS	60–89	Specified	Linear and planimetric	83
Spano et al. (1992)	29	11:18	69±8	53–84	36[b]	16:20	67±8	53–83	Specified	Volumetric	83
Willmer et al. (1993)	22		72±7	56–84	49		71±8	57–87	NINCDS-ADRDA	Linear	92

Notes:
NS, not specified
[a] Multiinfarct dementia/mixed dementia.
[b] 'Memory complainers'.

Table 3.2 *Discrimination between normal aging and mild AD*

Reference		AD				Controls				Method	Measurement	Discrimination (%)
	n	Male:female ratio	Mean age ± SD (years)	Age range (years)	*n*	Male:female ratio	Mean age ± SD (years)	Age range (years)				
Erkinjuntti et al. (1993)	34	16:18	70 ± 1		39	22:17	70 ± 1	40–83	MRI	Visual ratings: entorhinal cortex, Temporal neocortex Temporal horns	AUC 96 89 82
Förstl et al. (1995b)	14	22:18	67	54–81	40	22:18	67	54–81	CT	Volumetry: Left lateral ventricle Right lateral ventricle Left Sylvian fissure Right Sylvian fissure	AUC 88 92 84 85
Ichimaya et al. (1986)	6		61 ± 5		13	4:9	58 ± 7		CT	Volumetry	100
O'Brien et al. (1994)[a]	10		69 ± 7	60–70	10	4:6	73 ± 8	61–82 6:3	MRI	Visual ratings of anterior hippocampal atrophy	84

Notes:

AUC, area under curve

[a] Control subjects had major depression and mild cognitive impairment

et al. (1993) found that standardized visual ratings of temporal lobe structures attained high AUC (area under curve) values in specificity/sensitivity plots (receiver-operating characteristics (ROCs); ideal value=1). O'Brien *et al.* (1994) rated the atrophy of the anterior hippocampus and found that 84% of nine patients with mild AD and ten patients with depression and mild cognitive impairment were discriminated correctly, even though this measure was influenced by age and duration of dementia. Förstl *et al.* (1995b) found that volumetric CT scan measurements of lateral ventricular and Sylvian fissure size permitted a highly sensitive and specific distinction between aging and mild AD, similar to estimates of mediotemporal lobe atrophy using MRI (Table 3.2).

Figure 3.1 demonstrates the total estimates of intracranial CSF volumes in controls and in patients with mild, moderate and severe dementia, individually matched for gender and age (Förstl *et al.*, 1995b). The table demonstrates the significant degree of overlap between all stages of dementia and normal controls. As such, CT scanning merely represents the clinical equivalent of mild, moderate and severe dementia and adds little to the clinical impression. The relatively high discrimination rates in the literature belie the fact that selection of patients with mild AD (with demonstrable disease) or controls (who often are supranormal) tends to be biased.

Correlations between age and cognitive performance on the MMSE (Folstein, Folstein & McHugh, 1975) and a number of atrophy indices in AD are given in Table 3.3.

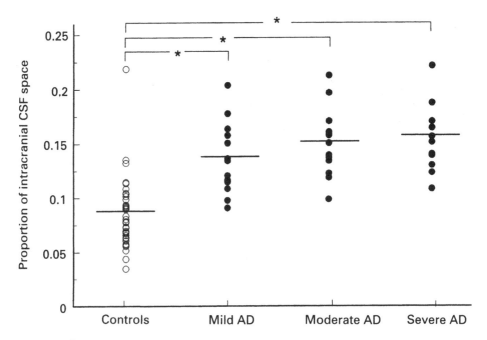

Figure 3.1 *A comparison between the proportion of intracranial CSF space in 40 healthy controls individually matched for age and gender with patients in the mild, moderate or severe stage of clinically diagnosed AD.* *$p<0.05$.

Table 3.3 *Correlations (Pearson's r) between quantitative indices of brain atrophy and age or MMSE in AD*

Reference	Method	n	Male:female ratio	Mean age ±SD (years)	Age range (years)	Index of brain atrophy	Correlation with	
							Age	MMSE
Burns et al. (1991)	CT	138		80	64–93	VBR	0.1	−0.3
						Third ventricle	0.2	−0.3
						Left Sylvian fissure	0.1	−0.3
						Right Sylvian fissure	0.2	−0.3
Förstl et al. (1991)	CT	60	14:46	75	66–82	Third ventricle	0.2	−0.2
						Left anterior horn	0.1	−0.5
						Right anterior horn	0.0	−0.3
Förstl et al. (1995b)	CT	84	32:52	69 ± 9	54–81	Total CSF space	0.4	−0.5
						Left lateral ventricle	0.3	−0.3
						Right lateral ventricle	0.2	−0.4
						Third ventricle	0.4	−0.3
						Anterior fissure	0.2	−0.3
						Left Sylvian fissure	0.5	−0.3
						Right Sylvian fissure	0.3	−0.4
Kumar et al. (1994)	MRI	34	17:17	66 ± 9		Total CSF space	–	−0.4
						Total ventricular volume	–	−0.3
						Left lateral ventricle	–	−0.2
						Right lateral ventricle	–	−0.3
Murphy et al. (1993b)	MRI	19	19:0	68 ± 9		Total CSF space	–	−0.5
Pearlson et al. (1992)	CT	13	4:9	71 ± 2		Ventricular:brain ratio	–	−0.6
Sullivan et al. (1993)	CT	117	63:54	69 ± 8	55–84	Total ventricular space	−0.4	−0.4
						Third ventricular sulci:	−0.3	−0.1
						Vertex	−0.4	−0.0
						Frontal	−0.4	−0.4
						Sylvian	−0.5	−0.5
						Parietooccipital	−0.4	−0.4

Age is positively correlated with ventricular and fissure size; cognitive performance is negatively related. Ventricular size correlates less well with age than does sulcal atrophy. The results of different studies are fairly consistent irrespective of whether CT, MRI or planimetric or volumetric estimates are used.

Estimates of total CSF space, ventricular or sulcal CSF in aging and AD from different studies using CT or MRI are presented in Table 3.4. In the control groups, MRI yielded higher values of sulcal and total CSF space than CT. On average, the patients in the CT scan studies were more severely demented than the patients in the MRI studies. This may explain the larger ventricular volume and the greater proportional enlargement of total CSF space in the patients compared with controls from the CT studies. In spite of this, the sulcal CSF estimates are smaller than in the MRI analyses, both in the AD and control groups. This underlines the disadvantages of the CT scanner, which are caused by partial volume effects in the vicinity of structures with high radiodensity. MRI scans are free from these deficits and have a number of other advantages, such as a higher resolution and greater freedom in image reconstruction. The latter has been used to visualize subtle changes in the mediotemporal lobe.

Mediotemporal lobe

Neuropathological studies have shown that the entorhinal cortex is affected early in AD (Braak & Braak, 1991). Changes in this area are observed in most nondemented elderly individuals (Bouras et al., 1994), whereas neuronal loss in the hippocampal area CA1 is largely restricted to patients suffering from AD (West et al., 1994). Golomb et al. (1993; 1994) demonstrated that an impairment of delayed secondary memory (delayed recall of paragraphs, lists, paired associates) is correlated with hippocampal atrophy in the MRI of elderly individuals. MRI has shown the participation of mediotemporal lobe structures in the 'normal' aging process (Jernigan et al., 1991; Sandor et al., 1990). Figure 3.2 illustrates that the hippocampus and parahippocampal structures can be seen adequately by CT if the horizontal slices are tilted at an angle of 20° negative to the canthomeatal line. Jobst et al. (1992b) found that in 44 patients with AD the minimum width of the medio temporal lobe was approximately half that in controls. The possibility was considered by the authors that this measurement might serve as an early diagnostic test for AD (Burns, 1993). Recent results from the CERAD study have shown that temporal lobe atrophy on CT and MRI scanning correlated with hippocampal atrophy assessed neuropathologically (Davis et al., 1995).

The ability of several linear, planimetric or volumetric estimates of mediotemporal brain atrophy to discriminate AD, normal aging and degenerative brain diseases has been examined with varying success (CT: Aylward et al., 1991 Kido et al., 1989; Willmer et al., 1993; MRI: Howieson et al., 1993; Murphy et al., 1993b). Coronal MR imaging has been recommended for a demonstration of early hippocampal and perihippocampal changes (de Leon, 1993; Jack et al., 1992; Kesslak, Nalcioglu & Cotman, 1991; Seab et al., 1988). However, the reported rates of correct classification hardly ever exceeded the 80%

Table 3.4 *Volumetric differences between elderly, nondemented controls and patients with clinically diagnosed AD*

	AD				Controls				Method	Total CSF[a] AD/C (%)	Ventricular CSF[a] AD/C (%)	Sulcal CSF[a] AD/C (%)
	n	Male:female ratio	Mean age ±SD (years)	Age range (years)	n	Male:female ratio	Mean age ±SD (years)	Age range (years)				
Förstl et al. (1995b)	40	22:18	67	54–81	40	22:18	67	54–81	CT	14.7/8.6 *** 171%	7.2/3.1 *** 232%	7.5/5.5 *** 136%
Kumar et al. (1994)	34	17:17	66 ± 9		29	12:17	67 ± 9		MRI	18.8/13.2 *** 142%	3.7/2.3 *** 161%	15.0/10.9 *** 138%
Murphy et al. (1993a)	19	19:0	68 ± 9		18	18:0	70 ± 8		MRI	16.2/11.4 ** 143%	3.9/1.4 *** 279%	12.3/9.9 n.s. 124%

[a] The individual estimates are given as proportions of intracranial volumes. The ratios of these estimates in AD/C controls are given as a percentage.

margin described in most of the earlier CT scan studies (Table 3.1; George *et al.*, 1990; Sandor *et al.*, 1992). It will be important to demonstrate the predictive power of medio-temporal lobe changes and their superiority over more conventional estimates of brain atrophy in order to establish their position as early markers of AD (de Leon, 1993). Simple quantitative measurements of brain atrophy, for example the ventricular: brain ratio (VBR) may also be helpful in predicting the development of cognitive deterioration in patients who do not satisfy criteria for a diagnosis of dementia but fulfill criteria for age-associated memory impairment or benign senescent forgetfulness at the time of their initial examination (Förstl *et al.*, 1995a).

White matter changes of the cerebral hemispheres and corpus callosum in AD have

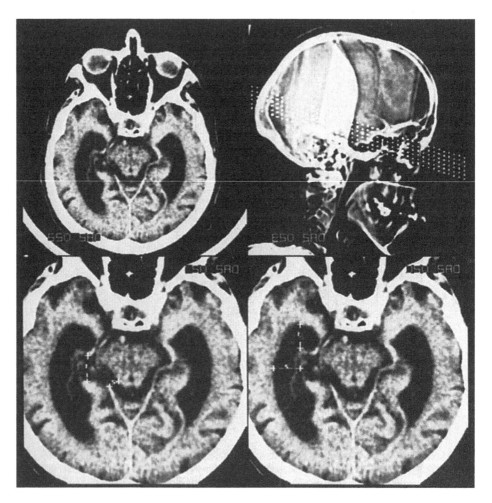

Figure 3.2 *Atrophy of hippocampus and parahippocampal structures with enlargement of the perihippocampal CSF spaces demonstrated by cranial CT (angle – see scout view).*

been the subject of extensive investigation. Sagittal MRI planes show a decrease of the callosal area that is related to dementia severity and patterns of cortical damage (Yamauchi *et al.*, 1993). Atrophy of the genu appears to be characteristic of AD, whereas the body of the corpus callosum is also reduced in normal aging (Biegon *et al.*, 1994).

The nature of hemispheric white matter changes or 'leukoaraiosis' is still a matter of debate. Subcortical white matter lesions seem to be primarily age related; periventricular lesions are more closely associated with cognitive decline and are more typical for AD (Matsubayashi *et al.*, 1992; McDonald *et al.*, 1991). MRI is more sensitive in detecting leukoaraiosis than CT, but because of very different technical methods and standards of evaluation the reported prevalence rates in AD are also highly variable, ranging from 40% (Diaz *et al.*, 1991) to more than 60% (Kobari *et al.*, 1990) in CT scan studies, and from 17% (Kozachuk *et al.*, 1990) to 66% in MRI studies (Mirsen *et al.*, 1991). It has been suggested that the occurrence and severity of white matter change in AD is associated with cognitive impairment (Bondareff *et al.*, 1990; Diaz *et al.*, 1991; Harrell *et al.*, 1991), more specifically with deficits of attention and comprehension (Almkvist *et al.*, 1992; Kertesz, Polk & Carr, 1990). This influence has not been confirmed by other authors (Aharon-Peretz, Cummings & Hill, 1988; Kozachuk *et al.*, 1990; Lopez *et al.*, 1992). Several groups demonstrated a correlation of leukoaraiosis with age (Almkvist *et al.*, 1992; Kobari *et al.*, 1990; Kozachuk *et al.*, 1990; Kumar *et al.*, 1992; Scheltens *et al.*, 1992). There is an association with higher blood pressure (Almkvist *et al.*, 1992, Bondareff *et al.*, 1990) and evidence that leukoaraiosis may herald the development of additional cerebrovascular disease (Matsubayashi *et al.*, 1992).

Functional neuroimaging: SPET, PET and QEEG

Numerous SPET studies have shown a temporoparietal hypoperfusion that is typically asymmetric (Burns *et al.*, 1989b; Curran *et al.*, 1993; Goldenberg *et al.*, 1989; Montaldi *et al.*, 1990; Prohovnik *et al.*, 1988). A temporoparietal : cerebellar perfusion ratio below 0.85 has been considered suggestive of AD (Weinstein *et al.*, 1991) but the ratio may be normal in the early stages of the illness (Reed *et al.*, 1989).

SPET may contribute to the discrimination of normal aging, AD, frontal lobe degeneration and vascular forms of dementia (Frisoni *et al.*, 1994; Osimani *et al.*, 1994), and it may be superior to MRI in distinguishing AD from vascular dementia (Ebmeier *et al.*, 1987). Pearlson *et al.* (1992) reported a 100% discrimination between AD and normal aging based on combined volumetric MRI measurements of the left amygdala and entorhinal cortex together with a SPET measurement of left temporoparietal blood flow. Not all patients with AD show temporoparietal hypoperfusion, but AD can be accompanied by a great variety of perfusion patterns, depending on the cognitive findings or the severity of illness (McMurdo *et al.*, 1994; Waldemar *et al.*, 1994).

Several authors have found significant correlations between regional hypoperfusion and the patterns of cognitive impairment (Besson et al., 1990; Burns et al., 1989a; Reed, Jagust & Coulter, 1993). Some of these studies are listed in Table 3.5. Perfusion patterns are influenced by premorbid factors, including education (Stern et al., 1992, using Xenon-133inhalation methods), dementia severity (Waldemar et al., 1994) and other features, such as insight into illness (Reed et al., 1993).

PET has yet to gain the same clinical importance for the diagnosis of AD as any of the other methods mentioned in this chapter, but its potential to measure cerebral metabolism directly is of great significance. Similar to the typical hypoperfusion pattern visualized by SPET, PET can be used to demonstrate a reduced cortical oxygen consumption or glucose metabolism, which is most pronounced and often asymmetric in the temporal and parietal areas (Haxby et al., 1990; Salmon et al., 1994; Table 3.6). The difference between frontal and parietal hypometabolism appears to remain stable over time (Jagust et al., 1988). It has been suggested that the reduction of glucose metabolism exceeds what would be expected from the degree of brain atrophy (Smith et al., 1992).

The suggestive metabolic pattern has been observed in more than 90% of the patients from one series (Salmon et al., 1994) and it has been shown that PET may detect this typical distribution slightly more often than SPET (Messa et al., 1994). Two reports mention that 87% of the patients with AD were discriminated correctly from controls (Azari et al., 1993; Szelies et al., 1992). A variety of task-dependent differences that may aid case identification have been described in memory and perceptual tasks (Buchsbaum et al., 1991; Grady et al., 1993; Riddle et al., 1993).

The observed metabolic changes are correlated with test performance (Nybäck et al., 1991), the severity of illness (Szelies et al., 1992) and the duration of illness (Kwa et al., 1993). They were more severe in patients with early-onset disease (Small et al., 1989), but there was no difference between so-called 'familial' and 'sporadic' cases (Guze et al., 1992). Mesial temporal lobe metabolism decreases with age, but a decrease in the ratio mesial: neocortical temporal lobe is characteristic of AD and can already be found in the mild stage. The decrease of this ratio is more severe with greater memory impairment and less severe in patients with predominent visuospatial deficits (Jagust et al., 1993). A disproportionate frontal/parietal hypometabolism was associated with discrepancies between visuospatial and language impairment and with other clinical deficits (Haxby et al., 1988; 1990). Frontal hypometabolism can be observed in frontal lobe degeneration, but also in neuropathologically verified AD (Salmon et al., 1994). It may predict a faster progression of illness (Mann et al., 1992). On follow-up, the most severe metabolic decline is usually observed in the areas that showed the most severe deficits during the initial examination (McGeer et al., 1990). Asymmetric temporoparietal hypometabolism may signal the development of cognitive impairment in previously nondemented patients, but there is no clear evidence that the hypometabolism generally precedes the development of clinical deficits; instead the metabolic and clinical deficits appear to develop parallel to one another (Haxby et al., 1990; Pietrini et al., 1993). Therefore, standard analysis of resting glucose metabolism may not be useful for the reliable early diagnosis of AD.

Table 3.5 *SPET studies on patients with clinically diagnosed Alzheimer's disease satisfying NINCDS-ADRDA criteria*

Reference	n	Male:Female ratio	Mean age ±SD	Age range (years)	Neuroimaging	Correlations
Besson et al. (1990)	13 of 21	3:18	69	57–76	Tc-HMPAO [+MRI], visual rating	Significant correlations between focal perfusion deficits and focal cognitive deficits were found.
Burns et al. (1989a)	20	7:13	70 ± 10		Tc-HMPAO (+CT), visual rating	Praxis scores were correlated with posterior parietal, memory with left temporal and language with total left hemisphere perfusion
DeKosky et al. (1990)	19		68 ± 2		^{123}I-HIPDM	Highest correlations between regional perfusion and scores on cognitive tests were found in the parietal area (>occipital>temporal>frontal)
Eberling et al. (1993)	50	16:24	70 ± 7	56–86	^{123}I-IMP, computer assisted	Right orbitofrontal perfusion associated with 'frontal', right parietal perfusion associated with visuoconstructive function
Goldenberg et al. (1989)	23	7:16	71 ± 5	58–75	Tc-HMPAO, computer assisted	Frontal/temporoparietal dichotomy
Jagust et al. (1990)	26	13:13	71 ± 4		^{123}IMP	Left frontal hypoperfusion in presenile, but not in senile AD
Jobst et al. (1992a)	23				Tc-HMPAO (+CT), visual rating	Hippocampal atrophy was associated with decreased temporoparietal blood flow in all patients with neuropathologically verified AD
Montaldi et al. (1990)	26	9:17	76	54–90	Tc-HMPAO (+CT), computer assisted	'Numerous' – nonspecific – correlations between tests scores and rCBF
Reed et al. (1993)	10	3:7	72 ± 12		^{123}I-IMP, computer assisted	Anosognosia was associated with diminished relative dorsolateral frontal lobe perfusion
Riddle et al. (1993)	10	3:7	72 ± 12		TC labeled	Successful performance in patients was correlated with activation of dorsolateral frontal and parietal cortex on the left side

Note:
Tc-HMPAO, technetium-labeled hexamethylpropyleneamine oxime; ^{123}I-IMP. [^{123}I] *n*-isopropyl-*p*-iodoamphetamine.

Table 3.6 *PET studies on 10 or more patients with clinically diagnosed AD satisfying NINCDS-ADRDA or DSM-IIIR criteria*

Reference	AD			Controls		Neuroimaging	Areas with decreased metabolism
	n	Male:Female ratio	Age (years)[a]	n	Male:Female ratio		
Azari et al. (1993)	19	12:7	52–81	22	14:8	FDG	Most regions with the exception of occipital and subcortical regions; two complex discriminant functions correctly classified 87% of patients and controls
Friedland et al.(1989)	16	9:7	66 ± 7	7	2:5	FDG	The temporoparietal cortex upon a background of widespread cortical metabolic impairment
Goto et al. (1993)	14	–	58 (42–68)	5	–	FDG(+CT or MRI)	The frontal, temporal, parietal, occipital and sensory motor cortex
Guze et al. (1992)	15	8:7	68 ± 6	8	6:2	FDG	Multiple cortical areas; no difference between familial and sporadic cases
Haxby et al. (1988)	32	18:14	67 ± 9	31	26:5	FDG	Parietal, lateral temporal lobe (mild dementia); parietal, premotor area (moderate dementia); all regions apart from the occipital cortex (severe dementia)
Haxby et al. (1990)	32	19:13	67 ± 9	31	26:5	FDG	Asymmetric in the association cortex
Mann et al. (1992)	21	12:9	66 ± 3	–	–	FDG	Temporoparietal cortex
Nybäck et al. (1991)	13	4:9	65 (51–78)	9	4:5	C2DG (+CT)	The posterior parietal and temporal cortex (down to 60% of the control level)
Small et al. (1989)	24	15:9	Early/late onset	–	–	FDG	Left parietal lobe, more severe in early-onset than in late-onset cases
Smith et al. (1992)	45	23:22	68 ± 9	20	7:13	C2DG (+CT)	The temporoparietal association areas that show metabolic deficits cross-sectionally also show further deficits longitudinally; the reduction of glucose metabolism is greater than would be expected from the degree of brain atrophy
Szelies et al. (1992)	42	14:28	67 ± 8	15	9:6	FDG (+EEG)	Temporoparietal cortex (a correct diagnostic classification by PET was achieved in 87% – and by EEG in 86%)

Notes:
FDG, ^{18}F-labeled deoxyglucose; C2DG, [^{14}C$_2$] deoxyglucose.
[a] Age given as a range or as a mean±SD.

The strength of EEG is its time resolution, not the spatial resolution, which is in the range of several centimeters for a scalp EEG. In this respect, EEG does not stand comparison with the neuroimaging methods mentioned above, even though technically impressive displays of topographic EEGs seem to suggest the opposite. The classical observations of Berger (1937), who described an unspecific slowing of the background activity with dementia, have been confirmed with quantitative EEG power analysis. Changes found in mild AD are listed in Table 3.7. In comparison with normal aging, there is a decrease of the mean frequency (Brenner *et al.*, 1986) of the dominant occipital activity (Prinz & Vitiello, 1989), of the alpha : theta ratio (Penttilä *et al.*, 1985) and an increase of the relative (Coben, Danziger & Berg, 1983) or absolute theta power, whereas delta power increases in the later stages of illness (Prichep *et al.*, 1994). These parameters are not independent from one another and partly reflect different mathematical approaches to interwoven phenomena. The change or disorganization of EEG topography in AD is more difficult to handle statistically (Dierks *et al.*, 1993). Other, more complex analyses, revealed significant differencies between AD and normal aging, for example a decrease of EEG coherence or synchronicity and of dimensional complexity (Besthorn *et al.*, 1994; 1995; Leuchter *et al.*, 1987; Pritchard *et al.*, 1994).

Although a wealth of data can be derived from the EEG, the efficiency of standard parameters in discriminating mild AD from normal aging is inferior to morphological variables. The inclusion of nonlinear parameters (e.g. dimensional complexity) may improve the statistical distinction of aging from AD, even at early stages (Besthorn *et al.*, 1995; Pritchard *et al.*, 1994). The occipital : frontal alpha ratio was efficient in distinguishing AD from vascular forms of dementia, whereas the relative theta power proved more sensitive in discriminating AD from aging, approaching the efficiency of PET measurements (these analyses were not restricted to mild cases of illness: Szelies *et al.*, 1992; 1994). In this study, EEG and PET were considered as complementary methods investigating different aspects of AD.

Earlier work on EEG and CT did not reveal any consistent correlations between morphology and electrophysiology in AD (Merskey *et al.*, 1980; Roberts, McGeorge & Caird, 1978; Stefoski *et al.*, 1976). Förstl and colleagues (1996a) found a significant correlation between alpha power and the size of the interhemispheric fissure. This is in line with earlier findings of a preserved alpha activity with intact parietal lobe function, demonstrated by neuropsychychology and PET (Sheridan *et al.*, 1988). Earlier onset of illness, longer duration and greater severity are associated with a decreased alpha and an increased theta or delta activity (Schreiter-Gasser, Gasser & Ziegler, 1994). Correlations between the MMSE and power data from different locations are listed in Table 3.8. Inverse correlations with delta or theta power and positive correlations with the alpha power have been demonstrated consistently; the largest coefficients were observed over the temporoparietal and also the occipital lobes.

Table 3.7 *Differences in QEEG parameters between normal aging and AD*

	AD				Controls					Difference compared with controls
Reference	n	Male:Female ratio	Mean age ±SD (years)	Age range (years)	n	Male:Female ratio	Mean age ±SD (years)	Age range (years)		
Brenner et al. (1986)	11				61	24:37	67 ± 7			↓ mean frequency; 4 of 11 patients classified correctly (36% sensitivity; 93% specificity)
Coben et al. (1983)	40	19:21	–	64–83	40	19:21	–	64–83		↓ mean frequency, ↓ relative Beta power, ↑ relative theta power
Dierks et al. (1991)	9				14	2:12	73 ± 7	64–85		↓peak frequency; the topography of the peak frequency was a better discriminator than the peak frequency
Penttilä et al. (1985)	11		70 ± 7		11		73 ± 7			↑ relative theta power, ↓ alpha:theta ratio, ↓ mean frequency
Prichep et al. (1994)	48	25:23	71 ± 9	54–87	40	13:27	69 ± 7	56–82		↑ relative and absolute theta power
Prinz & Vitiello (1989)	41	18:23	71 ± 8		50	19:31	68 ± 7			↓ dominant occipital frequency
Pritchard et al. (1994)	14	5:9	72 ± 10	53–85	25	9:16	69 ± 6	61–83		85% classified correctly (77% jack-knifed; 92% neuronal net)

Note:
↑, increase; ↓, decrease.

Table 3.8 *Correlations between delta, theta, alpha and beta power or mean frequency (MF) with the MMSE scores in AD*

Reference	n	Male:Female ratio	Mean age ±SD (years)	Age range (years)	Correlations with MMSE[a]
Brenner et al. (1986)	35	12:23	67 ± 7	51–89	Delta −0.5 Theta −0.6
Elmstahl, Rosen & Gullberg (1994)	10	0:10	85 ± 5		MF 0.7 Theta −0.7 (posterior)
Gueguen et al. (1988)	28	11:17	74	54–82	Alpha/theta 0.4 (T5, T6) MF>0.4 (T5, T6, P4, P3, O2, O1)
Leuchter et al. (1987)	12	5:7	75		18–22 Hz/2–6 Hz=0.6 (left temporal)
Primavera et al. (1990)	21	13:8	61 ± 7		Delta −0.6 (F7, O1, O2) Alpha>0.4 (O1, O2, T5, T6) Beta 0.5 (F7) MF 0.6
Sloan & Fenton (1993)	40		74 ± 9		Delta-1<−0.4 (T4–T6, T3–T5, P4–O2) Delta-2<−0.4 (T4–T6, T3–T5, F4–C4, F3–C3, P4–O2, P3–O1) Alpha>0.4 (T4–T6, T3–T5, P3–O1, P4–o2, F4–C4, F3–C3) Beta 0.4 (T3–T5)

Note:
[a] Only Pearson coefficients greater or equal to 0.4 are given. The electrode positions according to the 10/20 system are shown in brackets.

Discussion

Brain imaging offers a unique perspective of cerebral function and structure. The work summarized in this chapter suggests that imaging has an identifiable and worthwhile contribution to make to the differential diagnosis of dementia, the accurate identification of AD and the beginnings of understanding the pathophysiological processes occurring in the dementias. The correlations between clinical symptomatology, pathology, function and neuroimaging findings are encouraging and serve as an essential validator of the techniques. However, there is a need to evaluate critically the techniques lest they should become the sole driving force of research – they must serve the clinical questions or run the risk of leading researchers into blind alleys. With regard to diagnosis, success rates for the accurate prediction of AD remains stubbornly at around 85% whether pathological or neuroimaging studies are included. The remaining 15% may represent the tail end of diagnostic inaccuracy that inevitably involves all medical conditions, especially psychiatric disorders.

Areas that probably will bear fruit in the future include the combination of structural and functional scans (already available in many bespoke software imaging packages), longitudinal changes in scan appearances extending imaging to presymptomatic screening, and identification of patients likely to respond to particular classes of drug. Two prerequisites to allow meaningful interpretation of imaging studies are, first, the need to obtain biological verification of imaging changes whether these be pathological or chemical and, second, the need to conduct studies on representative populations of patients with dementia rather than relying on secondary or tertiary referrals. At the same time, the rapid development of techniques such as functional MRI will greatly add to the investigative armamentarium available to clinical neuroimagers.

References

Aharon-Peretz, J., Cummings, J.L., & Hill, M.A. (1988). Vascular dementia and dementia of the Alzheimer type – cognition, ventricular size, and leukoaraiosis. *Archives of Neurology*, 45, 719–721.

Albert, M., Naeser, M.A., Levine, H.L. & Garvey A.J. (1984). Ventricular size in patients with presenile dementia of the Alzheimer's type. *Archives of Neurology*, 41, 1258–1263.

Almkvist, O., Wahlund, L.-O., Andersson-Lundman, G., Basun, H. & Bäckman, L. (1992). White-matter hyperintensity and neuropsychological functions in dementia and healthy aging. *Archives of Neurology*, 49, 626–632.

Arai, H., Kobayashi, K., Ikeda, K., Nagao, Y., Ogihara, R. &

Kosaka K. (1983). A computed tomography study of Alzheimer's disease. *Journal of Neurology*, 229, 69–77.

Aylward, E.H., Karagiozis, H., Pearlson, G. & Folstein, M.F. (1991). Suprasellar cistern measures as a reflection of dementia in Alzheimer's disease but not Huntington's disease. *Journal of Psychiatric Research*, 25, 31–47.

Azari, N.P., Pettigrew, K.D., Schapiro, M.B. *et al.* (1993). Early detection of Alzheimer's disease: a statistical approach using positron emission tomographic data. *Journal of Cerebral Blood Flow and Metabolism*, 13, 438–447.

Berger, H. (1937). On the electroencephalogram of man: twelfth report. *Archiv für Psychiatrie und Nervenkrankheiten*, 106, 165–187.

Besson, J.A.O., Crawford, J.R., Parker, D.M. et al. (1990). Multimodal imaging in Alzheimer's disease – the relationship between MRI, SPECT, cognitive and pathological changes. *British Journal of Psychiatry*, 157, 216–220.

Besthorn, C., Förstl, H., Geiger-Kabisch, C., Sattel, H., Gasser, T. & Schreiter-Gasser, U. (1994). EEG coherence in Alzheimer disease. *Electroencephalography and Clinical Neurophysiology*, 90, 242–245.

Besthorn, C., Sattel, H., Geiger-Kabisch, C., Zerfass, R. & Förstl, H. (1995). Parameters of EEG dimensional complexity in Alzheimer's disease. *Electroencephalography and Clinical Neurophysiology*, 95, 84–89.

Biegon, A., Eberling, J.L., Richardson, B.C. et al. (1994). Human corpus callosum in aging and Alzheimer's disease: a magnetic resonance imaging study. *Neurobiology of Aging*, 15, 393–397.

Bondareff, W., Raval, J., Woo, B., Hauser, D.L. & Colletti, P.M. (1990). Magnetic resonance imaging and the severity of dementia in older adults. *Archives of General Psychiatry*, 47, 47–51.

Bouras, C., Hof, P.R., Giannakopoulos, P., Michel, J.P. & Morrison, J.H. (1994). Regional distribution of neurofibrillary tangles and senile plaques in the cerebral cortex of elderly patients: a quantitative evaluation of a one-year autopsy population from a geriatric hospital. *Cerebral Cortex*, 4, 138–150.

Braak, H. & Braak, E. (1991). Neuropathological stageing of Alzheimer-related changes. *Acta Neuropathologica*, 82, 239–259.

Brenner, R.P., Ulrich, R.F., Spiker, D.G. et al. (1986). Computerized EEG spectral analysis in elderly normal, demented and depressed subjects. *EEG Clinical Neurophysiology*, 64, 483–492

Buchsbaum, M.S., Kesslak, P., Lynch, G. et al. (1991). Temporal and hippocampal metabolic rate during an olfactory memory task assessed by positron emission tomography in patients with dementia of the Alzheimer type and controls. *Archives of General Psychiatry*, 48: 840–847.

Burns, A. (1991). The clinical diagnosis of Alzheimer's disease. *Dementia*, 2, 186–194.

Burns, A. (1993). The current literature: CT in the early diagnosis of Alzheimer's disease. *British Journal of Psychiatry*, 163, 809–812.

Burns, A. & Förstl, H. (1994). The clinical diagnosis of Alzheimer's disease. In *Dementia*. ed. A. Burns & R. Levy, pp. 309–326. London: Chapman & Hall.

Burns, A., Jacoby, R., Philpot, M. & Levy, R. (1989a). Computerized tomography in Alzheimer's disease – methods of scan analysis, comparison with normal controls and clinical/radiological association. *British Journal of Psychiatry*, 159: 609–614.

Burns, A., Philpot, M.P., Costa, D.C., Ell, P.J. & Levy, R. (1989b). The investigation of Alzheimer's disease with single photon emission tomography. *Journal of Neurology, Neurosurgery and Psychiatry*, 52, 248–253.

Coben, L.A., Danziger, W.L. & Berg, L. (1983). Frequency analysis of the resting awake EEG in mild senile dementia of Alzheimer type. *Electroencephalography and Clinical Neurophysiology*, 55, 372–380.

Coffey, C.E., Wilkinson, W.E., Parashos, I.A. et al. (1992). Quantitative cerebral anatomy of the aging human brain: a cross-sectional study using magnetic resonance imaging. *Neurology*, 42, 527–536.

Curran, S.M., Murray, C.M., van Beck, M. et al. (1993). A single photon emission computerised tomography study of regional brain function in elderly patients with major depression and with Alzheimer-type dementia. *British Journal of Psychiatry*, 163, 155–165.

Damasio, H., Eslinger, P., Damasio, A.R., Rizzo, M., Huang, H.K. & Demeter, S. (1983). Quantitative computed tomographic analysis in the diagnosis of dementia. *Archives of Neurology*, 40, 715–719.

Davis, P., Gearing, M., Gray, L. et al. (1995). The CERAD experience, part VIII: neuroimaging–neuropathology correlates of temporal lobe changes in Alzheimer's disease. *Neurology*, 45, 178–179.

Davis, P.C., Gray, L., Albert, M. et al. (1992). The consortium to establish a registry for Alzheimer's disease (CERAD). Part III. Reliability of a standardized MRI evaluation of Alzheimer's disease. *Neurology*, 42, 1676–1680.

de Leon, M.J. (1993). Hippocampal formation atrophy in ageing and the prediction of Alzheimer's disease. In *Ageing and Dementia*. ed. A. Burns, pp. 103–124. Chichester: Edward Arnold.

DeKosky, S.T., Shih, W.J., Schmitt, F.A., Coupal, J. & Kirkpatrick, C. (1990). Assessing utility of single photon emission computed tomography (SPECT) scan in Alzheimer disease: correlation with cognitive severity. *Alzheimer's Disease and Associated Disorders*, 4, 14–23.

Diaz, J.F., Merskey, H., Hachinski, V.C. et al. (1991). Improved recognition of leukoaraiosis and cognitive impairment in Alzheimer's disease. *Archives of Neurology*, 48, 1022–1025.

Dierks, T., Ihl, R., Frölich, L. & Maurer, K. (1993). Dementia of the Alzheimer type: effects on the spontaneous EEG described by dipole sources. *Psychiatry Research*, 50, 151–162.

Dierks, T., Perisic, I., Frölich, L., Ihl, R. & Maurer, K. (1991). Topography of the quantitative electroencephalogram in dementia of the Alzheimer type: relation to severity of dementia. *Psychiatry Research*, 40, 181–194.

Drayer, B.P. (1988). Imaging of the aging brain, part I. Normal findings. *Radiology*, 166, 785–796.

Eberling, J.L., Reed, B.R., Baker, M.G. & Jagust, W.J. (1993). Cognitive correlates of regional cerebral blood flow in Alzheimer's disease. *Archives of Neurology*, 50, 761–766.

Ebmeier, K.P., Besson, J.A.O., Crawford, J.R. et al. (1987). Nuclear magnetic resonance imaging and single photon emission tomography with radio-iodine labelled compounds in the diagnosis of dementia. *Acta Psychiatrica Scandinavica*, 75, 549–556.

Elmstahl, S., Rosen, I. & Gullberg, B. (1994). Quantitative EEG in elderly patients with Alzheimer's disease and healthy controls. *Dementia*, 5, 119–124.

Erkinjuntti, T., Lee, D.H., Gao, F. *et al.* (1993). Temporal lobe atrophy on magnetic resonance imaging in the diagnosis of early Alzheimer's disease. *Archives of Neurology*, 50, 305–310.

Eslinger, P.J., Damasio, H., Graff-Radford, N. & Damasio, A.R. (1984). Examining the relationship between computed tomography and neuropsychological measures in normal and demented elderly. *Journal of Neurology, Neurosurgery and Psychiatry*, 47, 1319–1325.

Ettlin, T.M., Staehelin, H.B., Kischka, U. *et al.* (1989). Computed tomography, electroencephalography, and clinical features in the differential diagnosis of senile dementia – a prospective clinicopathologic study. *Archives of Neurology*, 46, 1217–1220.

Folstein, M.F., Folstein, S.E. & McHugh, P.R. (1975). 'Mini-mental state', a practical method of grading the cognitive state of patients for the clinician. *Journal of Psychiatric Research*, 12, 189–198.

Förstl, H., Besthorn, C., Sattel, H. *et al.* (1996a). Volumetric estimates of brain atrophy and quantitative EEG in normal ageing and Alzheimer's disease. *Nervenarzt*, 67, 53–61.

Förstl, H., Burns, A., Jacoby, R., Eagger, S. & Levy, R. (1991). Quantitative CT-scan analysis in senile dementia of the Alzheimer type I. II. radioattenuation of grey and white matter. *International Journal of Geriatric Psychiatry*, 6, 709–713; 715–719.

Förstl, H. & Fischer, P. (1994). Diagnostic confirmation, severity, and subtypes of Alzheimer's disease: a short review on clinico-pathological correlations. *European Archives of Psychiatry and Clinical Neuroscience*, 244, 252–260.

Förstl, H., Sattel, H., Besthorn, C. *et al.* (1996b). Longitudinal cognitive, electroencephelographic and morphological brain changes in ageing and Alzheimer's disease. *British Journal of Psychiatry*, 168, 280–286.

Förstl, H., Hentschel, F., Geiger-Kabisch, C. *et al.* (1995a). Age-associated memory impairment and early Alzheimer's disease. *Drug Research*, 45, 394–397.

Förstl, H., Zerfass, R., Geiger-Kabisch, C., Sattel, H., Besthorn, C. & Hentschel, F. (1995b). Brain atrophy in normal ageing and Alzheimer's disease: volumetric discrimination and clinical correlations. *British Journal of Psychiatry*, 167, 739–746.

Friedland, R.P., Jagust, W.J., Huesman, R.H. *et al.* (1989). Regional cerebral glucose transport and utilization in Alzheimer's disease. *Neurology*, 39, 1427–1434.

Frisoni, G.B., Pizzolato, G., Bianchetti, A. *et al.* (1994). Single photon emission computed tomography with (^{99}Tc)-HM-PAO and (^{123}I)-IBZM in Alzheimer's disease and dementia of frontal type: preliminary results. *Acta Neurologia Scandinavica*, 89, 199–203.

George, A.E., de Leon, M.J., Stylopoulos, L.A. *et al.* (1990). CT diagnostic features of Alzheimer disease: importance of the choroidal/hippocampal fissure complex. *American Journal of Neuroradiology*, 11, 101–107.

Goldenberg, G., Podreka, I., Suess, E. & Deecke, L. (1989). The cerebral localization of neuropsychological impairment in Alzheimer's disease: a SPECT study. *Journal of Neurology*, 236, 131–138.

Golomb, J., de Leon, M.J., Kluger, A., George, A.E., Tarshish, C. & Ferris S.H. (1993). Hippocampal atrophy in normal aging – an association with recent memory impairment. *Archives of Neurology*, 50, 967–973.

Golomb, J., Kluger, A., de Leon, M.J. *et al.* (1994). Hippocampal formation size in normal human aging: a correlate of delayed secondary memory performance. *Learning and Memory*, 1, 45–54.

Goto, I., Taniwaki, T., Hosokawa, S. *et al.* (1993). Positron emission tomographic (PET) studies in dementia. *Journal of the Neurological Sciences*, 114, 1–6.

Grady, C.L., Haxby, J.V., Horwitz, B. *et al.* (1993). Activation of cerebral blood flow during a visuoperceptual task in patients with Alzheimer-type dementia. *Neurobiology of Aging*, 14, 35–44.

Gueguen, B., Filipovic, S., Derouesne, C. *et al.* (1988). *Senile Dementia*. London: J. Libbey.

Guze, B.H., Hoffman, J.M., Mazziotta, J.C., Baxter, L.R. & Phelps, M.E. (1992). Positron emission tomography and familial Alzheimer's disease: a pilot study. *Journal of the American Geriatrics Society*, 40, 120–123.

Harrell, L.E., Duvall, E., Folks, D.G. *et al.* (1991). The relationship of high-intensity signals on magnetic resonance images to cognition and psychiatric state in Alzheimer's disease. *Archives of Neurology*, 48, 1136–1140.

Haxby, J.V., Grady, C.L., Koss, E. *et al.* (1988). Heterogeneous anterior-posterior metabolic patterns in dementia of the Alzheimer type. *Neurology*, 38, 1853–1863.

Haxby, J.V., Grady, C.L., Koss, E. *et al.* (1990). Longitudinal study of cerebral metabolic asymmetries and associated neuropsychological patterns in early dementia of the Alzheimer type. *Archives of Neurology*, 47, 753–760.

Howieson, J., Kaye, J.A., Holm, L., & Howieson, D. (1993). Interuncal distance: marker of aging and Alzheimer disease. *American Journal of Neuroradiology*, 14, 647–650.

Ichimaya, Y., Kobayashi, K., Arai, H., Ikeda, K. & Kosaka, K. (1986). A computed tomography study of Alzheimer's disease by regional volumetric and parenchymal density measurements. *Journal of Neurology*, 233, 164–167.

Jack, C.R., Petersen, R.C., O'Brien, P.C. & Tangalos, E.G. (1992). MR-based hippocampal volumetry in the diagnosis of Alzheimer's disease. *Neurology*, 42, 183–188.

Jacoby, R.J. & Levy, R. (1980). Computed tomography in the elderly 2. Senile dementia: diagnosis and functional impairment. *British Journal of Psychiatry*, 136, 256–269.

Jagust, W.J., Eberling, J.L., Richardson, B.C. *et al.* (1993). The cortical topography of temporal lobe hypometabolism in early Alzheimer's disease. *Brain Research*, 629: 189–198.

Jagust, W.J., Friedland, R.P., Budinger, T.F., Koss, E. & Ober, B. (1988). Longitudinal studies of regional cerebral metabolism in Alzheimer's disease. *Neurology*, 38, 909–912.

Jagust, W.J., Reed, B.R., Seab, J.P. & Budinger, T.F. (1990). Alzheimer's disease – age at onset and single-photon emission computed tomographic patterns of regional cerebral blood flow. *Archives of Neurology*, 47, 628–633.

Jernigan, T.L., Archibald, S.L., Berhow, M.T. *et al.* (1991). Cerebral structure on MRI, part I: localization of age-related changes. *Biological Psychiatry*, 29, 55–67.

Jobst, K.A., Smith, A.D., Barker, C.S. *et al.* (1992a). Association of atrophy of the medial temporal lobe with reduced blood flow in the posterior parietotemporal cortex in patients with a clinical and pathological diagnosis of Alzheimer's disease. *Journal of Neurology, Neurosurgery and Psychiatry*, 55, 190–194.

Jobst, K., Smith, A.D., Szatmari, M. *et al.* (1992b). Detection in life of confirmed Alzheimer's disease using a simple measurement of medial temporal lobe atrophy by computed tomography. *Lancet*, 340, 1179–1183.

Kertesz, A., Polk, M. & Carr, T. (1990). Cognition and white matter changes on magnetic resonance imaging in dementia. *Archives of Neurology*, 47, 387–391.

Kesslak, J.P., Nalcioglu, O. & Cotman, C.W. (1991). Quantification of magnetic resonance scans for hippocampal and parahippocampal atrophy in Alzheimer's disease. *Neurology*, 41, 51–54.

Kido, D.K., Caine, E.D., LeMay, M. *et al.* (1989). Temporal lobe atrophy in patients with Alzheimer's disease: a CT study. *American Journal of Neuroradiology*, 10, 551–555.

Kobari, M., Stirling Meyer, J. & Ichijo, M. (1990). Leuko-araiosis, cerebral atrophy, and cerebral perfusion in normal aging. *Archives of Neurology*, 47, 161–165.

Kozachuk, W.E., DeCarli, C., Schapiro, M.B. *et al.* (1990). White matter hyperintensities in dementia of Alzheimer's type and in healthy subjects without cerebrovascular risk factors. *Archives of Neurology*, 47, 1306–1310.

Kumar, A., Newberg, A., Alavi, A. *et al.* (1994). MRI volumetric studies in Alzheimer's disease – Relationship to clinical and neuropsychological variables. *American Journal of Geriatric Psychiatry*, 2, 21–31.

Kumar, A., Yousem, D., Souder, E. *et al.* (1992). High-intensity signals in Alzheimer's disease without cerebrovascular risk factors: a magnetic resonance imaging evaluation. *American Journal of Psychiatry*, 149, 248–250.

Kwa, V.I.H., Weinstein, H.C., Posthumus Meyjes, E.F. *et al.* (1993). Spectral analysis of the EEG and 99m-Tc-HMPAO SPECT-Scan in Alzheimer's disease. *Biological Psychiatry*, 33, 100–107.

Leuchter, A.F., Spar, J.E., Walter, D.O. & Weiner, H. (1987).

Electroencephalographic spectra and coherence in the diagnosis of Alzheimer type and multiinfarct dementia. *Archives of General Psychiatry*, 44, 993–998.

Lopez, O.L., Becker, J.T., Rezek, D. *et al.* (1992). Neuropsychiatric correlates of cerebral white-matter radiolucencies in probable Alzheimer's disease. *Archives of Neurology*, 49, 828–834.

Mann, U.M., Mohr, E., Gearing, M. & Chase, T.N. (1992). Heterogeneity in Alzheimer's disease: progression rate segregated by distinct neuropsychological and cerebral metabolic profiles. *Journal of Neurology, Neurosurgery and Psychiatry*, 55, 956–959.

Matsubayashi, K., Shimada, K., Kawamoto, A. & Ozawa, T. (1992). Incidental brain lesions on magnetic resonance imaging and neurobehavioral functions in the apparently healthy elderly. *Stroke*, 23, 175–180.

McDonald, W.M., Krishnan, K.R.R., Murali Doraiswamy, P. *et al.* (1991). Magnetic resonance findings in patients with early-onset Alzheimer's disease. *Biological Psychiatry*, 29, 799–810.

McGeer, E.G., Peppard, R.P., McGeer, P.L. *et al.* (1990). 18-Fluorodeoxyglucose positron emission tomography studies in presumed Alzheimer cases, including 13 serial scans. *Canadian Journal of Neurological Sciences*, 17, 1–11.

McKhann, G., Drachman, D., Folstein, M. *et al.* (1984). Clinical diagnosis of Alzheimer's disease: report of the NINCDS-ADRDA work group under the auspices of Department of Health and Human Services Task Force on Alzheimer's Disease. *Neurology*, 34, 939–944.

McMurdo, M.E.T., Grant, D.J., Kennedy, N.S.J., Gilchrist, J., Findlay, D. & McLennan, J.M. (1994). The value of HMPAO SPECT scanning in the diagnosis of early Alzheimer's disease in patients attending a memory clinic. *Nuclear Medicine Communications*, 15, 405–409.

Merskey, H., Ball, M.J., Blume, W.T. *et al.* (1980). Relationships between psychological measurements and cerebral organic changes in Alzheimer's disease. *Canadian Journal of Neurological Sciences*, 7, 45–49.

Messa, C., Perani, D., Lucignani, G. *et al.* (1994). High-resolution technetium-99m-HMPAO SPECT in patients with probable Alzheimer's disease: comparison with fluorine-18–FDG PET. *Journal of Nuclear Medicine*, 35, 210–216.

Mirsen, T.R., Lee, D.H., Wong, C.J. *et al.* (1991). Clinical correlates of white-matter changes on magnetic resonance imaging scans of the brain. *Archives of Neurology*, 48, 1015–1021.

Montaldi, D., Brooks, D.N., McColl, J.H. *et al.* (1990). Measurements of regional cerebral blood flow and cognitive performance in Alzheimer's disease. *Journal of Neurology, Neurosurgery and Psychiatry*, 53, 33–38.

Murphy, D.G.M., Bottomley, P.A., Salerno, J.A. *et al.* (1993a). An in vivo study of phosphorus and glucose metabolism in Alzheimer's disease using magnetic resonance spectroscopy and PET. *Archives of General Psychiatry*, 50, 341–349.

Murphy, D.G.M., DeCarli, C.D., Daly, E. et al. (1993b). Volumetric magnetic resonance imaging in men with dementia of the Alzheimer type: correlations with disease severity. *Biological Psychiatry*, 34, 612–621.

Nybäck, H., Nyman, H., Blomqvist, G., Sjögren, I. & Stone-Elander, S. (1991). Brain metabolism in Alzheimer's dementia: studies of ^{11}C- deoxyglucose accumulation, CSF monoamine metabolites and neuropsychological test performance in patients and healthy subjects. *Journal of Neurology, Neurosurgery and Psychiatry*, 54, 672–678.

O'Brien, J.T., Desmond, P., Ames, D., Schweitzer, I., Tuckwell, V. & Tress B. (1994). The differentiation of depression from dementia by temporal lobe magnetic resonance imaging. *Psychological Medicine*, 24, 633–640.

Osimani, A., Ichise, M., Chung, D.G., Pogue, J.M. & Freedman, M. (1994). SPECT for differential diagnosis of dementia and correlation of rCBF with cognitive impairment. *Canadian Journal of Neurological Sciences*, 21, 104–111.

Pearlson, G.D., Harris, G.J., Powers, R.E. et al. (1992). Quantitative changes in mesial temporal volume, regional cerebral blood flow, and cognition in Alzheimer's disease. *Archives of General Psychiatry*, 49, 402–408.

Penttilä, M., Partanen, J.V., Soininen, H. & Riekkinen, P.J. (1985). Quantitative analysis of occipital EEG in different stages of Alzheimer's disease. *Electroencephalography and Clinical Neurophysiology*, 60, 1–6.

Pietrini, P., Azari, N.P., Grady, C.L. et al. (1993). Pattern of cerebral metabolic interactions in a subject with isolated amnesia at risk for Alzheimer's disease: a longitudinal evaluation. *Dementia*, 4, 94–101.

Prichep, L.S., John, E.R., Ferris, S.H. et al. (1994). Quantitative EEG correlates of cognitive deterioration in the elderly. *Neurobiology of Aging*, 15, 85–90.

Primavera, A., Novello, P., Finocchi, C., Canevari, E. & Corsello, L. (1990). Correlation between mini-mental state examination and quantitative electroencephalography in senile dementia of Alzheimer type. *Neuropsychobiology*, 23: 74–78.

Prinz, P.N. & Vitiello, M.V. (1989). Dominant occipital (alpha) rhythm frequency in early stage Alzheimer's disease and depression. *Electroencephalography and Clinical Neurophysiology*, 73, 427–432.

Pritchard, W.S., Duke, D.W., Coburn, K.L. et al. (1994). EEG-based, neural-net predictive classification of Alzheimer's disease versus control subjects is augmented by non-linear EEG measures. *Electroencephalography and Clinical Neurophysiology*, 91, 118–130.

Prohovnik, I., Mayeux, R., Sackeim, H.A. et al. (1988). Cerebral perfusion as a diagnostic marker of early Alzheimer's disease. *Neurology*, 38, 931–937.

Reed, B.R., Jagust, W.J. & Coulter, L. (1993). Anosognosia in Alzheimer's disease: relationships to depression, cognitive function, and cerebral perfusion. *Journal of Clinical and Experimental Neuropsychology*, 15, 231–244.

Reed, B.R., Jagust, W.J., Seab, J.P. & Ober, B.A. (1989). Memory and regional cerebral blood flow in mildly symptomatic Alzheimer's disease. *Neurology*, 39, 1537–1539.

Riddle, W., O'Carroll, R.E., Dougall, N. et al. (1993). A single photon emission computerised tomography study of regional brain function underlying verbal memory in patients with Alzheimer-type dementia. *British Journal of Psychiatry*, 163, 166–172.

Roberts, M.A., McGeorge, A.P. & Caird, F.I. (1978). Electroencephalography and computerised tomography in vascular and non-vascular dementia in old age. *Journal of Neurology, Neurosurgery and Psychiatry*, 41, 903–906.

Salmon, E., Sadzot, B., Maquet, P. et al. (1994). Differential diagnosis of Alzheimer's disease with PET. *Journal of Nuclear Medicine*, 35, 391–398.

Sandor, T., Albert, M., Stafford, J. & Kemper, T. (1990). Symmetrical and asymmetrical changes in brain tissue with age as measured on CT scans. *Neurobiology of Aging*, 11, 21–27.

Sandor, T., Jolesz, F., Tieman, J., Kikinis, R., Jones, K. & Albert, M. (1992). Comparative analysis of computed tomographic and magnetic resonance imaging scans in Alzheimer patients and controls. *Archives of Neurology*, 49, 381–384.

Scheltens, P.H., Barkhof, F., Valk, J. et al. (1992). White matter lesions on magnetic resonance imaging in clinically diagnosed Alzheimer's disease. *Brain*, 115, 735–748.

Schreiter-Gasser, U., Gasser, T. & Ziegler, P. (1994). Quantitative EEG analysis in early onset Alzheimer's disease: correlations with severity, clinical characteristics, visual EEG and CCT. *Electroencephalography and Clinical Neurophysiology*, 90, 267–272.

Seab, J.P., Jagust, W.J., Wong, S.T.S. et al. (1988). Quantitative NMR measurements of hippocampal atrophy in Alzheimer's disease. *Magnetic Resonance in Medicine*, 8, 200–208.

Sheridan, P.H., Sato, S., Foster, N. et al. (1988). Relation of EEG alpha background to parietal lobe function in Alzheimer's disease as measured by positron emission tomography and psychometry. *Neurology*, 38, 747–750.

Sloan, E.P. & Fenton, G.W. (1993). EEG power spectra and cognitive change in geriatric psychiatry: a longitudinal study. *Electroencephalography and Clinical Neurophysiology*, 86, 361–367.

Small, G.W., Kuhl, D.E., Riege, W.H. et al. (1989). Cerebral glucose metabolic patterns in Alzheimer's disease. *Archives of General Psychiatry*, 46, 527–532.

Smith, G.S., de Leon, M.J., George, A.E. et al. (1992). Topography of cross-sectional and longitudinal glucose metabolic deficits in Alzheimer's disease. *Archives of Neurology*, 49, 1142–1150.

Spano, A., Förstl, H., Almeida, O.P. & Levy, R. (1992).

Neuroimaging and the differential diagnosis of early dementia: quantitative CT-scan analysis in patients attending a memory clinic. *International Journal of Geriatric Psychiatry*, 7, 879–883.

Stefoski, D., Bergen, D., Fox, J., Morrell, F., Huckman, M. & Ramsey, R. (1976). Correlation between diffuse EEG abnormalities and cerebral atrophy in senile dementia. *Journal of Neurology, Neurosurgery and Psychiatry*, 39, 751–755.

Stern, Y., Alexander, G.E., Prohovnik, I. & Mayeux, R. (1992). Inverse relationship between education and parietotemporal perfusion deficit in Alzheimer's disease. *Annals of Neurology*, 32, 371–375.

Sullivan, E.V., Shear, P.K., Mathalon, D.H. *et al.* (1993). Greater abnormalities of brain cerebrospinal fluid volumes in younger than in older patients with Alzheimer's disease. *Archives of Neurology*, 50, 359–373.

Szelies, B., Grond, M., Herholz, K. *et al.* (1992). Quantitative EEG mapping and PET in Alzheimer's disease. *Journal of the Neurological Sciences*, 110, 46–56.

Szelies, B., Mielke, R., Herholz, K. & Heiss, W.D. (1994). Quantitative topographical EEG compared to FDG PET for classification of vascular and degenerative dementia. *Electroencephalography and Clinical Neurophysiology*, 91, 131–139.

Waldemar, G., Bruhn, P., Kristensen, M., Johnsen, A., Paulson, O.B. & Lassen, N.A. (1994). Heterogeneity of neocortical cerebral blood flow deficits in dementia of the Alzheimer type: a (99mTc)-d,l-HMPAO SPECT study. *Journal of Neurology, Neurosurgery and Psychiatry*, 57, 285–295.

Weinstein, H.C., Haan, J., van Royen, E.A. *et al.* (1991). SPECT in the diagnosis of Alzheimer's disease and multiinfarct-dementia. *Clinical Neurology and Neurosurgery*, 93, 39–43.

West, M.J., Coleman, P.D., Flood, D.G. & Troncoso, J.C. (1994). Differences in the pattern of hippocampal neuronal loss in normal ageing and Alzheimer's disease. *Lancet*, 344, 769–772.

Willmer, J., Carruthers, A., Guzman, D.A., Collins, B., Pogue, J. & Stuss, D.T. (1993). The usefulness of CT scanning in diagnosing dementia of the Alzheimer type. *Canadian Journal of Neurological Sciences*, 20, 210–216.

Yamauchi, H., Fukuyama, H., Harada, K. *et al.* (1993). Callosal atrophy parallels decreased cortical oxygen metabolism and neuropsychological impairment in Alzheimer's disease. *Archives of Neurology*, 50, 1070–1074.

4 Vascular dementia

Hiroo Kasahara and Kazuo Hasegawa

Introduction

Vascular dementia is a type of dementia resulting from cerebrovascular disorder. It is not rare that cerebral stroke (infarction or hemorrhage) is followed by typical vascular dementia. There are, however, some patients with vascular dementia who have no preceding episodes of evident cerebrovascular disorder such as stroke or transient cerebral ischemia.

Arteriosclerotic dementia and multiinfarct dementia are terms used for pathological conditions similar to vascular dementia. Although the former term commonly has been used to describe dementing diseases in the elderly, it is very obscure in definition, as if covering every ambiguous dementing condition.

Multiinfarct dementia is a concept proposed in 1974 by Hachinski, Lassen & Marshall, who criticized the existing tendency for dementing disease in the elderly to be over-diagnosed as cerebrovascular dementia. According to Hachinski and colleagues (1974), dementia should be classified in terms of the cause into senile dementia of Alzheimer type and multiinfarct dementia. The former, which is predominant, occurs along with aging changes in the brain, and the latter is caused by cerebrovascular disorder. They stated, on the basis of studies of CBF, that dementia related to cerebral vascular lesions is caused by multiple development of infarcts varying in size, rather than simply by the presence of cerebral arteriosclerosis. This opinion became widely accepted, with an understanding of the concept that the lesion responsible for dementia is not arteriosclerosis itself, but the resultant infarct(s).

Later, however, it was pointed out that cerebrovascular dementia attributable to pathological conditions other than infarction accounts for a substantial proportion of all cases of vascular dementia. Such cases include those resulting from cerebral hemorrhage or from incomplete softening of the white matter, as in Binswanger's disease. Cerebrovascular lesions causative of dementia do not fall into a single category named multiple infarction, indicating that the term 'vascular dementia' is better suited to these conditions. Hence this term, vascular dementia, is now more commonly used.

Patients with such dementia often have a history of hypertension and cerebral stroke, accompanied by neurological signs and symptoms consistent with these conditions and exhibit the presence of infarct(s) or local enlargement of a cerebral sulcus on CT and MRI. SPET and PET often show macular areas of hypometabolism. An autopsy finding characteristic of this disease is the presence of many degenerative areas distributed over the entire cerebral hemisphere.

Characteristic features of vascular dementia

Vascular dementia shows a wide variety of disease type, with its clinical symptoms varying according to the location, size and distribution of the lesion(s). The clinical course also differs from one patient to another. In this aspect, this condition makes a clear contrast with dementia caused by AD, which is characterized by relatively uniform clinical course and symptoms. However, there are some general features common to vascular dementia as a whole. These features should be understood accurately. Table 4.1 shows a comparison of the characteristic features of vascular dementia and AD and Table 4.2 shows the clinical picture of vascular dementia reported by Hachinski et al. (1975). These clinical features are correlated with the CBF, and their usefulness in differentiation from multiinfarct dementia has been demonstrated in pathological studies. The history of the patient is characterized by the presence of hypertension, previous episode(s) of cerebrovascular disorder, abrupt onset, stepwise aggravation and localized neurological signs. A right–left difference and pseudobulbar paralysis found on neurological examination suggest the presence of multiple infarctions underlying the dementia. In most patients, rigidity, spasticity, hyperreflexia, plantar extension reflex and gait disturbance occur bilaterally, often showing a right–left difference in their manifestation.

Previous studies on changes in the mental symptoms of vascular dementia have disclosed that cortical infarction is likely to induce aphasia, amnesia and visuospatial agnosia, while multiple subcortical infarctions tend to induce psychomotor inhibition and memory and cognitive disturbance. In patients with vascular dementia, personality is relatively well maintained, and depression is often seen. Although a paranoid state may be found, it is less obvious in patients with multiinfarct dementia than in those with AD. Epidemiological features distinguishing between patients with vascular dementia and those with AD are earlier onset and predominance of males in the former group (Hasegawa et al., 1980; 1982; Hasegawa, Homma & Imai, 1986).

Table 4.1 *Distinguishing features of vascular dementia and AD*

Features	Vascular dementia	AD
Time of onset	The incidence increases with age, but the proportion of young patients is greater than among those with AD	The incidence increases markedly with age
Clinical course	The progress of disease is slow – but sometimes acute and stepwise	Slow and insidious onset and continuous progression
Subjective Symptoms	Headache, vertigo, numbness, insomnia, subjective memory impairment and depressed mood may occur in the initial stage	None
Psychiatric Symptoms	1. Personality, judgement and common sense are relatively well maintained until the terminal stage 2. Patchy dementia 3. Symptoms are labile, but may be fixed occasionally	1. Distinct deterioration of personality 2. Global dementia 3. Symptoms are less labile and progress gradually
Cerebral focal symptoms	May appear according to the site of the lesion	Present, but not as conspicuous in cases of AD
Neurological symptoms	Accompanying hemiplegia, parkinsonism, apraxia of gait or pseudobulbar palsy appears in the early stage	Absent in the early stage; muscular rigidity and myoclonus may appear in the advanced stage
Systemic disease	Complications such as hypertension, diabetes mellitus, hyperlipidemia and cardiac disease are common	Not remarkable
Consciousness of disease	Insight is maintained to some extent until the terminal stage	Insight is lacking
Others	Affective incontinence and focal symptoms are present; a depressive stage may occur; forced crying and laughing (+)	Euphoria, polyogia; forced crying and laughing (−)
CT findings	1. Multiinfarct dementia: many low-density areas of middle or small size are present in the region covered by the cortical branch or penetrating branch 2. Encephalopathy of Binswanger type: ventricular distension; extensive low density in the white matter areas	Symmetrical dilatation of the sulci and ventricular distention; no marked changes in the early stage; cerebral atrophy becomes conspicuous according to the advance of stage of the disease

Table 4.2 *Hachinski's cerebral ischemic scores*

Feature	Score
Abrupt onset	2
Stepwise deterioration	1
Fluctuating course	2
Nocturnal confusion	1
Relative preservation of personality	1
Depression	1
Somatic complaints	1
Emotional incontinence	1
History of hypertension	1
History of strokes	2
Evidence of associated atherosclerosis	1
Focal neurological symptoms	2
Focal neurological signs	2
Vascular dementia	Score of 7 or more
Dementia of Alzheimer type	Score of 4 or less

From Hachinski, *et al.* (1975)

Classification of vascular dementia

Vascular dementia results from cerebrovascular lesions. The focus involves destruction of the brain tissue generally on a scale of more than 50 ml, or of a part of the brain pivotal for the maintenance of cognitive function on a smaller scale (Hasegawa & Imai, 1991). In the former, medium or greater infarction or hemorrhage may cause dementia even if there is only a single lesion. Multiple occurrence of small infarcts and hemorrhage may also cause dementia. Extensive degeneration of the cerebral white matter in cases of encephalopathy of Binswanger type causes severe dementia. The clinical course and symptoms of cerebrovascular dementia vary largely according to the site, type and cause of the lesion(s).

Classification of vascular dementia allows a better understanding of this disease. Table 4.3 shows such classification by Matsushita (1984). His classification is characterized by primary grouping of the underlying lesions into ischemic (infarction) and hemorrhagic, followed by subgrouping of extensive, multiple and special localized lesions. Since this classification shows good agreement with underlying diseases and risk factors (Table 4.4), it is clinically helpful (Meyer *et al.*, 1986; Matsubayashi *et al.*, 1988).

Table 4.3 *Classification of vascular dementia*

Types		Characteristics
Ischemic lesions[a]	1.	Extensive lesions involving the cortex and white matter Obstruction of the major arteries in the brain base or their cortical branches (thrombosis, embolism)
	2.	Multiple infarcts of middle or small size Obstruction of penetrating arteries, long penetrating cortical branches supplying the white matter (thrombosis)
	3.	Extensive lesions localized in the white matter Encephalopathy of Binswanger type (chronic circulatory failure of long penetrating cortical branches supplying the white matter)
	4.	Localized lesions in the area pivotal to the formation of dementia (thalamus, temporal lobe, parietal lobe, etc.)
Hemorrhagic lesions[a]	1.	Hemorrhage of moderate or greater scale at thalamus, putamen, cerebral lobe (hypertensive in most cases, with some cases of amyloid angiopathy)
	2.	Multiple lobular hemorrhage (amyloid angiopathy in most cases)
	3.	Focal hemorrhage (thalamus, temporal lobe)
Special types not clearly distinguishable from consciousness disturbance	1.	Apallic syndrome
	2.	Akinetic mutism
	3.	Other types of prolonged consciousness disturbance

Note:
[a] Ischemic lesions (mainly thrombosis) and hemorrhagic lesions may appear in the same patient.

Table 4.4 *Causative diseases and risk factors for cerebral stroke*

Causes	Risk factors
Cerebral thrombosis	Cerebral arteriosclerosis, hypertension, diabetes mellitus, hyperlipidemia, polyemia, hyperfibrinogenemia, hypercoagulability (e.g. through the use of oral contraceptives)
Cerebral embolism	Atrial fibrillation, cardiac valve disease, myocardial infarction, cardiovascular surgery, air embolism (including diver's disease), fat embolism, atrial myxoma, cervical arterial atherosclerosis, bacterial and nonbacterial endocarditis
Cerebral hemorrhage	Hypertension, hemorrhagic diathesis, blood disease, use of antiplatelet or anticoagulant agents, amyloid angiopathy (advanced age, familial cerebrovascular amyloidosis on rare occasions)
Subarachnoid hemorrhage	Cerebral aneurysm, cerebral arteriovenous malformation, hemorrhagic diathesis (leukemia, purpura, hemophilia, use of anticoagulant agents)

Types of vascular dementia

Vascular dementia can be classified into a number of types according to the clinicopathological features (Table 4.3) (Tohgi, 1983; 1984; 1988; Tohgi et al., 1985).

Extensive ischemia type involving the cortex and white matter

This extensive ischemia type of vascular dementia is the basic type, showing the major characteristic features of vascular dementia described in the previous section. With regard to the etiology, although cerebral thrombosis as a result of cerebral arteriosclerosis is the predominant cause, cerebral embolism derived from cardiac disease accounts for a substantial proportion. In cases of cerebral thrombosis, severe arteriosclerosis is present in the internal carotid artery, basilar artery, their cortical and penetrating branches and arterioles in the cerebral parenchyma. The region of the infarcts varies from small to large in size, often involving the cortex and white matter. At the same time, infarcts of small or medium size occur in a multiple fashion in the deep white matter, basal ganglia and thalamus, accompanied by thinning of the callosal body. Infarcts are located most frequently in the areas supplied by the middle cerebral artery, followed by those supplied by the posterior cerebral artery and anterior cerebral artery. Extensive infarction involving the cortex and white matter is likely to occur in the border zone among the regions supplied by the anterior, middle and posterior cerebral arteries. Obstruction of the internal carotid artery induces atrophy and incomplete softening extending to the entire cerebral hemisphere. Cerebral embolism usually takes the form of cortical branch infarction. Since cerebral embolism is likely to cause infarction of medium or larger size, resultant severe mental hypofunction is not uncommon even if there is a single lesion.

In cases of the extensive ischemia type involving the cortex and white matter, CT reveals low-density areas of various sizes including the cortex and white matter in the regions supplied by the major cerebral arteries and their cortical branches or in their border zone. Small or medium-sized low-density areas are also frequently found in the deep white matter, basal ganglia and brain stem. When the focus is located in the left hemisphere, there is concomitant aphasia, Gerstmann's syndrome or apraxia in many cases, whereas a focus in the right hemisphere is often accompanied by left unilateral spatial disorientation or personality change (Figs. 4.1 and 4.2). The location where infarcts occur in the next highest frequency is the border zone between the middle and anterior or posterior cerebral artery. The infarcts are medium in size.

Obstruction of the posterior cerebral artery is likely to cause delirium, while obstruction of the anterior cerebral artery may cause hypobulia and personality change.

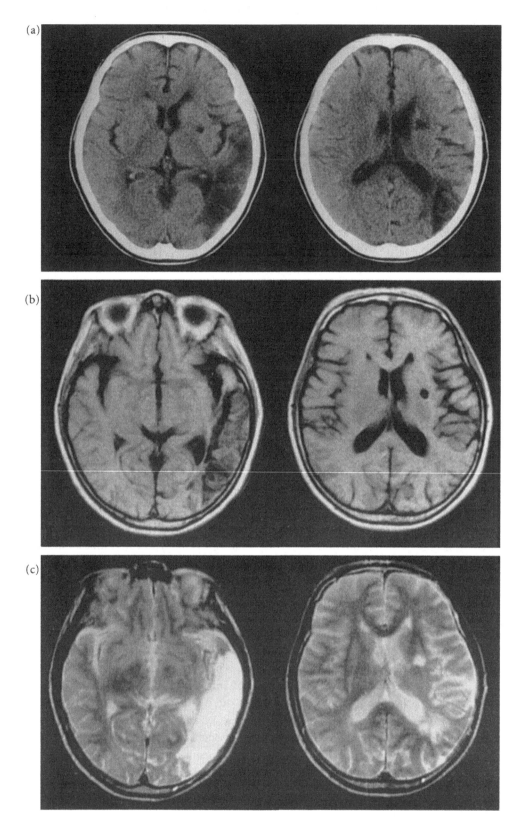

Figure 4.1 *Multiinfarct dementia caused by infarction in branches of the cortical artery and penetrating branches of artery. (a) CT; (b) MRI T₁-weighted image; (c) MRI T₂-weighted image.*

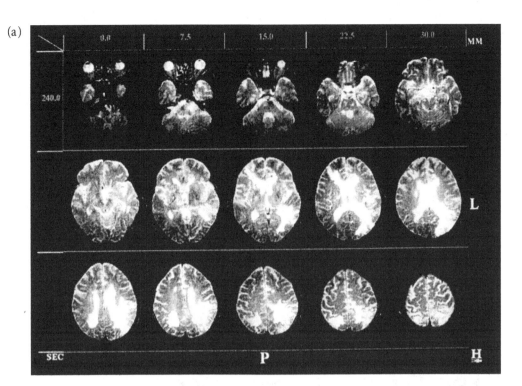

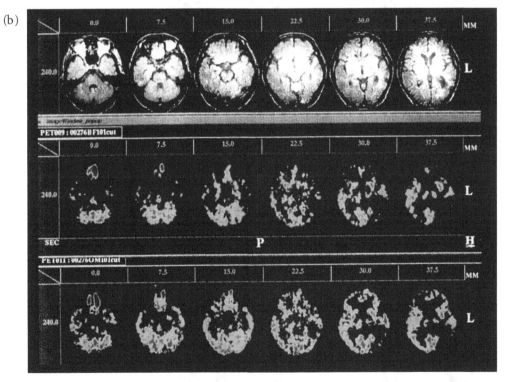

Figure 4.10 *(a, b) Brain PET image of a patient with vascular dementia acquired with ^{18}F-FDG. FDG uptake is lower in bilateral frontal and left temporoparietal regions.*

A colour version of this image is available for download from www.cambridge.org/9780521112475.

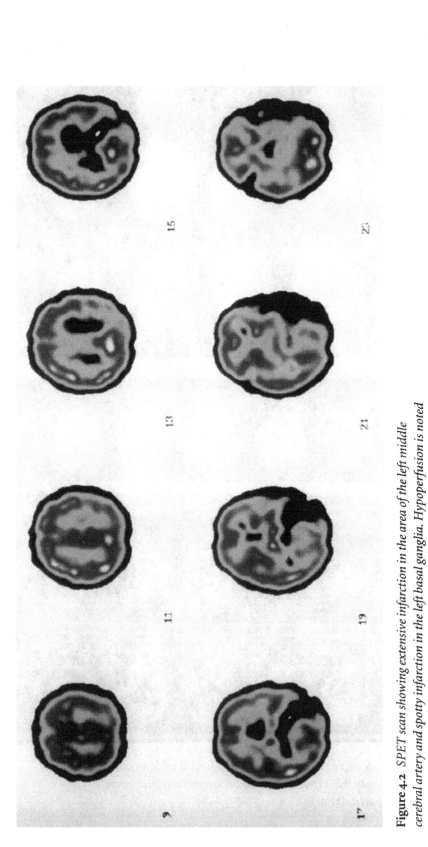

Figure 4.2 *SPET scan showing extensive infarction in the area of the left middle cerebral artery and spotty infarction in the left basal ganglia. Hypoperfusion is noted in left temporoparietal area.*

A colour version of these images are available for download from www.cambridge.org/9780521112475.

Multiple small infarction type involving the deep white matter

Vascular dementia caused by multiple small infarcts occurs through obstruction of the penetrating arterial branches, mostly caused by thrombosis. Small or medium-sized infarcts develop in a multiple fashion in the basal ganglia, thalamus and deep white matter of the cerebrum. Concomitant lacunar infarcts (small infarcts measuring 5mm or less in diameter) are often found in the brain stem (pons). Dementia is often accompanied by neurological symptoms such as hemiplegia, tiny step gait, parkinsonian syndrome, pseudobulbar paralysis (disturbance of swallowing and articulation), affective incontinence, forced crying and laughing, and urinary incontinence (Figs. 4.3 and 4.4).

Extensive ischemia and multiple small infarctions cause the two types of cerebrovascular dementia that represent the pathological condition called multiinfarct dementia.

Binswanger type encephalopathy

Extensive degeneration and demyelination occurs in the cerebral white matter in Binswanger type encephalopathy and this results in severe dementia. CT shows diffuse low-density areas in the white matter surrounding the cerebral ventricles: WMHI or leukoaraiosis. Leukoaraiosis means rarefaction of the white matter and is visualized as an extensive area of high-intensity signal localized in the white matter in T_2-weighted

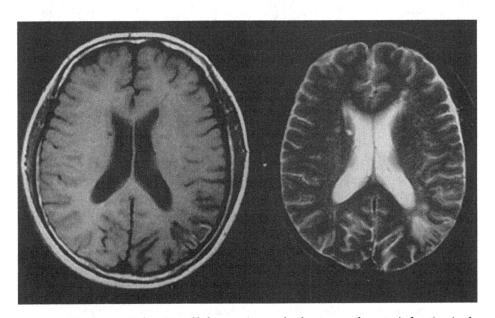

Figure 4.3 *Infarction of left posterior cerebral artery and spotty infarction in the right caudate nucleus and putamen. MRI shows an old infarction in the left occipitoparietal region.*

images of MRI (Fig. 4.5). There is also a transitional type of damage lying between this type and the multiple small infarction type. Although the mechanism of occurrence of this condition remains to be clarified, it is speculated that chronic circulatory failure of the most distal penetrating artery of the cortex branch supplying the cerebral white matter is responsible. In recent years, attention has been focused on the relation with nocturnal hypertension. Severe and gradually progressive dementia occurs in patients with Binswanger's disease (Bennett *et al.*, 1990).

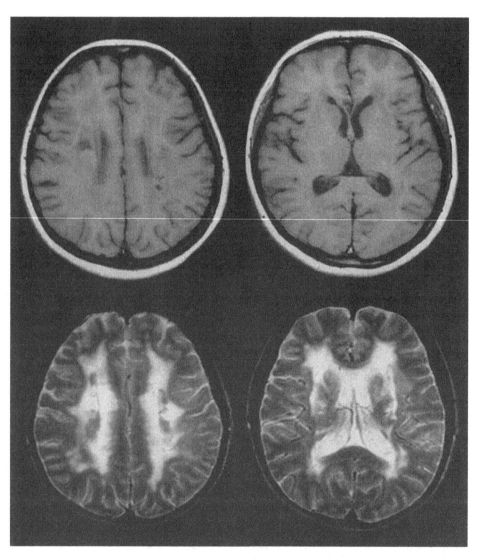

Figure 4.4 *Multiple small infarcts of the deep white matter. Multiple old infarcts noted in bilateral centrum semiovale, paraventricular region and PVH.*

Dementia caused by focal lesions located at a particular site

When the focus of damage is located in a part of the brain pivotal for maintaining cognition or intelligence, dementia occurs even if the focus is small and localized. Since characteristic features such as those described below are present regardless of whether the responsible focus is infarction or hemorrhage, observation of the clinical symptoms allows inference of the lesion site.

Thalamic dementia
Marked decrease in retention, decreased volition and acathexis occur when the antero-medial region of the thalamus is affected. Although the focus is more frequently located on the left side, the right side may also be affected. The former case is often accompanied by speech disorder, and the latter by cognitive disorder (Fig. 4.6).

Occipital dementia
Occipital dementia occurs as a result of obstruction of the posterior cerebral artery. This condition is characterized by the manifestation of prolonged delirium in addition to retention disorder and hemianopia. It is not rare that accompanying pseudopsia or delusions are present.

Marginal dementia
In marginal dementia, severe retention disorder occurs as a result of a focus on the medial side of the lateral lobe or in the hippocampus in the cerebral limbic system. The

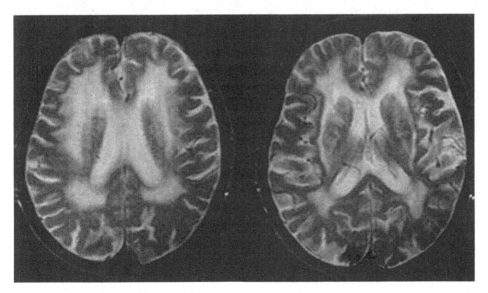

Figure 4.5 *Binswanger type encephalopathy. The MRI T_2-weighted image shows extended high signal intensity area in periventricular regions.*

cause is obstruction of the posterior cerebral artery in most cases. The left side alone or both sides are usually involved.

Angular syndrome

Angular syndrome is caused by a left angular focus, resulting in fluent aphasia, aphasic agraphia, Gerstmann's syndrome and constructional apraxia. It is not uncommon for this condition to be accompanied by diminished general intellectual function. Since the

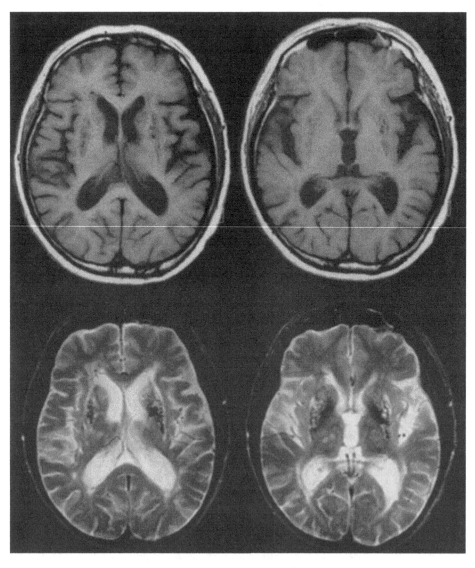

Figure 4.6 *Dementia in bilateral thalamic infarction. Multiple old infarctions in both basal ganglia, pons and centrum semiovale noted on MRI.*

signs and symptoms of this condition resemble those of dementia of Alzheimer type, particular caution is necessary in differential diagnosis.

Dementia caused by cerebral hemorrhage

The most frequent cause of cerebral hemorrhage in elderly patients is hypertension, followed by amyloid angiopathy.

Hypertensive cerebral hemorrhage
The hypertensive cerebral hemorrhage is frequently located in the thalamus (medial hemorrhage), putamen (lateral hemorrhage), tegmental region of the pons, and cerebellum (Fig. 4.7). Thalamic hemorrhage is likely to induce thalamic dementia or a decreased conscious level. Hemorrhage in the putamen causes dementia accompanied by hemiplegia or aphasia if its extent is moderate or greater. In recent years, the introduction of MRI has raised the detection rate of old cerebral hemorrhage, demonstrating that the coexistence of hemorrhage and infarction in the same patient is not necessarily rare (Figs. 4.8 and 4.9).

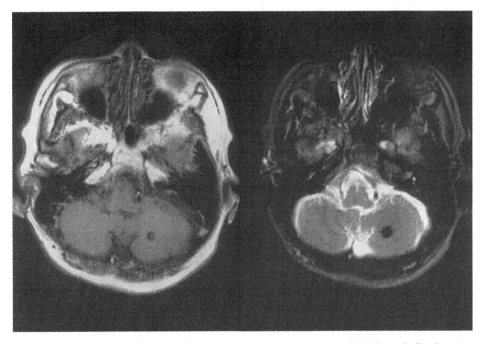

Figure 4.7 *Dementia caused by an old hemorrhage in the left cerebellar hemisphere. A very low intensity area is seen in the left cerebeller hemisphere on T$_1$- and T$_2$-weighted images as a result of the old hemorrhage.*

(a)

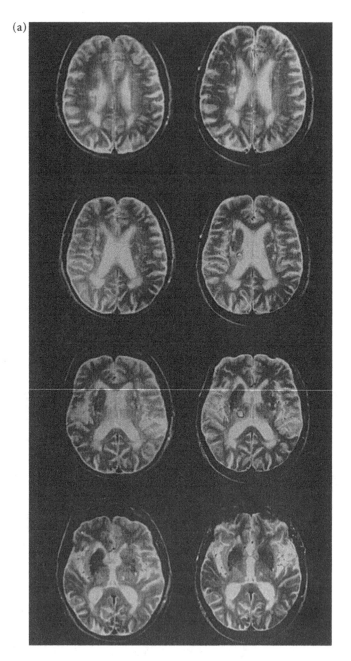

Figure 4.8 *Dementia caused by hemorrhage from ischemic region. (a) MRI T$_2$-weighted images before hemorrhage on the left and after hemorrhage on the right. Several spotty infarctions are scattered in both basal ganglia, centrum semiovale and left thalamus on the prehemorrhage image. Small hemorrhage of the right thalamus is seen in the weighted image after hemorrhage. (b) Hemorrhage noted in right thalamus in MRI T$_1$-weighted image.*

(b)

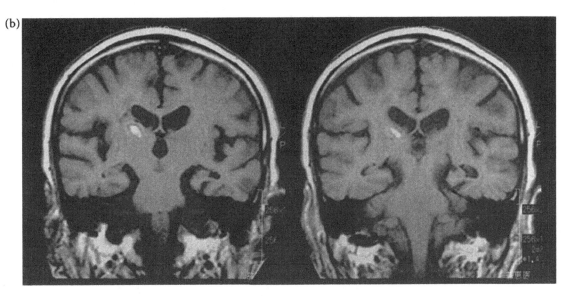

Figure 4.8 (*cont.*)

Although pontine hemorrhage and cerebellar hemorrhage themselves are not the direct causes of dementia, they may secondarily result in dementia if the aqueduct of the midbrain or the fourth ventricle is obstructed or narrowed by a hematoma, followed by hydrocephalus or a decrease in conscious level resulting from circulatory disturbance of the CSF.

Hemorrhage caused by amyloid angiopathy

Hemorrhage caused by amyloid angiopathy has been attracting attention recently as a type of cerebral hemorrhage common in the elderly. This condition accounts for a high proportion of patients with cerebral hemorrhage over 70 years of age. In contrast to hypertensive cerebral hemorrhage, recurrent and multiple hemorrhage (subcortical hemorrhage) characteristically occurs near to the cerebral surface. Since bleeding occurs just beneath the cortex of the parietal, frontal, occipital or temporal lobe, this condition is also called cerebral lobe-type hemorrhage. Although movement disorder is relatively mild, dementia occurs along with neuropsychological symptoms corresponding to the site of hemorrhage, and advances every time an additional episode occurs.

Transitional type changing to prolonged disturbance of consciousness

When a large area of the brain is affected by major infarction, massive bleeding or multiple lesions, or when diffuse lesions have developed in the brain as the result of general cerebral ischemia or anoxic encephalopathy, severe disturbance of consciousness occurs in the acute stage. In the chronic stage, the patients open their eyes and are apparently awake but do not show any spontaneous expression of consciousness nor significant response to stimuli, being in the state of prolonged disturbance of consciousness characterized by akinetic mutism or apallic syndrome.

Pathogenesis of vascular dementia

Clinicopathological correlates

Cerebral lesions causative of vascular dementia can be localized lesions in a particular part of the brain or diffuse lesions in the white matter. Whether localized lesions cause dementia depends on their size and site. If the lesion is large, the probability of dementia is high. Even if the infarct is middle-sized, it can cause dementia if located at a site

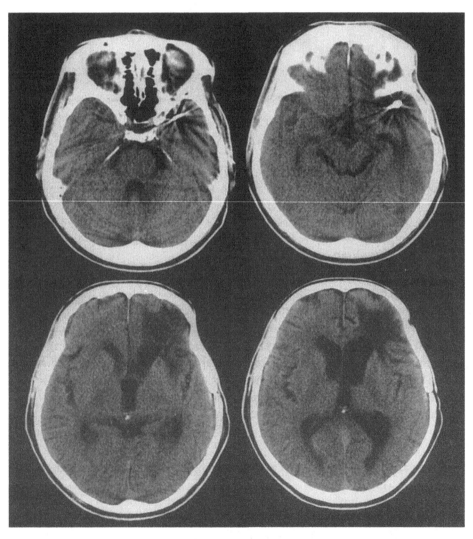

Figure 4.9 *Dementia caused by intracranial and subarachnoid hematoma.*
Postaneurysmal clipping and left frontal old infarction region noted on CT.

influential to the general cerebral function, for example the medial side of the frontal lobe, thalamus and its ascending projection, and limbic system. Multiinfarct dementia is a type of dementia occurring as a result of multiple development of infarcts of varying size; it does not necessarily mean dementia caused by the multiple occurrence of only small infarcts. Leukoaraiosis (Hachinski, Potter & Merskey, 1987) is rarefaction of the white matter as visualized by diagnostic imaging procedures such as CT and MRI and is not necessarily accompanied by dementia.

Dementia resulting from localized lesions occurs secondary to an episode of cerebral infarction caused by cerebral thrombosis or embolism, and its etiology is the same as in cerebral infarction. By comparison Binswanger's disease is not accompanied by discrete episodes of cerebral infarction and shows gradual manifestation of dementia. Its etiology should be examined from an angle different from that for localized cerebral infarction.

Reported risk factors for vascular dementia include hypertension, diabetes mellitus, cardiac disease, hyperlipidemia and heavy smoking. Controlling these risk factors may improve the symptoms of dementia (Meyer et al., 1986). A comparison of patients with multiinfarct dementia and those with multiple infarction without dementia revealed that the level of total cholesterol tended to be lower, systolic pressure was significantly lower and the arteriosclerosis index tended to be higher in the former group. There were, however, no intergroup differences in hematocrit, serum blood urea nitrogen, creatinine, uric acid, atrial fibrillation, hypercardia, ejection fraction on echocardiography, ischemic cardiac disease, diabetes mellitus, hypertension and blood oxygen partial pressure (Matsubayashi et al., 1988).

Attempts have been made to predict directly the onset of dementia on the basis of the morphological and functional state of the brain as determined on CT, MRI and examination of cerebral circulation, in order to take prophylactic measures. Rogers et al. (1986) carried out a seven year prospective study from the aspect of cerebral circulation. They observed 181 healthy subjects aged 50–90 years (mean 70.6 years) divided into 88 persons with risk factors for cerebrovascular disorder and 93 without such factors; they noted the occurrence of senile dementia in six (3.3%) persons and vascular dementia in ten (5.5%) during the seven years. Although the six patients with senile dementia included only one individual who had risk factors, all ten patients with vascular dementia had some risk factor. Therefore, dementia occurred in 10 (11.4%) of 88 subjects who had risk factors for cerebral stroke. Eight (80%) of the ten patients with vascular dementia were heavy smokers, while the proportion of heavy smokers to total subjects was 18%.

Hypertension is an important risk factor for vascular dementia of Binswanger type, being found in about 80% of all patients with this condition. Among hypertensive patients with multiinfarct dementia, the prognosis was favorable in those who had a systolic pressure of 135–150mmHg, whereas neurological symptoms and cognitive function were aggravated in those who had a lower systolic pressure (Meyer et al., 1986). It has been reported that both casual systolic pressure and mean daily systolic pressure were lower in patients with multiinfarct dementia (114 ± 25mmHg and 121 ± 15mmHg, respectively) than in patients with multiple infarction without dementia (137 ± 18mmHg, 140 ± 17mmHg, respectively) (Matsubayashi *et al.*, 1988).

Although there are many problems regarding the treatment of hypertension in the elderly, it is true that excessive lowering can cause chronic hypoperfusion in the brain. The systolic pressure should be kept not lower than 130mmHg, usually at 140–150mmHg.

It has long been known that not only hypertension but also variations in blood pressure are important for the development of hypertensive vascular lesions. Although it is generally more common in the elderly than in the young that the blood pressure decreases during sleep, this is particularly conspicuous in patients with vascular dementia of Binswanger type.

Since the activity of autoregulation of cerebral blood vessels is decreased in elderly patients who have cerebrovascular lesions, hypoperfusion may occur with decreased blood pressure during sleep, possibly contributing to the manifestation of dementia.

Old hemorrhagic foci are found in the brain in many patients with vascular dementia of Binswanger type. Including hematoma and minor hemorrhage (ball hemorrhage), such findings are obtained in 73% of hypertensive patients and in 37% of normotensive patients. This suggests that there is some common basis for the development of hemorrhagic lesions and vascular lesions of the white matter.

Nonvalvular atrial fibrillation (NVAF) is common in the elderly and is an important cause of cerebral embolism. This condition is attracting attention mainly as a cause of relatively large cortical infarction and has also been cited as a risk factor for vascular dementia (Peterson *et al.*, 1987).

Vascular lesions

Sclerosis of arterioles in the cerebral parenchyma has been attracting attention as a type of vascular lesion characteristic of Binswanger's disease. Abnormalities in cerebrovascular permeability also have been found in patients with this disease.

Koyama *et al.* (1988) determined the CSF : serum ratios of albumin and immunoglobulin G in patients with Binswanger's disease or cortical infarction and in controls. The CSF : serum ratios of both were significantly higher in patients with Binswanger's disease.

Tohgi, Chiba & Sasaki (1988) examined plasminogen activator in the vascular wall. Focusing attention on each lacuna, they found that there are usually microvessels surrounded by spaces, which are further surrounded by degenerated nerve tissues.

These histological findings suggest the possibility that, in addition to ischemia, a certain substance exuding from the blood vessel induces cerebral disorder. When the activity of plasminogen activator at the lesion site was examined histochemically, using the fibrin slide method, it was found to be increased, centering on microvessels in the cerebral white matter, in patients with vascular dementia of Binswanger type in comparison with controls.

Yamanouchi *et al.* (1988) examined 22 autopsy cases and found that stenosis of the delta branch of the anterior, middle or posterior cerebral artery was predominant. In many cases, there were concomitant lesions of not only arterioles but also of relatively thick arteries in the areas from the brain base to the trunk of the white matter. Such arteriosclerosis in the cerebral trunk seems to be involved in circulatory disorder of the periphery.

Cerebral circulation

Like patients with AD, patients with vascular dementia show a decrease in CBF in proportion to the grade of cognitive function disorder. However, with regard to the distribution of local CBF, the decrease is patchy or limited to within the border zone in the frontal lobe or thalamus in many cases (Kitagawa et al., 1984; Loeb, Gandolfo & Bino, 1987). In contrast, in patients with AD, a decrease in blood flow in the parietal lobe is predominant. This discrepancy leads to the difference in clinical symptoms between vascular dementia and the dementia of AD.

Clinical features characteristic of vascular dementia of Binswanger type include decreased spontaneity, slow movement, articulation disorder, tiny step gait, affective incontinence and grasp reflex; most of which are frontal signs. A decreased blood flow in the frontal lobe can explain these clinical features. This is also consistent with the pathological finding that white matter lesions accompanied by lacunae are predominant in the frontal lobe (Ishii, Nishihara & Imamura, 1986).

SPET revealed a further decrease in blood flow in the deep gray matter of the cerebrum. This may reflect in part a decrease in blood flow in the basal ganglia, which are associated with a high incidence of lacunae in the putamen, or may indicate secondary hypofunction of the thalamus as a result of hypofunction of the frontal lobe.

When the regional CBF and cognitive function were examined at three monthly intervals in patients with vascular dementia, the range of variation in these parameters was wider than in normal elderly subjects or in patients with AD (Meyer et al., 1988). Vascular dementia is known to be characterized by wide variation in its symptoms. The large variation in CBF seems to explain this clinical feature of vascular dementia.

It should be noted that the mean CBF in the gray matter in both cerebral hemispheres decreases in parallel with the manifestation of symptoms in patients with AD, whereas such a decrease precedes the manifestation of symptoms by two years in those with vascular dementia. This indicates that decreased CBF plays an important role in the etiology of vascular dementia and suggests prophylactic measures may be possible.

Neurotransmitters

It has been demonstrated in an experimental model of cerebral ischemia that dopamine, DOPAC and homovanillic acid increase in the acute stage of cerebral ischemia (Nakamura, Iijima & Tsuji, 1988). A study of clinical cases in the acute stage of cerebral stroke has revealed that the blood levels of catecholamines, which are normal just after onset, increase to reach a peak after three days and decrease thereafter. The blood norepinephrine level increases again to show a second peak about 11–13 days later (Komatsumoto *et al.*, 1982a). The serum dopamine β–hydroxylase activity increases in an early stage after onset, followed by a decline lasting up to seven days. The poorer the prognosis, the more rapid was the decline (Komatsumoto, Gotoh & Shimazu, 1982b).

In a study of catecholamines and their metabolites in CSF after an episode of cerebral stroke, Meyer *et al.* (1973; 1974) found that the synthesis, release and reuptake of neuro-transmitters were disturbed.

However, transmitters in CSF are also reported to decrease in patients in the chronic stage. According to Hachinski *et al.* (1978), homovanillic acid in CSF decreases in cases of brain stem infarction, whereas its level varies widely according to the patient in cases of cortical infarction, showing no consistent trend. Nakamura & Kameyama (1986) carried out a detailed study of transmitters in CSF and obtained the following findings. The CSF level of homovanillic acid was lower in patients with multiple infarction (31.8 ± 18.9 ng/ml), particularly those who showed pathological crying and laughing (24 ± 19 ng/ml), than in controls (44.3 ± 16.4 ng/ml) (Nakamura &Kameyama, 1986). Among patients with multiple infarction, there was no difference in the CSF level of homo-vanillic acid between those who had dementia and those who did not.

Characteristic findings on diagnostic imaging

CT

Atrophy of the brain progresses with aging. Cognitive function deteriorates with pro-gression of brain atrophy when it exceeds the physiological limit. In cases of dementia, enlargement of the inferior horn of the lateral ventricle is conspicuous in addition to the atrophy of the overall brain. Whereas patients with AD show marked brain atrophy, various vascular lesions as well as brain atrophy are found in cases of vascular dementia.

CT findings are similar to those seen in neuropathologic studies, some patients show atrophy, various infarction foci and old hemorrhagic foci in the cortex, while others show small infarcts in the basal ganglia. There may be WMHI. With regard to the clinical course of vascular dementia, an obvious cerebral stroke is followed by dementia in some patients, while in other patients dementia develops with deteriorated activities of daily living against a background of hypertension and cardiac disease although there is no obvious cerebral stroke. In the latter group, the lacunar type and Binswanger type are common. Thus, CT findings of vascular dementia are extremely diverse, without showing any specificity.

MRI

High signal intensity areas begin to appear in T_2-weighted images with aging. This seems to be related to systemic arteriosclerotic changes. Enlargement of the cerebral sulcus centering on the frontal or temporal lobe and enlargement of the lateral ventricles are found in patients with vascular dementia and AD. Findings of cerebrovascular lesions are similar to CT findings.

After Press, Amaral & Squire (1989) reported the relation of atrophy of the hippocampus with amnesia, a similar relationship with dementia was pointed out. There is a report documenting that the hippocampus was reduced in volume by 40% in patients with AD in comparison with healthy persons, although it was not correlated with the severity of dementia (Seab et al., 1988). Atrophy of the hippocampus is a characteristic feature of both vascular dementia and AD.

Such atrophy is apparent in patients with vascular dementia, as shown in T_1-weighted images sectioned in parallel with the hippocampus.

High signal intensity in T_2-weighted images is found in the subcortical white matter, deep part white matter, basal ganglia and periventricular areas. The pathological implications of this include *état criblé*, atrophy owing to perimicrovascular demyelination, gliosis, thinning of myelin, demyelination, loss of axons, increased water content and lacunar infarction (Awad et al.,1986; Drayer, 1988; Kertesz, Polk & Carr, 1990).

PET

Since PET visualizes *in vivo* physiologic and biochemical information and allows its quantitative evaluation, it is extremely useful for evaluating the function of the human brain and for diagnosis of disease. PET is, however, disadvantageous in that it requires costly equipment (see Chapter 1(c)). In addition, the examination is time-consuming and requires a team of specialists in medicine, pharmacology, chemistry and engineering. Therefore, it is difficult to employ PET in routine examination.

In cases of vascular dementia and AD, the relationship between the severity of disease and CBF, oxygen removal or metabolic rate for oxygen has been investigated using the equilibrium method (Frackowiak et al., 1980; Frackowiak, Pozzilli & Legg, 1981). Available data show that, although the blood flow and metabolic rate for oxygen decrease in parallel with the severity of disease in both vascular dementia and AD, there is no detectable increase in oxygen removal, a characteristic finding of ischemia. A marked decrease in blood flow and oxygen metabolism is present in the temporal and parietal lobes (Meguro et al., 1990).

For determination of the cerebral metabolic rate for glucose, [^{18}F]FDG is used as a tracer. The radiolabel is transferred into the brain tissue as a glucose analog and phosphorylated there but does not serve as a substrate for phosphohexose isomerase. Therefore, it accumulates in tissue, not entering the subsequent glycolytic pathway.

Using this characteristic feature of $[^{18}F]FDG$, the cerebral metabolic rate for glucose is calculated according to the model proposed by Sokoloff et al. (1977).

In patients with vascular dementia, brain metabolism is decreased mainly in the transitional zone of the temporal, parietal and occipital lobes. Although metabolism in the frontal lobe may also be decreased, it is often accompanied by small infarcts in the basal ganglia and hence decreased metabolism in the basal ganglia. In addition, it is not rare that a decrease in metabolism owing to a distant effect (diaschisis) occurs contra-laterally in the cerebellum or cerebral hemisphere according to the site of infarction. As a result, glucose metabolism in vascular dementia mostly shows asymmetric diverse patterns reflecting regional abnormalities, although the basis of this is decreased metabolism in the transitional zone of the temporal, parietal and occipital lobes (Duara et al., 1989; Meguro et al., 1991) (Fig. 4.10 (facing p. 129)).

SPET

SPET differs from PET in that it uses gamma ray-emitting radioisotopes while PET uses positron-emitting radioisotopes. (See Chapter 1(c) for a full discussion of the relative merits of these techniques.)

Labeling compounds used for the measurement of the CBF with SPET include ^{123}I-IMP, ^{99m}Tc-HMPAO and xenon-133 (see Chapter 1(c)). Although ^{99m}Tc-labeled HMPAO is suitable for gamma encephalography, ^{123}I-IMP is most commonly used because it is a neutral substance and is incorporated at a high rate after intravenous injection, shows stable distribution, and because ^{123}I has a half-life of 13 hours it can be quantified. With regard to differences in sensitivity among labeling compounds, ^{123}I-IMP is reported to allow more accurate detection of lesions than does ^{99m}Tc-HMPAO (Gemmell et al., 1988), indicating that IMP would be the more useful compound.

The CBF in patients with AD has been determined by SPET in various facilities. The data thus obtained are basically the same as those yielded by PET. Namely, there is a bilateral decrease in blood flow in the transitional zone of the temporal, parietal and occipital lobes, with an additional decrease in blood flow in the frontal lobe in severe cases. The decrease in blood flow in the parietal lobe and other areas is more conspicuous in patients with AD than in patients with vascular dementia, and its relation with the severity of disease is clearer in the former type of dementia (Jagust, Budinger & Reed, 1987).

Conclusion

Characteristic findings of vascular dementia obtained by imaging procedures have been described in relation to the lesion site, giving an outline of what information CT, MRI,

SPET and PET can provide. It is expected that morphological information obtained by CT and MRI in combination with information of circulatory metabolism provided by SPET and PET will help more accurately to diagnose dementia.

The authors have previously reported that small silent infarcts were found on CT in 15% of healthy elderly volunteers (Kasahara *et al.*, 1990), indicating that they may result in depression, delirium, consciousness disturbance, hallucinations, delusions, dementia and convulsive seizures (Kasahara *et al.*, 1993). The subcortical high signal intensity areas observed on MRI were distributed along long noncollateral penetrating branches, representing the loss of cerebral parenchyma accompanied by an increase in tissue water content. This finding partly corresponds to a former concept of *état criblé*. Asymptomatic subcortical high signal intensity areas are attributable to cerebral hypoperfusion and arteriolar disease. As etiological factors, hypotension, cardiac disease, hypoxia, hypertension and aging have been cited. These high signal intensity areas are also observed in cases of vascular dementia. In the future, data obtained by imaging procedures may help clarify the pathology of vascular dementia and prevent the disease, in addition to helping in its diagnosis.

References

Awad, I.A., Johnson, P.C., Spetzler, R.E. & Hodak, J.A. (1986). Incidental subcortical lesions identified on magnetic resonance imaging in the elderly, II, Postmortem pathological correlations. *Stroke*, 17, 1090–1097.

Bennett, D.A., Wilson, R.S., Gilley, D.W. & Fox, J.H. (1990). Clinical diagnosis of Binswanger's disease. *Journal of Neurology, Neurosurgery and Psychiatry*, 53, 961–965.

Drayer, B.P. (1988). Imaging of the aging brain. Part I. Normal findings. *Radiology*, 166, 785–906.

Duara, R., Barker, W., Loewenstein, D., Pascal S. & Bowen B. (1989). Sensitivity and specificity of positron emission tomography and magnetic resonance imaging studies in Alzheimer's disease and multiinfarct dementia. *European Neurology*, 29 (Suppl. 3), 9–15.

Frackowiak, R.S., Lenzi, G.L., Jones, T. & Heather, J.D. (1980). Quantitative measurement of regional cerebral blood flow and oxygen metabolism in man using ^{15}O and positron emission tomography: theory, procedure, and normal values. *Journal of Computer Assisted Tomography*, 4, 727–736.

Frackowiak, R.S., Pozzilli, C. & Legg, N.J. (1981). Regional cerebral oxygen supply and utilization in dementia. A clinical and physiological study with oxygen-15 and positron tomography. *Brain*, 104, 753–778.

Gemmell, H.G., Sharp, P.F., Besson, J.A.O., Ebmeier, K.P. & Smith, F.W. (1988). A comparison of Tc-99m HM-PAO and I-123 IMP cerebral SPECT images in Alzheimer's disease and multiinfarct dementia. *European Journal of Nuclear Medicine*, 14, 463–466.

Hachinski, V.C., Iliff, L.D., Zihka, E. et al. (1975). Cerebral blood flow in dementia. *Archives of Neurology*, 32, 632–637.

Hachinski, V.C., Lassen, N.A., & Marshall, J. (1974). Multiinfarct dementia – a cause of mental deterioration in the elderly. *Lancet*, ii, 207–210.

Hachinski, V.C., Potter, P. & Merskey, H. (1987). Leukoaraiosis. *Archives of Neurology*, 44, 21–23.

Hachinski, V., Shibuya, M., Norris, J.W. et al. (1978). Cerebrospinal fluid homovanillic acid in cerebral infarction. *Journal of Neural Transmission* (Suppl.), 14, 45–50.

Hasegawa, K., Homma, A. & Imai, Y. (1986). An epidemiological study of age-related dementia in the community. *International Journal of Geriatric Psychiatry*, 1, 45–55.

Hasegawa, K., Homma, A., Imai, Y., Takubo, E., Kawamura, C. & Ichimura, H. (1982). Psychiatric investigation of the institutionalised elderly in Japan. *Japanese Journal of Gerontology*, 4, 89–110.

Hasegawa, K., Homma, A., Yook, M. et al. (1980). A gerontopsychiatric five-year follow-up on age-related dementia residing in the community. *Japanese Journal of Geriatrics*, 17, 630–638.

Hasegawa, K. & Imai, Y. (1991). Vascular dementia. In *Psychiatry in the Elderly*, ed. R. Jacoby & C. Oppenheimer, pp. 621–646. Oxford: Oxford University Press.

Ishii, N., Nishihara, Y. & Imamura, T. (1986). Why do frontal lobe symptoms predominate in vascular dementia with lacunes? *Neurology*, 36, 340–345.

Jagust, W.J., Budinger, T.F. & Reed, B.R. (1987). The diagnosis of dementia with single photon emission computed tomography. *Archives of Neurology*, 44, 258–262.

Kasahara, H., Tanno, M., Yamada, H. *et al.* (1993). MRI study of the brain in aged volunteers: T_2 high signal intensity lesions and high cortical function. *Japanese Journal of Geriatrics*, 30, 892–900.

Kasahara, H., Yamada, H., Endo, K. & Kobayashi, M. (1990). A follow-up study of computed tomography in the healthy Japanese elderly. In *Psychogeriatrics: Biomedical and Social Advances*, ed. K. Hasegawa & A. Homma, pp. 151–156. Tokyo: Excerpta Medica.

Kertesz, A., Polk, M. & Carr, T. (1990). Cognition and white matter changes on magnetic resonance imaging in dementia. *Archives of Neurology*, 47, 387–391.

Kitagawa, Y., Meyers, J.S., Tachibana, H., Mortel, K.F. & Rogers, R.L. (1984). CT-CBF correlations of cognitive deficits in multiinfarct dementia. *Stroke*, 15, 1000–1009.

Komatsumoto, M., Gotoh, F. & Araki, N. *et al.* (1982a). Catecholamine dynamics in cerebrovascular disease. *Nousocchu*, 4, 127–134.

Komatsumoto, M., Gotoh, F. & Shimazu, K. (1982b). Cerebrovascular disease and dopamine-ß-hydroxylase activity. *Nousocchu*, 4, 291–296.

Koyama, A., Atsumi, T., Kawakami, A. *et al.* (1988). Progressive subcortical vascular encephalopathy. *Nousocchu*, 10, 364–368.

Loeb, C., Gandolfo, C. & Bino, G. (1987). Correlations between the cerebral lesion and the demented state in patients with multiple infarcts. In *Cerebrovascular Disease 6*, ed. J.S. Meyer, H. Lechner, M. Reivich *et al.*, pp.00–00. Amsterdam: Excerpta Medica.

Matsubayashi, K., Matsumoto, M., Kawamoto, A. *et al.* (1988). Risk factors on cerebrovascular dementia. *Nichirouishi*, 25, 576–580.

Matsushita, M. (1984). Clinical or cerebrovascular dementia and its classification. *Geriatric Medicine*, 22, 1255.

Meguro, K., Doi, C., Ueda, M. *et al.* (1991). Decreased cerebral glucose metabolism associated with mental deterioration in multiinfarct dementia. *Neuroradiology*, 33, 305–309.

Meguro, K., Hatazawa, J., Yamaguchi, T. *et al.* (1990). Cerebral circulation and oxygen metabolism associated with subclinical periventricular hyperintensity as shown by magnetic resonance imaging. *Annals of Neurology*, 28, 378–383.

Meyer, J.S., Judd, B.W., Tawaklna, T., Rogers, R.I. & Mortel, K.F. (1986). Improved cognition after control of risk factors for multiinfarct dementia. *Journal of the American Medical Association*, 256, 2203–2209.

Meyer, J.S., Rogers, R.L., Judd, B.W. Mortel, K.F. & Sims. P. (1988). Cognition and cerebral blood flow fluctuate together in multiinfarct dementia. *Stroke*, 19, 163–169.

Meyer, J.S., Stoica, E., Pascu, I., Shimazu, K. & Hartmann, A. (1973). Catecholamine concentrations in CSF and plasma of patients with cerebral infarction and haemorrhage. *Brain*, 96, 277–288.

Meyer, J.S., Welch, K.M.A., Okamoto, S. & Shimazu, K. (1974). Disordered neurotransmitter function: demonstration by measurement of norepinephrine and 5–hydroxytryptamine in CSF of patients with recent cerebral infarction. *Brain*, 97, 655–664.

Nakamura, S., Iijima, T. & Tsuji, T. (1988). Cerebrovascular disease and neurotransmitters. *Shinkennosinpo*, 32, 259–270.

Nakamura, S. & Kameyama, M. (1986). Cerebral vascular disease and neurotransmitters. In *Internal Medicine*, ed. T. Oda, K. Hamaguchi, M. Homma *et al.*, pp. 45–48. Amsterdam: Elsevier Science.

Petersen, P., Madsen, E.B., Brun, B., Petersen, F., Gyldensted, C. & Boysen, G. (1987). Silent cerebral infarction in chronic atrial fibrillation. *Stroke*, 18, 1098–1100.

Press, G.A., Amaral, D.G. & Squire, L.R. (1989). Hippocampal abnormalities in amnesic patients revealed by high-resolution magnetic resonance imaging. *Nature*, 341, 54–57.

Rogers, R.L., Meyer, J.S., Mortel, K.F., Roderick, K., Mahurin, K.A. & Judd, B.W. (1986). Decreased cerebral blood flow precedes multiinfarct dementia, but follows senile dementia of Alzheimer's type. *Neurology*, 36, 1–6.

Seab, J.P., Jagust, W.J., Wong, S.T.S., Roos, M.S., Reed, B.R. & Budinger, T.F. (1988). Quantitative NMR measurements of hippocampal atrophy in Alzheimer's disease. *Magnetic Resonance Imaging*, 8, 200–208.

Sokoloff, L., Reivich, M., Kennedy, C. *et al.* (1977). The [^{14}C]deoxyglucose method for the measurement of local cerebral glucose utilization: theory, procedure, and normal values in the conscious and anesthetized albino rat. *Journal of Neurochemistry*, 28, 897–916.

Tohgi, H. (1983). Status lacunaris. *Brain and Nerve* (Tokyo), 35, 209–219.

Tohgi, H. (1984). Cerebrovascular dementia. *Rounenseii*, 43, 214–224.

Tohgi, H. (1988). Subcortical arteriosclerotic encephalopathy – so called Binswanger disease. *Medicina*, 25, 2202–2203.

Tohgi, H., Chiba, K. & Sasaki, K. (1988). Multiple infarctional dementia. *Shinkennoshinpo*, 32, 284–295.

Tohgi, H., Sasaki, K., Chiba, K. *et al.* (1985). Cerebrovascular dementia. *Nipponrinsho*, 43, 140–147.

Yamanouchi, H., Tomonaga, M., Yoshimura, M. *et al.* (1988). Pathological study on progressive subcortical vascular encephalopathy – Binswanger type. *Nousocchu*, 10, 404–411.

5   Other dementias

E. Jane Byrne and Stephen Simpson

Prevalence

It is difficult to estimate the frequency with which etiologies other than AD and cerebrovascular disease (vascular dementia) cause the dementia syndrome. There are problems in the uncritical acceptance of frequency estimates based on autopsy series (Byrne, Smith & Arie, 1991) as such samples are usually highly selected, and pathological diagnosis, until recently, has been less than reliable. Other factors such as the medical specialty from which the autopsy sample was derived have been shown to influence the frequency with which different etiologic causes for the dementia syndrome occur (Jellinger *et al.*, 1990). AD is more common in autopsy samples referred by psychiatrists, whereas Parkinson's disease is most frequently found in samples referred by geriatricians and physicians. Galasko *et al.* (1994), found that 12% of their sample of (predominantly) community residents with dementia who came to autopsy had non-AD, nonvascular dementia.

Epidemiological studies of dementia rarely consider differential diagnosis and those that do are largely limited to AD and vascular dementia (Hofman *et al.*, 1990). We do know the prevalence of some of the individual conditions that cause dementia and in some instances have information on how frequently this occurs. For example, the prevalence of Parkinson's disease is 2% of the population aged over 70 years (Schoenburg, 1987) and dementia arises in around 15–20% of these patients (Brown & Marsden, 1984; Mayeux *et al.*, 1988). Lishman (1987) lists 39 non-AD, nonvascular causes of dementia and McKeith (1994) lists 42 other dementias. It is likely that they constitute a greater proportion of clinical cases of the dementia syndrome than the 10% that are suggested on the basis of autopsy data (Brun, 1991; Galasko *et al.*, 1994).

This review is selective and includes the putatively common other dementias (dementia with cortical Lewy bodies, dementia of the frontal lobe type) and a selection of conditions that are either uncommon (Huntington's disease) or rather more common in elderly people than is generally assumed (multi-system atrophies and neuropsychiatric systemic lupus erythematosus). We have also chosen to include the controversial concept of 'the dementia of depression'.

Degenerative diseases

Parkinson's disease and dementia with cortical Lewy bodies

The prevalence of Parkinson's disease increases with age from 8 per 100 000 of those aged under 50 years to 2000 per 100 000 at age 70 years (Schoenburg, 1987). Increasing age in Parkinson's disease is also associated with increased likelihood of developing dementia. In patients with disease onset at an early age (onset at 20–39 years of age) dementia is very rare (Gibb & Lees, 1988), the prevalence rising with age to over 20% of those aged above 70 years (Godwin-Austen & Lowe, 1987; Mayeux *et al.*, 1988). It is likely that the dementia in Parkinson's disease is heterogeneous. In some patients AD coexists with Parkinson's disease (Yoshimura, 1988), whereas in others cortical Lewy bodies may be the cause (Lennox *et al.*, 1989) or cortical Lewy bodies and preclinical AD together may produce dementia (Quinn, Rossor & Marsden, 1986). It is also important to recognize that frontal lobe function is impaired in nondemented patients with Parkinson's disease (Lees & Smith, 1983; Taylor *et al.*, 1986). The heterogeneous nature of the pathology in Parkinson's disease with dementia probably explains the variation in findings in both structural and functional neuroimaging studies.

CT studies in Parkinson's disease have found few significant correlations between imaging parameters and cognitive function. Sroka *et al.* (1981) found that only patients with Parkinson's disease with dementia had abnormal CT scans, a finding largely accounted for by including atypical cases of Parkinson's disease (defined as patients with brain stem or cerebellar signs and an unusual course) in their series. Intellectual changes, which they described as organic mental impairment, were present in 68% of the atypical group, two-thirds of whom had ventricular enlargement.

In Parkinson's disease, Pearce *et al.* (1981) found no correlations between neuropsychologic tests (including the Wechsler Adult Intelligence Scale) and measurements of atrophy (including Evans' ratio). The degree of atrophy was only significantly greater in the 70–79 year age group with Parkinson's disease compared with controls.

MRI in Parkinson's disease has been similarly unrewarding in terms of identifying structural correlates of intellectual impairment. In a carefully matched study, Huber *et al.* (1990), found no difference in MRI findings (including ventricular measurement, surface area of the brain and signal intensity in the substantia nigra) in Parkinson's disease with dementia, Parkinson's disease without dementia and normal controls. This report contrasts with others who have found reduction in the width of the substantia nigra (pars compacta) in patients with Parkinson's disease compared with controls (Huber *et al.*, 1990; Pujol *et al.*, 1992).

MRI scans in patients with parkinsonism and intellectual change are useful in detecting causes other than Parkinson's disease for these symptoms (Drayer *et al.*, 1986) and one recent case report of postencephalitic parkinsonism showed reversible hyperintensity of the substantia nigra (pars compacta) on repeated MRI (Shen *et al.*, 1994).

Studies of Parkinson's disease using SPET have shown more significant abnormalities

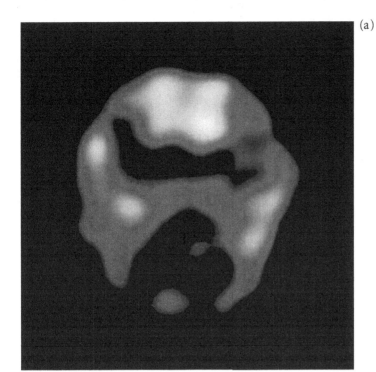

(a)

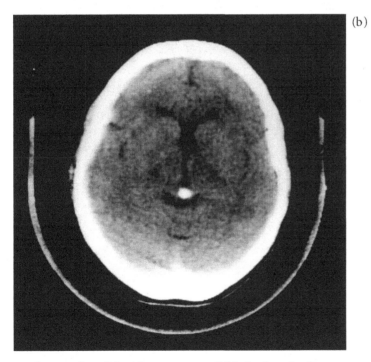

(b)

Figure 5.1 *A patient with treatment-resistant depression. This depressed patient with subcortical vascular disease was labeled 'treatment resistant'. (a) SPET scan shows hypofrontality caused by thalmic infarcts. (b) CT scan shows the thalmic infarcts.*

than seen in structural imaging (CT and MRI) studies. Goldenberg *et al.* (1989) studied neuropsychology and rCBF in 28 patients with Parkinson's disease without dementia, compared with normal controls. The neuropsychometry of Parkinson's disease showed frontal impairment but this correlated with rCBF in both frontal and parietal areas.

In a similar controlled study of nondemented Parkinson's disease patients, Jagust *et al.* (1992) found that those patients with Parkinson's disease who performed most poorly on neuropsychometry showed reduced rCBF in temporal lobes, with flow rates similar to AD patients. They found no difference between the groups in the frontal areas, but frontal lobe tests did correlate with rCBF reduction of frontal regions in Parkinson's disease. They also reported the important observation that depression scores predicted performance on frontal lobe neuropsychologic tests and dorsolateral frontal lobe perfusion. Others have noted this relationship between depression in Parkinson's disease and frontal hypometabolism (Mayberg *et al.*, 1990).

Sawada *et al.* (1992) compared rCBF in 13 demented Parkinson's disease patients with 13 age-matched nondemented Parkinson's disease 'controls'. They found that it was significantly reduced in the frontal and parietal areas bilaterally and the temporal area unilaterally in the demented Parkinson's disease patients compared with the controls. They also noted heterogeneity of rCBF in the demented group. In four patients, frontal hypoperfusion alone occurred, eight showed frontoparietal hypoperfusion and one had isolated parietal hypoperfusion. There are no published imaging findings in diffuse Lewy body disease (senile dementia of the Lewy body type).

Frontotemporal dementia

In 1994 the Lund and Manchester groups published their clinical and neuropathological criteria for frontotemporal dementia (FTD) (Lund & Manchester Groups, 1994). They described the clinical picture of behavioral and mood changes associated with early language disorder and incontinence that is associated with two main pathologic findings: frontal lobe degeneration and Pick-type degeneration (with or without Pick bodies) and occasionally with the amyotrophic form of motor neurone disease. There are a number of focal atrophic degenerative syndromes of non-AD type including progressive aphasia (Chawluk, *et al.*, 1986 Mesulam, 1982; Neary, Snowden & Mann, 1993) and posterior cortical atrophy (Benson, Davis & Snyder, 1988; Victoroff *et al.*, 1994). The latter is clinically and neuropathologically distinct from frontotemporal dementia, whereas the former may share clinical and histologic features (Neary *et al.*, 1993; Salmon *et al.*, 1994). Some patients with progressive aphasia, however, have been found at postmortem to have AD (Pogacar & Williams, 1984). Others have argued that this condition is and should remain Pick's disease (Hodges, 1994).

There are no published reports of the clinical prevalence of frontotemporal dementia. In some autopsy studies it is common (Brun, 1991) and in one consecutive series of SPET scans in 98 demented patients, reduced rCBF in frontotemporal areas was found in ten patients (Launes *et al.*, 1991). In histopathologically confirmed cases of Pick's disease, rCBF is reduced in frontotemporal areas (Ingvar et al., 1978; Risberg, 1987) and PET studies show frontal hypometabolism (Brion et al., 1988; Kamo et al., 1987).

In progressive aphasia, SPET studies have shown reduced rCBF in frontotemporal areas in patients with cognitive impairment and dominant temporal lobe reduction in rCBF in patients with aphasia alone (Neary et al., 1993). PET scans show a similar pattern of hypometabolism. In those with aphasia alone, the dominant temporal lobe (usually left) is affected (Chawluk et al., 1986; Tyrell et al., 1990) and in those with aphasia but who are relatively impaired in higher cortical function, the metabolic deficits are more widespread (Tyrell et al., 1990).

In patients with a clinical diagnosis of frontotemporal dementia, CT scan may show frontal and/or temporal lobe atrophy (Starkstein et al., 1994). SPET scans show reduced rCBF in anterior cerebral hemispheres (Neary et al., 1988) especially in frontotemporal areas and the basal ganglia (Starkstein et al., 1994). Salmon et al. (1994) found frontotemporal hypometabolism on PET scans of two patients with a histological diagnosis of Pick's disease, one of whom presented with progressive aphasia.

Huntington's disease

The reported prevalence of Huntington's disease varies widely (Chiu, 1994), from 0.11 per 100 000 in Japan (Kanazawa, 1983) to 700 per 100 000 in Venezuela (Avila-Giron, 1973). James et al. (1994) have studied late-onset Huntington's disease in south Wales, which has a point prevalence of 6.2 per 100 000 (86 affected individuals). Using the south Wales Huntington's disease register established in 1975, they identified 33 individuals whose onset of disease was later than 60 years (range 60–77 years, median 65 years). This study suggests that late-onset Huntington's disease is not uncommon but the diagnosis is not often made in life.

In Huntington's disease, a CT scan may show bilateral caudate atrophy (Kuhl et al. 1982; Myers et al., 1985; Terrence, Delaney & Alberts, 1977) that correlates with the extent of impaired cognitive function (Starkstein et al., 1988; Tanahashi et al., 1985). Various changes have been found on MRI scans, including reduced volumes of thalamus and medial temporal structures (Jernigan et al., 1991), increased bicaudate diameter and hyperintense signals in T_2-weighted images in the striatum (Olivia et al., 1993). Some of these differences may be explained by the appearance of striatal change in the akinetic-rigid variant of Huntington's disease (Olivia et al., 1993; Savoirdo et al., 1991). One early study found no changes on MRI scan or SPET (Sharp et al., 1986), but later SPET studies in Huntington's disease have shown reduced rCBF in the caudate nucleus (Gemmell et al., 1989; Kuhl et al., 1982; Reid et al., 1988; Smith et al., 1988), in parietal cortex (Goldberg et al., 1990) and in numerous other cortical regions (Tanahashi et al., 1985). The magnitude of these changes may be greater than that predicted by structural imaging (Smith et al., 1988).

Both SPET (Ichise et al., 1993; Tanahashi et al., 1985) and PET (Mazziota et al., 1987) have been used to study at-risk subjects. Caudate glucose metabolism is reduced in some at-risk subjects (Mazziota et al., 1987) and both [123I]–iodobenzamide (IBZM) dopamine D_2 receptor striatum-to-frontal cortex ratio and perfusion ratios (HMPAO) were reduced in some at-risk subjects (Ichise et al., 1993), whereas no changes in rCBF were found in at risk individuals by Tanahashi et al. (1985).

Progressive supranuclear palsy (the Steele–Richardson–Olszewski syndrome)

No information on the prevalence of progressive supranuclear palsy is available. Imaging studies are of interest in view of the disease as one of the causes of subcortical dementia (Albert, Feldman & Willis, 1974; Tolosa & Alvarez, 1992), a controversial concept.

Several PET studies of patients with progressive supranuclear palsy have shown frontal hypometabolism (Blin et al., 1990; D'Atona et al., 1985; Leenders, Frackowiak & Lees, 1988). Blin et al. studied 41 patients and found that frontal lobe tests (including Wisconsin card sorting test and verbal fluency) significantly correlated with frontal hypometabolism and that a high parkinsonian score correlated with low caudate and thalamic metabolism values. Striatal dopamine D_2 receptors have been shown to be reduced in progressive supranuclear palsy by both SPET (Chabriat et al., 1992) and PET (Baron et al., 1984).

Multiple system atrophy

Multiple system atrophy has three main clinical presentations: olivopontocerebellar atrophy, striatonigral degeneration and the Shy–Drager syndrome. These syndromes share a common histological feature: glial cytoplasmic inclusions (Lantos & Papp, 1994). The diagnosis is often missed in life, but Quinn (1989) has proposed clinical criteria that may assist. Neither the prevalence of the disorder nor the frequency with which it is associated with dementia is known. In patients with olivopontocerebellar atrophy cognitive function is usually only mildly impaired (Berent et al., 1990; Kish et al., 1988). MRI studies suggest both pontocerebellar and putamenal hyperintensities on T_2-weighted images, irrespective of the clinical classification (Schulz et al., 1994). Striatal dopamine (D_2) receptor loss has been shown with [123]IBZM – SPET (Schulz et al., 1994).

Infection, autoimmune and other disorders

Normal pressure hydrocephalus (communicating hydrocephalus)

The true prevalence of normal pressure hydrocephalus is unknown but it is probably rare in the very old. In (albeit highly selected) clinical investigations of dementia, it is common, accounting for between 10 and 20% of cases (Byrne, 1987).

In patients with normal pressure hydrocephalus, CT clearly shows ventricular enlargement, with rounding of the anterior horns of the lateral ventricles together with periventricular radiolucency (Black, 1980; Mori et al., 1977; Vanneste et al., 1993). In patients with concomitant sulcal widening, opinion has been divided as to whether this, in itself, is a predictor of poor outcome following shunt operations (Greenberg, Shenkin & Adam, 1977; Katzman, 1977).

Vanneste et al. (1993) have combined clinical and CT data to predict the clinical outcome for shunt operations. Their criteria for shunt-responsive normal pressure hydrocephalus are clinical – predominance of gait disturbances, a mild-to-moderate mental impairment and absence of another cause for the symptoms – and CT – rounded frontal horns, at least moderate ventriculomegaly, absence of moderate or severe cortical atrophy and absence of moderate or severe WMHI. These criteria have a sensitivity of 0.54, specificity of 0.84 and predictive accuracy of 0.75. Golomb et al. (1994) studied with MRI a group of sixteen very old patients (age range 70–87) who were thought to have possible normal pressure hydrocephalus. They examined the correlation between MMSE (Folstein, Folstein & McHugh, 1975) scores and MRI measures of hippocampal size and CSF volume. They found that hippocampal size strongly correlated with MMSE scores whereas CSF volume did not. They suggest that some of their patients may have AD and that an MRI scan may assist in the investigation of normal pressure hydrocephalus.

Two PET studies (Jagust, Friedland & Budinger, 1985; Salmon et al., 1994) have also addressed this issue. They both found that patients with normal pressure hydrocephalus had more global metabolic abnormalities than the largely parietotemporal abnormalities seen in AD.

Cognitive change and alcohol abuse

Alcohol abuse in elderly people is not uncommon. Community surveys report prevalence rates of between 0.01% and 3.6% in men and 3.2% in women (Iliffe et al., 1991; Livingston & King, 1993).

In a comprehensive review of alcoholism in old people, Beresford & Gordis (1992) commented that prevalence rates are dependent on the mode of case identification and that estimates based on the quantity of alcohol consumed may underestimate the size of the problem among the elderly (who are less tolerant of alcohol). There is also a continuing debate as to whether alcohol abuse leads to dementia or whether the cognitive changes are consistent with the Wernicke–Korsakoff syndrome (Joyce, 1994; Lishman, 1990).

Few imaging studies of alcohol abuse include many very old people. CT scans show varying degrees of cerebral atrophy, which is greater than that found in age-matched controls (Byrne, 1982) and may be partially reversible (Carlen & Wilkinson, 1980; Jacobson, 1986).

SPET scan studies in chronic alcoholism suggest a reduction in rCBF in the frontal lobe (Hunter et al., 1989; Nicolas et al., 1993). Nicolas et al. (1993) found a correlation between neuropsychological tests of frontal function and rCBF in the frontal lobes ($n =$ 40, mean age 44 ± 10 years, range 26–63 years), but these were independent of atrophy on CT scan.

Vitamin B_{12} deficiency

Vitamin B_{12} deficiency is not uncommon in elderly people. However, it is rare as the sole etiological cause of the dementia syndrome (Byrne, 1987; Hector & Burton, 1988). Probably because of this there are no imaging studies in B_{12} 'dementia' in elderly people. One early study of CBF in pernicious anemia included four people aged more than 65 years. It found increased CBF and reduced cerebral glucose metabolism in subjects versus controls (Scheinberg, 1951).

Creutzfeldt–Jakob disease

Because Creutzfeldt–Jakob disease is rare, most prevalence estimates are in terms of annual mortality rates, with values of 0.26 per million in the USA (Masters *et al.*, 1979) 0.31 per million in Chile (Galvez, Masters & Gajdusek, 1980) and 0.49 per million in the UK (Cousens *et al.*, 1990). CT scan may be normal or may show varying degrees of atrophy or focal hypodense lesions (Barboriak, Provenzale & Boyko, 1994; Chapman *et al.*, 1993; Galvez & Cartier, 1984). MRI scans almost always show hyperintense signal abnormalities in the basal ganglia on T_2-weighted images (Barboriak *et al.*, 1994; Gertz, Henks & Cervos-Navarro, 1988; Hilton *et al.*, 1991), with occasional reports of cortical lesions (Gertz *et al.*, 1988).

PET scans show hypometabolism in various cortical regions of people with Creutzfeldt–Jakob disease. All three pathologically proven cases reported by Salmon *et al.*, (1994) had different patterns of cortical hypometabolism: one temporoparietal, one frontal and temporoparietal and one diffuse cortical.

Neuropsychiatric systemic lupus erythematosus

Recent epidemiologic studies suggest that neuropsychiatric systemic lupus erythomatosus (SLE) in the elderly is not as uncommon as previously reported; two studies (Gudmunsson & Steinsson, 1990; Jonsson *et al.*, 1990) found the peak prevalence to be in the 50–74 and 55–74 age groups, respectively.

The condition may account for 1–2% of all elderly psychiatric admissions (Dennis *et al.*, 1992; Hopkinson, Bendall & Powell, 1992). Dennis (1994) has reviewed the clinical and immunological findings in neuropsychiatric SLE in the elderly and stresses the inadequacy of revised American Rheumatism Association criteria for SLE (Tan *et al.*, 1982) in this age group.

CT has proved relatively insensitive in neuropsychiatric SLE, at times failing to show focal abnormalities even in patients with clear focal signs (Carette *et al.*, 1982; Kaell *et al.*, 1986). Mild cerebral atrophy and occasional focal vascular lesions are reported by others (Dennis *et al.*, 1992).

MRI scans are much more sensitive, revealing both diffuse and focal changes. Diffuse changes are manifest on MRI by high signal intensity on spin density and T_2-weighted images especially in the subcortical white matter of the occipital lobes, and less frequently, in parietal and frontal lobes (Bell *et al.*, 1991; Sibbitt *et al.*, 1989). These changes are reversed with treatment. Bell *et al.* (1991) found that patients with focal neuropsychiatric SLE were older than those with diffuse disease and that focal lesions were in regions corresponding to the territory of a major cerebral artery.

The dementia of depression and 'pseudodementia'

The dementia spectrum of depression has been a subject of contention since the early 1950s. Traditional views hold that the elderly person with depression may be cognitively normal, or have the reversible dementia of depression (DOD), as described by the Americans (Folstein & McHugh, 1978; Rabins, 1983); this is termed 'pseudodementia' by the British. Baldwin (1991) has identified at least three ways in which the term 'pseudodementia' is applied, and neuropsychologists have found that in so-called pseudodementia recovery from cognitive deficits is frequently incomplete (Sahakian, 1991).

The term pseudodementia was first used in 1952 by Madden *et al.* to encompass all causes of reversible dementia. In 1983 McAllister noted that patients with depressive pseudodementia were significantly older than patients with pseudodementia owing to other psychiatric illness. The US–UK diagnostic study (Duckworth & Ross, 1975) demonstrated that elderly patients were more likely to be diagnosed as demented by the Americans and as depressed by the British. Kendell (1974) stressed the importance of accurate diagnosis of these individuals by showing that patients initially diagnosed as having dementia were often rediagnosed as depressed at follow-up. A simplified modern definition of pseudodementia has been used by Pearlson, Rabins & Burns (1991) to describe cases of DSM–IIIR depression with MMSE scores below 24 which increase to above 27 after treatment. (Patients must be judged to be accessible, mentally alert and performing with full effort during neuropsychologic evaluation.)

Continuum of depression and dementia

It may be more useful to look upon some cases of depression as being on a continuum with dementia. There is evidence from CT neuroimaging research that depression with onset in later life has more in common with a dementing disorder than depression with a younger age of onset (Alexopoulos, Young & Shindledecker, 1992). Bieliauskas (1993) stated that in pseudodementia the emotional influence on cognitive function is overrated and that disease-based factors are more important. Neuroimaging with CT has supported this notion. Pearlson *et al.* (1991) analyzed CT attenuation values in centrum semiovale gray and white matter. Amongst their patients there were 14 cases of DOD (or pseudodementia). They found abnormalities on a continuum that was progressively more apparent from normals to depressed cognitively normal to DOD, and then to dementia. Abas, Sahakian & Levy (1990) have approached the problem from a neuropsychologic angle and combined this with CT changes. Neuropsychology applied to depressed people not thought to be cognitively impaired reveals a high rate of abnormalities. Thirty percent remained impaired after treatment of depression and these cases were associated with larger lateral ventricles.

The variability in both cognitive and depressive features of some cases of late-life depression may be evidence of a spectrum disorder of depression– dementia (especially subcortical vascular dementia).

Findings in late-life depression

The anatomical MRI findings in cognitively normal depressed elderly are well established (see Chapter 7 and Baldwin, 1993); there is a higher prevalence of subcortical gray and white matter abnormalities than in normal old people. These abnormalities are probably the result of vascular changes but their significance in relation to both pseudodementia and reversibility of depression remains to be established.

In patients referred for electroconvulsive therapy, these MRI abnormalities were more severe and included lacunar infarcts in subcortical gray matter (Coffey *et al.*, 1990). The finding of a weak association between normal or adequate subcortical rCBF perfusion (SPET) and favorable 6–18 month outcome for depression (Curran *et al.*, 1993) would support the notion that normal or adequate subcortical functioning is an important factor in predicting the reversibility of depression. In Manchester, a series of patients have been studied who have developed an irreversible depressive character change as a result of mild subcortical vascular disease. The reduced subcortical frontal lobe functioning was confirmed with neuropsychology and SPET and resulted from subcortical cerebrovascular disease, as shown in the patient with thalamic dementia (Fig. 5.1).

Reversibility of depression in the elderly

Research into dementia with depression area has focused largely on cerebrovascular disease, and indeed one of the items in Hachinski's ischemic scale for vascular dementia includes the presence of depression (Hachinski, Lassen & Marshall, 1974). Starkstein, Robinson & Price (1987) used CT in multiinfarct dementia to show that there was a strong correlation between depression and proximity of stroke lesions (both cortical and subcortical) to the left frontal pole. It is likely that subcortical vascular disease is not only a risk factor for developing depressive illness but, like other dementias, it can confound the clinical assessment of depression (Katona, 1993).

References

Abas, M.A., Sahakian, B.J. & Levy, R. (1990). Neuropsychological deficits and CT changes in elderly depressives. *Psychological Medicine*, 20, 507–520.

Albert M.L., Feldman, R.G. & Willis, A.L. (1974). The subcortical dementia of progressive supranuclear palsy. *Journal of Neurology, Neurosurgery and Psychiatry*, 37 121–130.

Alexopoulos, G.S., Young, R.C. & Shindledecker, R.D. (1992). Brain computed tomography findings in geriatric depression and primary degenerative dementia. *Biological Psychiatry*, 31, 591–599.

Avila-Giron, R. (1973). Medical and social aspect of Huntington's chorea in the state of Lulia, Venezuela. *Advances in Neurology*, 1, 261–266.

Baldwin, R. (1991). Depressive illness. In *Psychiatry in the Elderly*, ed. R. Jacoby & C. Oppenheimer, pp. 676–719. Oxford: Oxford Medical Publications.

Baldwin, R. (1993). Late life depression and structural brain changes: a review of recent magnetic resonance imaging research. *International Journal of Geriatric Psychiatry*, 8, 115–123.

Barboriak, D.P., Provenzale, J.M. & Boyko O.B. (1994). MR diagnosis of Creutzfeldt–Jakob disease: significance of high signal intensity of basal ganglia. *American Journal of Roentgenology*, 162, 137–140.

Baron, J.C., Maziere, B., Loc'H, C., Sgouropoulos, P., Bonnet, A.M. & Agid, Y. (1984). Progressive supranuclear palsy: loss of striatal dopamine receptors demonstrated in vivo by position emission tomography. *Lancet*, i, 1163–1164.

Bell, C.L., Partington, C., Robbins, M., Graziano, F., Tski, P. & Korngath, S. (1991). Magnetic resonance imaging of central nervous system lesions in patients with lupus erythematosus. *Arthritis and Rheumatism*, 34, 432–441.

Benson, F., Davis, R.J. & Snyder, B.D. (1988). Posterior cortical atrophy. *Archives of Neurology*, 45, 789–793.

Berent, S., Giordani, B., Gilman, S. et al. (1990). Neuropsychological changes in olivopontocerebellar atrophy. *Archives of Neurology*, 47, 997–1001.

Beresford, T.P. & Gordis, E. (1992). Alcoholism and the elderly patient. In *Oxford Text Book of Geriatric Medicine*, ed. J.G. Evans & T.F. Williams, pp. 639–645. Oxford: Oxford Medical Publications.

Bieliauskas, L.A. (1993). Depressed or not depressed? *Journal of Clinical and Experimental Neuropsychology*, 15, 119–134.

Black, P.M. (1980). Idiopathic normal-pressure hydrocephalus. *Journal of Neurosurgery*, 52, 371–377.

Blin, J., Baron, J.C., Dubois, B. et al. (1990). Positron emission tomography study in progressive supranuclear palsy. Brain hypometabolic pattern and clinicometabolic correlations. *Archives of Neurology*, 47, 747–752.

Brion, S., Mikol, J., Bavon, J.C., Plas, J., Guerin, R. & Bessac, J.F. (1988). Neuroimaging in Pick's disease with histological data. *Journal of Neurology*, 235 (Suppl. 1), 15–22.

Brown, R.G. & Marsden, C.D. (1984). How common is dementia in Parkinson's disease? *Lancet*, ii, 1262–1265.

Brun, A. (1991). Structural and topographic aspects of degenerative dementia: diagnostic considerations. *International Journal of Psychogeriatrics*, 3, 75–83.

Byrne, E.J. (1982). The early detection of brain damage in alcoholics. *Australian and New Zealand Journal of Psychiatry*, 16, 211–214.

Byrne, E.J. (1987). Reversible dementia. *International Journal of Geriatric Psychiatry*, 2, 73–81.

Byrne, E.J., Smith, C.W. & Arie, T. (1991). The diagnosis of dementia. A, clinical and pathological criteria: a review of the literature. *International Journal of Geriatric Psychiatry*, 6, 199–208.

Carette, S., Urowtz, M., Grosman, H. & St Louis, E.L. (1982). Cranial computerised tomography in systemic lupus erythematosus. *Journal of Rheumatology*, 9, 855–859.

Carlen, P.L. & Wilkinson, D.A. (1980). Alcoholic brain damage and reversible deficits. *Acta Psychiatrica Scandinavica*, 62 (Suppl. 286), 103–118.

Chabriat, H., Levasseur, M., Vidalhet, M. et al. (1992). In vivo SPECT imaging of D_2 receptor with iodine-iodolisuride: results in supranuclear palsy. *Journal of Nuclear Medicine*, 33, 1481–1485.

Chapman, J., Brown, P., Goldforb, L.G., Amazoroff, A., Gajdusek, D.C. & Korczyn, A.D. (1993). Clinical heterogeneity and unusual presentations of Creutzfeldt–Jakob disease in Jewish patients with the PRNP codon 200 mutation. *Journal of Neurology, Neurosurgery and Psychiatry*, 56, 1109–1112.

Chawluk, J.B., Mesulum, M.-M., Hurtig, H. et al. (1986).

Slowly progressive aphasia without generalised dementia: studies with positron emission tomography. *Annals of Neurology*, 19, 68–74.

Chiu, E. (1994). Huntington's disease. In *Dementia*, ed. A. Burns & R. Levy, pp. 735–762. London: Chapman & Hall.

Coffey, C.E., Figiel, G.S., Djang, W.T. & Wiener, R.D. (1990). Subcortical hyperintensities on magnetic resonance imaging: a comparison of normal and depressed elderly subjects. *American Journal of Psychiatry*, 147, 187–189.

Cousens, S.N., Harries-Jones, R., Knight, R., Will, R.G., Smith, P.G. & Matthews, W.B. (1990). Geographical distribution of cases of Creutzfeldt–Jakob disease in England and Wales 1970–84. *Journal of Neurology, Neurosurgery and Psychiatry*, 53, 459–465.

Curran, S.M., Murray, C.M., van Beck, M. *et al.* (1993). A single photon emission tomography study of regional brain function in elderly patients with major depression and with Alzheimer-type dementia. *British Journal of Psychiatry*, 163, 155–165.

D'Atona, R., Baron, J.C., Samson, Y. *et al.* (1985). Subcortical dementia. Frontal cortex hypometabolism detected by positron emission tomography in patients with progressive supranuclear palsy. *Brain*, 108, 785–799.

Dennis, M. (1994). Neuropsychiatric lupus erythematosus and the elderly. *International Journal of Geriatric Psychiatry*, 9, 97–106.

Dennis, M.S., Byrne, E.J., Hopkinson, N. & Bendall, P. (1992). Neuropsychiatric lupus erythematosus in elderly people: a case series. *Journal of Neurology, Neurosurgery and Psychiatry*, 55, 1157–1161.

Drayer, B.P., Olanow, W., Burger, P., Johnson, G.A., Herfkens, R. & Reiderer, S. (1986). Parkinson plus syndrome: diagnosis using high-field MR imaging of brain iron. *Radiology*, 159, 493–498.

Duckworth, G.S. & Ross, H. (1975). Diagnostic differences in psychogeriatric patients: Toronto, New York, London England. *Canadian Medical Association Journal*, 112, 847–851.

Folstein, M.F., Folstein, S.E. & McHugh, P.R. (1975). Mini mental state: a practical method for grading the psychiatric state of patients for the physician. *Journal of Psychiatric Research*, 12, 189–198.

Folstein, M.F. & McHugh, P.R. (1978). Dementia syndrome of depression. In *Alzheimer's Disease: Senile Dementia and Related Disorders*, ed. R. Katzman, R.D. Terry & K.L. Bick. New York: Raven Press.

Galasko, D., Hansen, L.A., Katzman, R. *et al.* (1994). Clinical-neuropathological correlations in Alzheimer's disease and related dementias. *Archives of Neurology*, 51, 888–895.

Galvez, S. & Cartier, L. (1984). Computer tomography findings in 15 cases of Creutzfeldt–Jakob disease with histological verification. *Journal of Neurology, Neurosurgery and Psychiatry*, 47, 1244–1246.

Galvez, S., Masters, C. & Gajdusek, D.C. (1980). Descriptive epidemiology of Creutzfeldt–Jakob disease in Chile. *Archives of Neurology*, 37, 11–14.

Gemmell, H., Sharp, P., Smith, E. *et al.* (1989). Cerebral blood flow measured by SPECT as a diagnostic tool in the study of dementia. *Psychiatry Research*, 29, 327–329.

Gertz, H.J., Henks, H. & Cervos-Navarro, J.C. (1988). Creutzfeldt–Jakob disease: significance of high signal intensity of basal ganglia. *American Journal of Radiology*, 162, 137–140.

Gibb, W.R.G. & Lees, A.J. (1988). The relevance of the Lewy body to the pathogenesis of idiopathic Parkinson's disease. *Journal of Neurology, Neurosurgery and Psychiatry*, 51, 745–752.

Godwin-Austen, R.B. & Lowe, J.S. (1987). Two types of Parkinson's disease. In *Current Problems in Neurology, Vol. 6: Parkinson's Disease – Clinical and Experimental Advances*, ed. F.C. Rose, pp. 79–82. London: Libbey.

Goldberg, T.E., Bergman, K.F., Mohr, E. & Weinberger, D.R. (1990). Regional cerebral blood flow and cognitive function in Huntington's disease and schizophrenia. *Archives of Neurology*, 47, 418–422.

Goldenberg, G., Podreka, I., Müller, C. & Deecke, L. (1989). The relationship between cognitive deficits and frontal lobe function in patients with Parkinson's disease: an emission computerised tomography study. *Behavioural Neurology*, 2, 79–87.

Golomb, J., de Leon, M.J., George, A.E. *et al.* (1994). Hippocampal atrophy correlates with severe cognitive impairment in elderly patients with suspected normal pressure hydrocephalus. *Journal of Neurology, Neurosurgery and Psychiatry*, 57, 590–593.

Greenberg, J.O., Shenkin, H.A. & Adam, R. (1977). Idiopathic normal pressure hydrocephalus. *Journal of Neurology, Neurosurgery and Psychiatry*, 40, 336–341.

Gudmunsson, S. & Steinsson, K. (1990). Systemic lupus erythematosus in Iceland 1975 through 1984. A nationwide epidemiological study. *Journal of Rheumatism*, 7, 1162–1167.

Hachinski, V.C., Lassen, N.A. & Marshall, J. (1974). Multi-infarct dementia. *Lancet*, ii, 207–210.

Hector, M. & Burton, J.R. (1988). What are the psychiatric manifestations of vitamin B_{12} deficiency. *Journal of American Geriatrics Society*, 36, 1105–1112.

Hilton, W.J., Atlas, S.W., Lavi, E. & Mollman, J.E. (1991). Magnetic resonance imaging of Creutzfeldt–Jakob disease. *Annals of Neurology*, 29, 438–440.

Hodges, R.J. (1994). Pick's disease. In *Dementia*, ed. A. Burns & R. Levy, pp. 739–752. London: Chapman & Hall.

Hofman, A., Rocca, W.A. & Brayne, C. *et al.* (1990). The prevalence of dementia in Europe: a collaborative study of 1980–1990 findings. *International Journal of Epidemiology*, 20, 736–748.

Hopkinson, N.D., Bendall, P. & Powell, R.J. (1992). Screening of acute psychiatric admissions for previously undiagnosed systemic lupus erythematosus. *British Journal of Psychiatry*, 161, 107–109.

Huber, S.J., Chakeves, D.W., Paulson, G.W. & Khanna, R. (1990). Magnetic resonance imaging in Parkinson's disease. *Archives of Neurology*, 47, 435–437.

Hunter, R., McLuskie, R. & Wyper, D. *et al.* (1989). The pattern of function-related regional cerebral blood flow investigated by single photon emission tomography with 99m Tc-HMPAO in patients with presenile Alzheimer's disease and Korsakoff's psychosis. *Psychological Medicine*, 19, 847–855.

Ichise, M., Totama, H., Farnazzari, L., Ballenger, J.R & Kirsh, J.C. (1993). Iodine-123-IBZM dopamine D_2 receptor and technetium-99m-HMPAO brain perfusion and SPECT in the evaluation of patients with and subjects at risk for Huntington's disease. *Journal of Nuclear Medicine*, 34, 1274–1281.

Iliffe, S., Haines, A. & Booroof, A. *et al.* (1991). Alcohol consumption by elderly people: a general practice survey. *Age and Ageing*, 20, 120–123.

Ingvar, D.H., Brun, A., Hagberg, B. & Gustafson, L. (1978). Regional cerebral blood flow in the dominant hemisphere in confirmed cases of Alzheimer's disease, Pick's disease and multiinfarct dementia: relationships to clinical symptomatology and neuropathological findings. In *Alzheimer's Disease: Senile Dementia and Related Disorders*, ed. R. Cosmin, R.D. Terry & K.L. Bick, pp. 203–210. New York: Raven Press.

Jacobson, R.R. (1986). The contribution of sex and drinking history to the CT brainscan changes in alcoholics. *Psychological Medicine*, 16, 547–559.

Jagust, W.J., Friedland, R.P. & Budinger, T. (1985). Positron emission tomography with [^{18}F] fluorodeoxyglucose differentiates normal pressure hydrocephalus from Alzheimer type dementia. *Journal of Neurology, Neurosurgery and Psychiatry*, 48, 1091–1096.

Jagust, W.J., Reed, B.R., Martin, E.M., Eberling, J.L. & Nelson-Abbott, R.A. (1992). Cognitive function and regional cerebral blood flow in Parkinson's disease. *Brain*, 115 521–537.

James, C.M., Houlihan, G.D., Snell, R.G., Cheadle, J.P. & Harper, D.S. (1994). Late-onset Huntington's disease: a clinical and molecular study. *Age and Ageing*, 23, 445–448.

Jellinger, K., Danielczyk, W., Fischer, P. & Gabriel, E. (1990). Clinicopathological analysis of dementia disorders in the elderly. *Journal of Neurological Sciences*, 95, 239–258.

Jernigan, T.L., Salmon, D.P., Butters, N. & Hesselink, J.R. (1991). Cerebral structures on MRI, part II: specific changes in Alzheimer's disease and Huntington's disease. *Biological Psychiatry*, 29, 68–81.

Jonsson, H., Nived, O., Sturfelt, G. *et al.* (1990). Estimating the incidence of systemic lupus erythematosus in a defined population using multiple sources of retrieval. *British Journal of Rheumatism*, 29, 185–188.

Joyce, E.M. (1994). Dementia associated with alcohol. In *Dementia*, ed. A. Burns & R. Levy, pp. 681–693. London: Chapman & Hall.

Kaell, A.T., Shetty, M., & Lee, B.C.P. *et al.* (1986). The diversity of neurological events in systemic lupus erythematosus. *Archives of Neurology*, 43, 273–276.

Kamo, H., McGeer, P.L. & Harrop, R. *et al.* (1987). Positron emission tomography and histopathology in Pick's disease. *Neurology*, 37, 439–445.

Kanazawa, I. (1983). *Prevalence Rate of Huntington's Disease in Ibakari Prefecture. Annual Report of Research Committee of CNS Degenerative Disease*, pp. 151–156. Tokyo: Ministry of Health and Welfare, Japan.

Katona, C. (1993). The measurement of depression in old age. *Nordic Journal of Psychiatry*, 47 (Suppl. 28), 53–58.

Katzman, R. (1977). Normal pressure hydrocephalus. In *Dementia*, ed. C.E. Wells, pp. 69–92. Philadelphia, PA: F.A. Davies.

Kendell, R.E. (1974). The stability of psychiatric diagnoses. *British Journal of Psychiatry*, 124, 352–356.

Kish, S.J., El-Awar, M., Shut, L., Leach, L., Oscar-Berman, M. & Freedman, M. (1988). Cognitive deficits in olivopontocerebellar atrophy: implications for the cholinergic hypotheses of Alzheimer's dementia. *Annals of Neurology*, 24, 200–206.

Kuhl, D.E., Phelps, M.E., Markham, C.H. *et al.* (1982). Cerebral metabolism and atrophy in Huntington's disease determined by F-18 DG and computed tomography. *Annals of Neurology*, 12, 325–434.

Lantos, P.L. & Papp, M.I. (1994). Cellular pathology of multiple system atrophy: a review. *Journal of Neurology, Neurosurgery and Psychiatry*, 57, 129–133.

Launes, J., Sulkava, R., Erkinjuntti, T. *et al.* (1991). ^{99}Tc^m-HMPAO SPECT in suspected dementia. *Nuclear Medicine Communications*, 12, 757–765.

Leenders, K.L., Frackowiak, R.S. & Lees, A.J. (1988). Steele–Richardson–Olszewski syndrome. Brain energy metabolism, blood flow and fluoro-dopa uptake measured by position emission tomography. *Brain*, 111, 615–630.

Lees, A.J. & Smith, E. (1983). Cognition deficits in the early stages of Parkinson's disease. *Brain*, 106, 257–270.

Lennox, G., Lowe, J., Landon, M., Byrne, E.J., Mayer, R.J. & Godwin-Austen, R. (1989). Diffuse Lewy body disease: correlative neuropathology using anti-ubiquitin immunocytochemistry. *Journal of Neurology, Neurosurgery and Psychiatry*, 52, 1236–1247.

Lishman, W.A. (1987). *Organic Psychiatry*, 2nd edn, pp. 126–133. Oxford: Blackwell.

Lishman, W.A. (1990). Alchohol and the brain. *British Journal of Psychiatry*, 156, 635–644.

Livingston, G. & King, M. (1993). Alcohol abuse in an inner city elderly population: the Gospel Oak Study. *International Journal of Geriatric Psychiatry*, 8, 511–514.

Lund & Manchester Groups – Burns, A., Englund, B., Gustafson, L. (1994). Clinical and neuropathological criteria for frontotemporal dementia. *Journal of Neurology Neurosurgery and Psychiatry*, 57, 416–418.

Madden, J.J., Luhan, J.A., Kaplan, L.A. & Manfredi, H.H.

(1952). Non-dementing psychoses in older persons. *Journal of the American Medical Association*, 150, 1567–1570.

Masters, C.L., Harris, J.O., Gajdusek, C., Gibbs, C.J., Bernoulli, C. & Asher, D.M. (1979). Creutzfeldt–Jakob disease: patterns of worldwide occurrence and the significance of familial and sporadic clustering. *Annals of Neurology*, 5, 177–188.

Mayberg, H.S., Starkstein, S.E., Sadzot, B. *et al.* (1990). Selective hypometabolism in the inferior frontal lobe in depressed patients with Parkinson's disease. *Annals of Neurology*, 28, 57–64.

Mayeux, R., Stern, Y., Rosentein, R. *et al.* (1988). An estimate of the prevalence of dementia in idiopathic Parkinson disease. *Archives of Neurology*, 45, 260–262.

Mazziotta, J.C., Phelps, M., Pahl, J. *et al.* (1987). Reduced cerebral glucose metabolism in asymptomatic subjects at risk for Huntington's disease. *New England Journal of Medicine*, 316, 357–362.

McAllister, T.W. (1983). Overview: pseudodementia. *American Journal of Psychiatry*, 140, 528–533.

McKeith, I.G. (1994). The differential diagnosis of dementia. In *Dementia*, ed. A. Burns & R. Levy, pp. 39–57. London: Chapman & Hall.

Mesulam, M.-M. (1982). Slowly progressive aphasia without generalised dementia. *Annals of Neurology*, 11, 592–598.

Mori, K., Murata, T., Nakano, Y. & Handa, H. (1977). Proventricular lucency in hydrocephalus in computerised tomography. *Surgical Neurology*, 8, 337–340.

Myers, R.H., Sax, D., Schoenfeld, M. *et al.* (1985). Late onset of Huntington's disease. *Journal of Neurology, Neurosurgery and Psychiatry*, 48, 530–534.

Neary, D., Snowden, J.S. & Mann, D.M.A. (1993). Familial progressive aphasia: its relationship to other forms of lobar atrophy. *Journal of Neurology, Neurosurgery and Psychiatry*, 56, 1122–1125.

Neary, D., Snowden, J.S., Northen, B. & Gouldeng, P. (1988). Dementia of frontal lobe type. *Journal of Neurology, Neurosurgery and Psychiatry*, 51, 353–361.

Nicolas, J.M., Catafau, A.M., Estruch, R. *et al.* (1993). Regional cerebral blood flow – SPECT in chronic alcoholism: relation to neuropsychological testing. *Journal of Neurological Medicine*, 34, 1452–1459.

Olivia, D., Carella, F., Savoiardo, M. *et al.* (1993). Clinical and magnetic resonance features of the classic and akinetic-rigid variants of Huntington's disease. *Archives of Neurology*, 50, 17–19.

Pearce, J.M.S, Flowers, K., Pearce, I. & Pratt, A.E. (1981). Clinical, psychometric and CAT scan correlations in Parkinson's disease. In *Research Progress in Parkinson's Disease*, ed. F.C. Roase & R. Capildeo, pp. 43–52. London: Pitman.

Pearlson, G.D., Rabins, P.V. & Burns, A. (1991). Centrum semiovale white matter CT changes associated with normal ageing, Alzheimer's disease and late life depression with and without reversible dementia. *Psychological Medicine*, 21, 321–328.

Pogacar, S. & Williams, R.S. (1984). Alzheimer's disease presenting as slowly progressive aphasia. *Rhode Island Medical Journal*, 67, 181–185.

Pujol, J., Jungue, C., Vendrell, P., Grau, J.M. & Capdevil, A. (1992). Reduction of the substantia nigra width and motor decline in ageing and Parkinson's disease. *Archives of Neurology*, 49, 1119–1122.

Quinn, N. (1989). Multiple system atrophy – the nature of the beast. *Journal of Neurology, Neurosurgery and Psychiatry*, 52 (special supplement), 78–89.

Quinn, N.P., Rossor M.N. & Marsden, C.D. (1986). Dementia and Parkinson's disease – pathological and neurochemical considerations. *British Medical Bulletin*, 42, 86–90.

Rabins, P.V. (1983). Reversible dementia and the misdiagnosis of dementia: a review. *Hospital and Community Psychiatry*, 34, 830–835.

Reid, I.C., Besson, J.A.O., Best, P.V. *et al.* (1988). Imaging of cerebral flow markers in Huntington's disease using single photon emission computed tomography. *Journal of Neurology, Neurosurgery and Psychiatry*, 51, 1264–1268.

Risberg, J. (1987). Frontal lobe degeneration of non-Alzheimer type. III Regional cerebral blood flow. *Archives of Gerontology and Geriatrics*, 6, 223–225.

Sahakian, B.J. (1991). Depressive pseudodementia in the elderly. *International Journal of Geriatric Psychiatry*, 6, 453–458.

Salmon, E., Sadzot, B., Maquet, P. *et al.* (1994). Differential diagnosis of Alzheimer's disease with PET. *Journal of Nuclear Medicine*, 35, 391–398.

Savoiardo, M., Strada, L., Olivia, D., Girotti, F. & D'Incerti, L. (1991). Abnormal MRI signal in the rigid form of Huntington's disease. *Journal of Neurology, Neurosurgery and Psychiatry*, 54, 888–891.

Sawada, H., Udaka, F., Kameyama, M. *et al.* (1992). SPECT findings in Parkinson's disease associated with dementia. *Journal of Neurology, Neurosurgery and Psychiatry*, 55, 960–963.

Scheinberg, P. (1951). Cerebral blood flow and metabolism in pernicious anaemia. *Blood*, 6, 213–227.

Schoenberg, (1987). Epidemiology of movement disorders. In *Movement Disorders 2*, ed. C.D. Marsden & S. Fahn, pp. 17–32. London: Butterworths.

Schulz, J.B., Klockgether, T., Petersen, D. *et al.* (1994). Multiple system atrophy: natural history, MRI morphology and dopamine receptor imaging with [123]IBZM-SPECT. *Journal of Neurology, Neurosurgery and Psychiatry*, 57, 1047–1056.

Sharp, P., Gemmell, G., Cherryman, J., Besson, J., Crawford, J. & Smith, F. (1986). Application of iodine-123-labelled isopropylamphetamine imaging to the study of dementia. *Journal of Nuclear Medicine*, 27, 761–768.

Shen, W.C., Ho, Y.J., Lee, S.K. & Lee, K.R. (1994). MRI of transient postencephalitic parkinsonism. *Journal of Computer Assisted Tomography*, 18, 155–156.

Sibbitt, W.L., Sibbitt, R.R., Griffey, R.H., Eckel, C. & Bankhurst, A.D. (1989). Magnetic resonance and computer tomographic imaging in the evaluation of acute neuropsychiatric disease in systemic lupus erythematosus. *Annals of the Rheumatic Diseases*, 48, 1014–1022.

Smith, F.W., Gemmell, H.G., Sharp, P.F. *et al.* (1988). Technetium-99m HMPAO imaging in patients with basal ganglia disease. *British Journal of Radiology*, 61, 914–920.

Sroka, H., Elizan, T.S., Yahr, M.D., Burger, A. & Mendazu, M.R. (1981). Organic mental syndrome and confusional states in Parkinson's disease. *Archives of Neurology*, 38, 339–342.

Starkstein, S.E., Brandt, J., Folstein, S. *et al.* (1988). Neuropsychologic and neuropathologic correlates in Huntington's disease. *Journal of Neurology, Neurosurgery and Psychiatry*, 51, 1259–1263.

Starkstein, S.E., Migliorelli, R., Teson, A. *et al.* (1994). Specificity of changes in cerebral blood flow in patients with frontal lobe dementia. *Journal of Neurology, Neurosurgery and Psychiatry*, 57, 790–790.

Starkstein, S.E., Robinson, R.G. & Price T.R.M. (1987). Comparison of cortical and subcortical lesions in the production of post stroke mood disorders. *Brain*, 110, 1045–1059.

Tan, E.M., Cohen, A.S., Fries, J.F. *et al.* (1982). The 1982 revised criteria for the classification of systemic lupus erythematosus. *Arthritis and Rheumatism*, 25, 1271–1277.

Tanahashi, N., Meyer, J.S., Ishikawa, Y. *et al.* (1985). Cerebral blood flow and cognitive testing correlate in Huntington's disease. *Archives of Neurology*, 42, 1169–1175.

Taylor, A.E., Saint-Cyr, J.A., Lang, A.E. & Kenny, F.T. (1986). Frontal lobe dysfunction in Parkinson's disease: the cortical focus of neostriatal out flow. *Brain*, 109, 845–883.

Terrence, C.F., Delaney, J.F. & Alberts, M.C. (1977). Computed tomography for Huntington's disease. *Neuroradiology*, 13, 173–175.

Tolosa, E.S. & Alvarez, R. (1992). Differential diagnosis of cortical versus subcortical dementia. *Acta Neurologica Scandinavica*, Suppl. 139, 47–53.

Tyrrell, P.J., Warrington, E.K., Frackowiak, R.S.J. & Rossor, M.N. (1990). Heterogeneity in progressive aphasia due to focal cortical atrophy. A clinical and PET study. *Brain*, 113, 1321–1326.

Vanneste, J., Augustijn, P., Tan, W.F. & Dirven, C. (1993). Shunting normal pressure hydrocephalus: the predictive value of combined clinical and CT data. *Journal of Neurology, Neurosurgery and Psychiatry*, 56, 251–256.

Victoroff, J., Ross, G.W., Benson, F., Verity, A. & Vinters, H.V. (1994). Posterior cortical atrophy neuropathologic correlations. *Archives of Neurology*, 51, 269–274.

Yoshimura, M. (1988). Pathological basis for dementia in elderly patients with idiopathic Parkinson's disease. *European Neurology*, 28 (Suppl. 1), 29–35.

6　Delirium

James Lindesay and Alastair Macdonald

Introduction

The classical syndrome of delirium has an abrupt onset. In the elderly, it involves a rapid cognitive decline from the preexisting level of functioning (whatever that might be) involving conscious level, orientation, attention, memory and concentration. The mental state fluctuates from minute to minute or hour to hour, often worse in the evenings than mornings. There are perceptual abnormalities (illusions, hallucinations and misrecognition), affective changes (apathy, lability, irritability, autonomic arousal), persecutory or terrifying ideas, behavioral changes (hypokinesis or hyperkinesis), and motor features – 'plucking' and pointing are common. It is an unpleasant state with a high mortality and a high risk of adverse iatrogenic consequences. In approximately 85% of recognised cases, one or more physical causes can be identified, for example infection, intoxication with prescribed drugs, and cardiovascular, respiratory and metabolic disease. In the other 15%, psychologic factors such as removal from home, grief, depression or acute psychotic illness are sufficient to precipitate delirium. The risk of delirium appears to rise with age and underlying cerebral disease.

　　The clinical diagnosis of delirium involves establishing that the syndrome is present and then identifying the underlying cause or causes. Delirium is common in elderly patients on medical and psychiatric wards; estimates vary widely, depending upon the setting and the methods of assessment and diagnosis, but recent studies of acute elderly medical inpatients suggest that 10–25% are delirious (Bowler *et al.*, 1994; Erkinjuntti *et al.*, 1986; Rockwood, 1989; Seymour *et al.*, 1980). Similar frequencies have been reported in studies of acute psychogeriatric admissions (Koponen *et al.*, 1989c). The rates of delirium in elderly surgical patients are even higher, particularly after procedures such as hip replacement (Gustafson *et al.*, 1988) and cardiothoracic surgery (Smith & Dimsdale, 1989). Despite the high prevalence of delirium in these settings, medical and nursing staff seem often to be unaware of its presence, or else they attribute the syndrome to dementia or depression (Bowler *et al.*, 1994; Cameron *et al.*, 1987; McCartney & Palmateer, 1985). This may be partly because of the presentation of delirium in elderly patients; it is often 'quiet', lacking the florid disturbances in perception, mood and behaviour usually seen in younger patients and enshrined in classical texts.

However, the preoccupation of hospital staff with the physical aspects of care in modern high-technology, fast-throughput medical environments also contributes to this lack of awareness; talking to the patient is very helpful in the identification of abnormal mental states, but this component of assessment and review is all too often ignored in modern hospital practice. Delirium is reversible if the underlying cause is identified and treated, so improved recognition results in better outcome and shorter hospital stays (Thomas, Cameron & Fahs, 1988). The consequences of missing reversible causes of cognitive impairment can be very serious, since patients who might have been able to manage at home if appropriately treated may be denied this opportunity and admitted to residential care, where institutionalization quickly removes any residual self-care capacity.

What contribution can neuroimaging techniques make to the understanding or management of delirium? There is very little published work in this area. The principal reason for this is not surprising; the necessity for stillness in most neuroimaging procedures apparently precludes the examination of patients with delirium. However, many elderly patients with delirium are hypoactive (Millar, 1981; Ross et al., 1991), so this is unlikely to be the only explanation. Unfortunately, clinical pessimism about the utility of imaging in elderly patients in general, and acutely ill ones in particular, may contribute more fundamentally to the paucity of both clinical and research data. This represents, of course, a fine example of 'Catch-22', since the clinical utility of neuroimaging can only be determined by studying its impact in practice. A substantial increase in social and academic interest in delirium will probably be necessary before researchers will be motivated to tackle the formidable practical and ethical obstacles to the clinical study of neuroimaging in this disorder.

The aim of this chapter is to examine the present clinical role of neuroimaging techniques in delirium, and the role of neuroimaging in research into the syndrome. The utility of imageless methods of assessing cerebral dysfunction in delirium will not be considered, nor will discussion be confined to studies in elderly populations, these being too few in number.

Clinical applications

Is it delirium?

Neuroimaging has the potential to contribute to both stages of the diagnostic process: the initial differentiation of delirium from other disorders and the subsequent identification of the cause. Delirium is a clinical syndrome and should be recognizable on the basis of the history and clinical features, provided that the clinician is alert to the possibility in the first place. However, in mild or atypical cases, or when other syndromes coexist (particularly depressive and delusional), specific investigations may be of value. The most established of these is EEG.

QEEG

EEG is one of the few useful diagnostic tools in mild and doubtful cases of delirium; decreased background frequency and increased disorganization is reliably associated with reduced arousal. However, there is generalized slowing of the alpha rhythm both with increasing age and in association with dementia, so the diagnostic value of EEG may be more limited in the elderly than it is in younger adults (Lipowski, 1983). The practical advantage of conventional EEG as an investigative procedure in delirium is that it is less reliant on the patient's cooperation than is neuroradiology, although it is still quite a lengthy procedure and the quality of the trace is significantly affected by movement arte-facts.

The development in recent years of QEEG, or brain area electrical mapping (BEAM) (see Chapter 1(d)), is potentially an advance on traditional EEG techniques for the investigation of delirious patients. QEEG uses digitally recorded EEG data to perform spectral analysis; it is much quicker and, therefore, much more practical to do with disturbed patients; the results are more accurate and reproducible and the pictorial output in the form of 'brainmaps' is easier to interpret by nonspecialists. In a comparison of delirious and nondelirious subjects using QEEG, Koponen *et al.* (1989b) found highly significant differences in the relative power, power ratios, occipital peak frequency and mean frequency in their EEG spectra; subjects with both delirium and dementia had the most abnormal findings. In a study examining the potential of both conventional EEG and QEEG to discriminate delirium, dementia and nonimpaired controls, Jacobson, Leuchter & Walter (1993) found that a combination of the MMSE score (Folstein, Folstein & McHugh, 1975) and the relative power in alpha correctly identified 94% of patients. The EEG/QEEG variables that distinguished best between delirium and dementia were relative power in delta and brainmap score according to a system devised by the authors; this achieved 93% accuracy in identification. The sample was small and retrospective, but the results are interesting and suggest that a discriminant function of selected EEG variables may be a useful and practical guide to diagnosis.

QEEG is also a promising technique for monitoring patients' progress. In a small study of three elderly patients (Leuchter & Jacobson, 1991), serial brainmaps were obtained. In two patients presenting with delirium, the brainmaps showed substantial changes from presentation to recovery, with EEG changes preceding clinical improvement. In the third patient, brainmaps taken before, during and after an episode of toxic delirium showed abnormalities specifically associated with the delirious episode. In all three cases, conventional EEG was relatively insensitive to these changes.

A number of important questions remain to be answered before QEEG can be confidently recommended as a clinical tool for diagnosis and monitoring in delirium. First, larger, prospective studies of the specificity and sensitivity of this technique in distinguishing delirium from other syndromes that can mimic it in elderly patients, (e.g. dementia, amnestic syndromes, affective disorders, panic and catatonia) need to be carried out. Second, assuming that QEEG is a reasonably specific and sensitive indicator of delirium, its cost-effectiveness as an aid to patient management will also need to be investigated. Third, which QEEG parameters are most discriminant in the differential diagnosis of delirium? Fourth, how vulnerable is QEEG to artefactual distortion, and how can this be identified and minimized? However, given the promising initial studies and the relative practicality of the technique, further evaluation of QEEG as an investigative procedure in delirium should be one of the priorities for research in this area.

CT

There is little evidence to suggest that either structural or functional neuroradiological procedures have much to offer in confirming the presence of a delirious syndrome, although, as we discuss below, much of the research in this area has been limited to neurologic and nonelderly samples. It is not surprising that structural imaging is unhelpful in delirium, as there is no neuropathologic evidence that delirium *per se* is associated with any measurable alterations in brain structure, with the possible exception of cases caused by focal lesions affecting specific areas (see below). CT studies have found that delirium is associated with increased cortical atrophy and focal lesions compared with nondelirious controls. Swigar *et al.* (1985) correlated psychopathologic features with CT scan findings in 50 elderly patients with various organic and functional disorders and found that those suggestive of delirium, such as 'disorientation', 'confusion/perplexity' and fluctuating mental state, were associated with left-sided temporoparietal atrophy. Another CT study of DSM-III delirium (delirium criteria: see American Psychiatric Association, 1987) in a small sample of elderly patients (Koponen *et al.*, 1987) found no evidence of increased cortical atrophy compared with controls, but delirious subjects had greater frontal horn and cella media indices, enlarged third ventricles, left-sided Sylvian fissures and an excess of focal infarcts. In a larger sample, Koponen *et al.* (1989a) found delirium to be associated with cortical atrophy, greater ventricular dilatation and an increased number of focal lesions, predominantly in the right hemisphere cortical association areas. In this study, hyperactive delirium was associated with right-sided parietooccipital lesions. This evidence of cortical atrophy and focal lesions associated with delirium supports clinical observations that brain-damaged and demented patients are at increased risk of developing delirium, but it is of no help in differentiating the syndrome from others. Similarly, anecdotal reports of delirium after subcortical (particularly thalamic) infarcts are unhelpful in the clinical task of distinguishing delirium from other syndromes – the specificity and sensitivity of these phenomena are likely to be appallingly low.

MRI

Similarly, MRI studies have found that subcortical disease is consistently associated with an increased risk of electroconvulsive therapy-induced and antidepressant-induced delirium in the depressed and psychotic elderly (Figiel *et al.*, 1989; 1990a; 1992; Figiel, Krishnan & Doraiswamy, 1990b; Krishnan, 1991), but, again, the positive and negative predictive values of these findings as indicators of delirium are unknown.

SPET and PET

So far as functional imaging is concerned, the evidence from the few published studies is contradictory. Trzepacz (1994) has reviewed PET and SPET studies of delirium, which have so far been confined to younger patients with hepatic encephalopathy, delirium tremens and traumatic brain injury emerging from coma. A case-study of bromide delirium found that this was associated with loss of normal hyperfrontality in measures of rCBF (Berglund, Nielsen & Risberg, 1977), but no correlation was found between rCBF and cognitive impairment in delirium tremens (Hemmingsen et al., 1988). If certain forms of delirium are associated with rCBF hypofrontality, this may potentially be of some diagnostic use, given that in AD rCBF is typically reduced in temporoparieto-occipital regions (Risberg, 1980), but further research is needed. In general, the results are inconclusive, and sample sizes are small or unitary; again, functional imaging is of no practical clinical use at present in confirming the presence of the delirium.

What is the underlying cause?

The principle that no investigation should be carried out if the result would not change the management of the patient is a sound one, provided the term 'management of the patient' is taken in a fairly broad sense, including dealing with patients' and relatives' anxieties and the natural human desire for explanations. Once the syndrome of delirium is recognized, and other confounding conditions relegated to low probability, the task is to identify the underlying causes. Again, neuroimaging ought to be helpful if there is clinical uncertainty as to the cause after the commonest (drugs, infection, metabolic disturbance) have been excluded. Structural neuroimaging is helpful to exclude gross focal intracerebral causes of delirium, such as subdural hematoma, stroke, cerebral abcess and other tumor. CT scanning will be sufficient to identify these lesions in most cases, but identification of small lesions in critical areas may require the better resolution possible with MRI (Eng et al., 1993). Delirium is rare after stroke (Benbadis, Sila & Cristea, 1994; Boiten & Lodder, 1989) but has been reported in association with right (nondominant) cerebral (middle cerebral artery) and thalamic infarcts, and also left posterior cerebral artery infarcts (Bogousslavsky et al., 1988; Martin, 1969; Medina, Rubino & Ross, 1977; Mesulam et al., 1976; Mori & Yamadori, 1987; Santamaria, Bleas & Tolosa, 1984; Verslegers et al., 1991).

EEG may also be of some limited use in identifying underlying causes. Rarely, postictal confusion, epilepsia partialis continua and periodic lateralized epileptiform discharges may present as clinical delirium, and some other causes of delirium such as hepatic encephalopathy and drug toxicity are associated with characteristic EEG abnormalities. It is not known if QEEG has anything specific to offer in this respect; brainmaps often show asymmetrical and focal features, but these are fluctuating and may not be related to any underlying localized structural lesion (Leuchter & Jacobson, 1991).

SPET may also be useful in resolving the side of intractable complex partial seizures (Duncan et al., 1993), which may, in the elderly, be manifest simply as a delirium. Occipital and parietal lobe seizures may provoke delirium (Sveinbjornsdottir & Duncan, 1993), when MRI may show underlying lesions not localized by clinical examination or EEG.

Will delirium recur?

This clinically important question needs an answer after the delirium has resolved. An individual, accurate prognosis is valuable in alerting the clinician to the need for preventative strategies (e.g. the management of cerebrovascular disease and hypertension), for continued surveillance and for the training of the patient, relatives and others (e.g. residential care staff) to be aware of risks such as changes in medication and infections. Part of the assessment of prognosis involves an estimate of the probability of further episodes, and it is here that imaging techniques are of particular value in clinical practice. Neuroradiologic evidence of deep white matter lesions suggestive of ischemia, or of cortical and subcortical infarcts, appears to be strongly indicative of increased risk of future delirium (e.g. Figiel *et al.* 1989; 1990a; 1992) and should focus attention on investigation of possible treatable causes; these lesions may not be apparent on CT scans. Alcoholic patients with frontal lobe atrophy on CT scans may be more prone to alcohol withdrawal delirium (Kato *et al.*, 1991).

The practicalities of investigating elderly delirious patients

The practical difficulties of obtaining useful neuroradiologic images and EEG records from disturbed, uncooperative delirious patients have already been alluded to. Since these procedures are sometimes necessary for complete investigation of the patient, it is worth considering what can be done to minimize these problems and increase the likelihood that the exercise is worthwhile. When one considers what is involved in obtaining, say, a CT or MRI scan, it is not surprising that delirious patients react badly to the procedure. First, in addition to being delirious, the patient is probably also previously cognitively impaired and physically ill and may well be suffering from significant sensory impairment and pain. The neuroradiology department is usually at some distance from the ward, perhaps even in another hospital, and the patient will have to travel by trolley or ambulance in order to have their scan. After the journey, they may be kept waiting in a strange, windowless room surrounded by strangers and then restrained with their head inside a frightening, noisy machine – the high-technology ambience of the average neuroradiology suite is totally outside the experience of most elderly patients. Finally, if contrast medium is needed, this will involve another bewildering assault. Seen from the delirious patient's perspective, the process is extremely distressing, and it is not surprising that many resist. However, an awareness of and sensitivity to the patient's experience can do much to lessen the impact of these procedures. First and foremost, it should be arranged for the time of day (or night) when the patient is usually at their most lucid and comprehending of the surroundings. This requires a degree of flexibility on the part of the neuroradiology department that can be difficult to arrange if it accords a low priority to elderly, 'difficult' cases. Patients should also be accompanied at all times by a familiar nurse or family member, and they should be given constant and repeated explanations of what is going on. In mildly delirious cases these precautions may be sufficient, but sometimes sedation is unavoidable and this needs to be chosen and administered with care if unnecessary aggravation of the delirium is to be avoided. Often, a light general anesthetic is preferable to the large doses of tranquillizing drugs that may otherwise be necessary to achieve the required immobility, provided that the patient's physical condition allows this. However carefully such procedures are carried out, ward staff caring for the patient on their return need to be aware that they will probably result in a temporary worsening of the patient's mental state and behavior, and they need to be prepared to manage this. Finally, it is worth mentioning that insensitive neuroradiologic investigations may even actually precipitate a delirium in previously nondelirious demented patients, so careful practice is required with all cognitively impaired subjects. Intravenous contrast media such as iopamidol may also cause delirium (Lucas, Colley & Gordon, 1992).

Neuroimaging in research into delirium

In order to examine the importance of neuroimaging in delirium research, it is necessary briefly to set the scene of delirium research at present, and to consider some of the more general obstacles to research in this area.

Case definition

The first obstacle is the possibility that the delirium syndrome, like many others before it, is a chimera. A syndrome is a 'characteristic' collection of phenomena (symptoms, signs, abnormalities on investigation) that, when recognized, leads the clinician to investigate possible causal hypotheses (the differential diagnosis) and then to try to interfere with the presumed process or processes (the disease or diseases). What symptoms and signs are 'characteristic' i.e. are excluded or included, and the degree of emphasis placed on each, is, in clinical practice, more a matter of taste than science. In clinical research, decisions are based at present on consensus criteria, principally DSM-IIIR (American Psychiatric Association, 1987) and its successor, DSM-IV (American Psychiatric Association, 1994), whether used directly or transformed into rating scales such as those produced by Trzepacz, Baker & Greenhouse (1988) and Inouye et al. (1990). These 'committee' criteria may be obstacles in themselves. For instance, in specifying recovery within six months, research based on ICD-10 criteria (World Health Organization, 1992) may exclude cases where recovery does not fall within this timeframe. Similarly, to exclude from delirium research patients with nonorganic etiology as would be suggested by DSM-IIIR, or those with dementia syndromes (Trzepacz, 1994) is likely to obscure rather than clarify our understanding.

These are circular problems that lie at the heart of all delirium research, but are particularly relevant to neuroimaging. On the one hand, if we have got the syndrome wrong (i.e. included or excluded criteria that are critical) then attempts to link the syndrome to neuroimaging findings will lead to incoherent results. There is some evidence that this might be the case (Johnson et al., 1990; Koponen & Riekkinen, 1993; Liptzin & Levkoff, 1992). We cannot, on the other hand, define the syndrome in terms of neuroimaging results since we do not know which are the crucial abnormalities. The authors (Lindesay, Macdonald & Starke, 1990) and others (Inouye, 1994; Lipowski, 1983; Trzepacz, 1994) have listed in general terms the research problems presented by delirium; but this particular nettle has yet to be grasped. One way forward might be to set aside temporarily the syndrome (a phenomenon of the sociology of medicine rather than a biologic entity) and focus instead on the clinical and investigative phenomenology of unselected samples in ways that are as free of preconceptions as is humanly possible. The syndrome could then be reassembled on a sound statistical basis.

Other methodological issues

Even if the characteristics of delirium syndromes were on a firmer footing, progress using neuroimaging techniques would require attention to many other methodologic issues. Some are general to all delirium research: choice of study populations, sampling and adequate sample size, refusals, consent, reliability of assessments (clinical and imaging), incident versus prevalent delirium, drop-outs, repeated measure biases, assessment of severity of physical illness, mortality and assessment of the cause of death. There are also those issues that are specifically pertinent to neuroimaging studies. Here only the latter will be considered.

Selection artefacts

Neuroimaging techniques are rarely available outside hospitals, and some (e.g. PET) in only a few centers, which may have a predominantly tertiary referral function. This means that the different populations of subjects with delirium (those at home, day hospital attenders, those on medical, surgical and psychiatric wards, those in intensive care units) will be differentially represented, depending on the center's access to neuroimaging services. This may introduce biases, especially in relation to the hypo/hyperactive issue (see below), or in any findings linked to problematic behavior.

Costs and numbers

Neuroimaging techniques are relatively costly, and the repeated clinical measures necessary in delirium research (because of its fluctuating nature) even more so. Economic pressures on researchers conspire to keep sample sizes to, or below, a bare minimum. However, delirium research is at a very primitive, exploratory stage, and in order to make progress (by, for instance, the development of fruitful hypotheses by post-hoc subgroup analysis) it is important to obtain substantial sample sizes. Most neuroimaging studies in delirium are of very small numbers of patients.

Ethical constraints

As we have described, neuroimaging involves disruption and discomfort for the patient, particularly if it involves transport to another site. Delirious patients are often disorientated, usually medically unwell, and although many are hypoactive, levels of distress may be very high (Cutting, 1987). Ethical and consent principles may preclude certain groups of delirious patients, depressing sample sizes still further.

Control groups

Controls should differ from cases only in the variable of interest, in this instance the presence of delirium. All too often in imaging studies, control groups are made up of patients that differ in many respects from the delirious subjects. This will not do; more precise matching is needed if the inevitably small-scale studies are to be efficient. This usually requires prospective rather than retrospective investigations.

Bearing in mind these constraints, what can be extracted from neuroimaging data in delirium research? So far, this research has focused on the imaging characteristics of clinical subtypes of delirium, the risk of delirium related to localized cerebral disease, and attempts to identify underlying mechanisms of delirium.

Elucidating clinical subtypes

The principal clinical division of delirium syndromes is into hyperactive ('activated') and hypoactive ('somnolent') states (Millar, 1981; Ross et al., 1991). Hemmingsen et al. (1988) used xenon-133 inhalation tomography and found a generalized increase in CBF in patients with delirium tremens, whilst others have found decreased flow in certain areas such as the right anterior cingulate region in hepatic encephalopathies (O'Carroll et al., 1991); these two conditions are said to reflect the poles of this clinical distinction. However, O'Carroll et al. (1991) also reported increased CBF in the basal ganglia and right occipital cortex. Nearly all the subjects in both studies were under 65 years of age, and the reliability of this distinction, and the relative importance of its poles, remains obscure. Suggestions that delirium with prominent psychotic phenomena (delusions, hallucinations) is more common with primarily right-hemisphere disturbance (Cutting, 1990) have not been followed up directly with imaging studies, and there have been no investigations of speed of onset and duration of delirium using neuroimaging.

Risk of delirium and localization of cerebral disease

The vexed distinction between cortical and subcortical function has attracted some interest in delirium – though not particularly in the elderly. Delirium following classical stroke revealed by CT scans has been reported as rare (Dunne, Leedman & Edis, 1986), although it seems more common when cerebrovascular accidents affect the nondominant parietal cortex (Boiten & Lodder, 1989; Koponen et al., 1989a). Brown et al. (1993) reported the results of 100 consecutive CT requests for patients referred with acute neurological problems on a geriatric ward. Twenty-one had 'acute confusional states', and of these, 11 had significant cerebral pathology. Most subdural hematomas were in the group with acute confusional states. However, the total number of delirious patients was small, delirium was not clinically defined and there may well have been a bias towards hyperactive delirium.

Studies of delirium after subcortical (particularly thalamic) infarcts have largely been confined to anecdotal single-case studies, although there is MRI evidence that subcortical and basal ganglia disease appears to be consistently associated with an increased risk of delirium (Figiel *et al.*, 1989; 1990a; 1990b; 1992; Krishnan, 1991). However, as Lipowski (1990) has warned, most cases of delirium are caused by diffuse and widespread disturbances of neuronal functioning, and we should be wary of simplistic localizationism. As noted above, CT studies of delirious samples do not even agree on whether it is the right or left cerebral hemisphere that is more involved (Koponen *et al.*, 1989a; Swigar *et al.*, 1985).

Identifying the underlying mechanisms

QEEG offers a means of visualizing cortical EEG activity with sampling times of as little as 30 seconds (Leuchter & Jacobson, 1991): a major advantage over all other imaging techniques in delirium. However, the maps produced cannot, at the time of writing, be used for localization; rather, the maps collapse large quantities of data for more reliable interpretation by a skilled interpreter. Jacobson *et al.* (1993) reported results on a sample of 15 delirious, 10 demented and 8 control subjects examined by repeated administration of the MMSE. They reported a high correlation between initial scores and ratings of relative and absolute power maps, the last also being associated with change in scores over time. However, sample sizes were, as ever, small, and the patients were selected because of overt delirium rather than from a screened population.

MRI T_1 relaxation time is a measure of brain water and has been used to evaluate the role of brain hydration in alcohol withdrawal; there was no correlation between T_1 relaxation and the severity of the withdrawal syndrome (Mander *et al.*, 1989).

SPET and PET offer theoretically interesting means of studying brain function in delirium, but the evidence to date is still very limited (Trzepacz, 1994).

Conclusion

In writing this chapter on neuroimaging in delirium, the authors have been very aware of the dangers of making too much of a small number of studies on small numbers of subjects. The findings to date are interesting and suggestive, but a much greater research effort is needed before signals can be reliably separated from the noise. There is much to be learned from the study of delirium, both about the syndrome itself and about the normal function of the brain. While neuroimaging techniques have yet to be established as useful clinical and scientific tools in this respect, they offer a promising window onto this little-understood condition.

References

American Psychiatric Association (1987). *Diagnostic and Statistical Manual of Mental Disorders*, 3rd edn (revised). Washington DC: American Psychiatric Association.

American Psychiatric Association (1994). *Diagnostic and Statistical Manual of Mental Disorders*, 4th edn. Washington DC: American Psychiatric Association.

Benbadis, S.R., Sila, C.A. & Cristea, R.L. (1994). Mental status changes and stroke. *Journal of General and Internal Medicine*, 9, 485–487.

Berglund, M., Nielsen, S. & Risberg, J. (1977). Regional cerebral blood flow in a case of bromide psychosis. *Archiv für Psychiatrie und Nervenkrankheit*, 223, 197–201.

Bogousslavsy, J., Ferrazzini, M., Regli, F., Assal, G., Tanabe, H. & Delaloye-Bischof, A. (1988). Manic delirium and frontal-like syndrome with paramedian infarction of the right thalamus. *Journal of Neurology, Neurosurgery and Psychiatry*, 51, 116–119.

Boiten, J. & Lodder, J. (1989). An unusual sequela of a frequently-occurring neurologic disorder: delirium caused by brain infarct. *Nederlands Tijdschrift voor Geneeskunde*, 133, 617–620.

Bowler, C., Boyle, A., Branford, M., Cooper, S., Harper, R. & Lindesay, J. (1994). Detection of psychiatric disorders in elderly medical in-patients. *Age and Ageing*, 23, 307–311.

Brown, G., Warren, M., Williams, J.E., Adam, E.J. & Coles, J.A. (1993). Cranial computed tomography of elderly patients: an evaluation of its use in acute neurological presentations. *Age and Ageing*, 22, 240–243.

Cameron, D.J., Thomas, R.I., Mulvihill, M. & Bronheim, H. (1987). Delirium: a test of the Diagnostic and Statistical Manual III criteria on medical inpatients. *Journal of the American Geriatrics Society*, 35, 1007–1010.

Cutting, J. (1987). The phenomenology of acute organic psychosis. Comparison with acute schizophrenia. *British Journal of Psychiatry*, 151, 324–332.

Cutting, J. (1990). *The Right Cerebral Hemisphere and Psychiatric Disorders*. Oxford: Oxford University Press.

Duncan, R., Patterson, J., Roberts, R., Hadley, D.M. & Bone, I. (1993). Ictal/postictal SPECT in the pre-surgical localisation of complex partial seizures. *Journal of Neurology, Neurosurgery and Psychiatry*, 56, 141–148.

Dunne, J.W., Leedman, P.J. & Edis, R.H. (1986). Inobvious stroke: a cause of delirium and dementia. *Australia and New Zealand Journal of Medicine*, 16, 71–78.

Eng, C., Cunningham, D., Quade, B.J. *et al.* (1993). Meningeal carcinomatosis from transitional cell carcinoma of the bladder. *Cancer*, 72, 553–557.

Erkinjuntti, T., Wikstrom, J., Palo, J. & Autio, L. (1986). Dementia among medical inpatients. Evaluation of 2000 consecutive admissions. *Archives of Internal Medicine*, 146, 1923–1926.

Figiel, G.S., Botteror, K., Zorumski, C.F., Jarvis, M.R., Doraiswamy, M. & Krishnan, R. (1992). The treatment of late age onset psychoses with electroconvulsive therapy. *International Journal of Geriatric Psychiatry*, 7, 183–189.

Figiel, G.S., Coffey, C.E., Djang, W.T., Hoffman, G. & Doraiswamy, P.M. (1990a). Brain magnetic resonance imaging findings in ECT-induced delirium. *Journal of Neuropsychiatry and Clinical Neurosciences*, 2, 53–58.

Figiel, G.S., Krishnan, K.R. & Doraiswamy, P.M. (1990b). Subcortical structural changes in ECT-induced delirium. *Journal of Geriatric Psychiatry and Neurology*, 3, 172–176.

Figiel, G.S., Krishnan, R., Nemeroff, C. *et al.* (1989). Radiologic correlates of antidepressant-induced delirium: the possible significance of basal-ganglia lesions. *Journal of Neuropsychiatry and Clinical Neurosciences*, 1, 188–190.

Folstein, M.F., Folstein, S.E. & McHugh, P.R. (1975). Mini-mental state – a practical method for grading the cognitive state of patients for the clinician. *Journal of Psychiatric Research*, 12, 189–198.

Gustafson, Y., Berggren, D., Brannstrom, B. *et al.* (1988). Acute confusional states in elderly patients treated for femoral neck fracture. *Journal of the American Geriatrics Society*, 36, 525–530.

Hemmingsen, R., Vorstrup, S., Clemmesen, L. *et al.* (1988). Cerebral blood flow during delirium tremens and related clinical states studied with xenon-133 inhalation tomography. *American Journal of Psychiatry*, 145, 1384–1390.

Inouye, S.K. (1994). The dilemma of delirium: clinical and

research controversies regarding diagnosis and evaluation of delirium in hospitalized elderly medical patients. *American Journal of Medicine*, 97, 278–288.

Inouye, S.K., van Dyck, C.H., Alessi, C.A., Balkin, S. & Siegal, A.P. (1990). Clarifying confusion: the confusion assessment method. A new method for detection of delirium. *Annals of Internal Medicine*, 113, 941–948.

Jacobson, S.A., Leuchter, A.F. & Walter, D.O. (1993). Conventional and quantitative EEG in the diagnosis of delirium among the elderly. *Journal of Neurology, Neurosurgery and Psychiatry*, 56, 153–158.

Johnson, J.C., Gottlieb, G.L, Sullivan, E. *et al.* (1990). Using DSM-III criteria to diagnose delirium in elderly general medical patients. *Journal of Gerontology*, 45, M113–119.

Kato, A., Tsuji, M., Nakamura, M. & Nakajima, T. (1991). Computerized tomographic study on the brain of patients with alcohol dependence. *Japanese Journal of Psychiatry and Neurology*, 45, 27–35.

Koponen, H., Hurri, L., Stenbäck, U., Mattila, E., Soininen, H. & Riekkinen, P.J. (1989a). Computed tomography findings in delirium. *Journal of Nervous and Mental Disease*, 177, 226–231.

Koponen, H., Hurri, I., Stenbäck, U. & Riekkinen, P.J. (1987). Acute confusional states in the elderly: a radiological evaluation. *Acta Psychiatrica Scandinavica*, 76, 726–731.

Koponen, H., Partanen, J., Paakkonen, A., Mattila, E. & Riekkinen, P.J. (1989b). EEG spectral analysis in delirium. *Journal of Neurology, Neurosurgery and Psychiatry*, 52, 980–985.

Koponen, H.J. & Riekkinen, P.J. (1993). A prospective study of delirium in elderly patients admitted to a psychiatric hospital. *Psychological Medicine*, 23, 103–109.

Koponen, H., Stenbäck, U., Mattila, E., Soininen, H., Reinikainen, K. & Riekkinen, P.J. (1989c). Delirium in elderly persons admitted to a psychiatric hospital: clinical course during the acute stage and one-year follow-up. *Acta Psychiatrica Scandinavica*, 79, 579–585.

Krishnan, K.R. (1991). Organic bases of depression in the elderly. *Annual Review of Medicine*, 42, 261–266.

Leuchter, A.F. & Jacobson, S.A. (1991). Quantitative measurement of brain electrical activity in delirium. *International Psychogeriatrics*, 3, 231–247.

Lindesay, J., Macdonald, A. & Starke, I. (1990). *Delirium in the Elderly*. Oxford: Oxford University Press.

Lipowski, Z.J. (1983). Transient cognitive disorders in the elderly. *American Journal of Psychiatry*, 140, 1426–1436.

Lipowski, Z.J. (1990). *Delirium: Acute Confusional States*. Oxford: Oxford University Press.

Liptzin, B. & Levkoff, S.E. (1992). An empirical study of delirium subtypes. *British Journal of Psychiatry*, 161, 843–845.

Lucas, L.M., Colley, C.A. & Gordon, G.H. (1992). Multisystem failure following intravenous iopamidol. *Clinical Radiology*, 45, 276–277.

Mander, A.J., Young, A., Chick, J.D., Ridgeway, J. & Best, J.J.

(1989). NMR T_1 relaxation time of the brain during alcohol withdrawal and its lack of relationship with symptom severity. *British Journal of Addiction*, 84, 669–672.

Martin, J.J. (1969). Thalamic syndromes. In *Handbook of Clinical Neurology*, ed. P.J. Vinken & G.W. Bruyn, Vol. 2, pp. 469–496. Amsterdam: North-Holland.

McCartney, J.R. & Palmateer, L.M. (1985). Assessment of cognitive deficits in geriatric patients: a study of physician behaviour. *Journal of the American Geriatrics Society*, 33, 467–471.

Medina, J.L., Rubino, F.A. & Ross, E. (1977). Agitated delirium caused by infarctions of the hippocampal formation and fusiform and lingual gyri: a case report. *Neurology*, 24, 1181–1183.

Mesulam, M.M., Waxman, S.G., Geschwind, N. & Sabrin, T.D. (1976). Acute confusional states with right middle cerebral artery infarctions. *Journal of Neurology, Neurosurgery and Psychiatry*, 39, 84–89.

Millar, H.R. (1981). Psychiatric morbidity in elderly surgical patients. *British Journal of Psychiatry*, 138, 17–20.

Mori, E. & Yamadori, A. (1987). Acute confusional state and acute agitated delirium. Occurrence after infarction in the right middle cerebral artery territory. *Archives of Neurology*, 44, 1139–1143.

O'Carroll, R.E., Hayes, P.C., Ebmeier, K.P. *et al.* (1991). Regional cerebral blood flow and cognitive function in patients with chronic liver disease. *Lancet*, 337, 1250–1253.

Risberg, J. (1980). Regional cerebral blood flow measurements by ^{133}Xe-inhalation: methodology and applications in neuropsychology and psychiatry. *Brain and Language*, 9, 9–34.

Rockwood, K. (1989). Acute confusion in elderly medical patients. *Journal of the American Geriatrics Society*, 37, 150–154.

Ross, C.A., Peyser, C.E., Shapiro, I. & Folstein, M.F. (1991). Delirium: phenomenologic and etiologic subtypes. *International Psychogeriatrics*, 3, 135–147.

Santamaria, J., Bleas, R. & Tolosa, E.S. (1984). Confusional syndrome in thalamic stroke. *Neurology*, 34, 1618.

Seymour, D.G., Henschke, P.J., Cape, R.D.T. & Campbell, A.J. (1980). Acute confusional states and dementia in the elderly: the role of dehydration/volume depletion, physical illness and age. *Age and Ageing*, 9, 137–146.

Smith, L.W. & Dimsdale, J.E. (1989). Postcardiotomy delirium: conclusions after 25 years? *American Journal of Psychiatry*, 146, 452–458.

Sveinbjornsdottir, S. & Duncan, J.S. (1993). Parietal and occipital lobe epilepsy: a review. *Epilepsia*, 34, 493–521.

Swigar, M.E., Benes, F.M., Rothman, S.L.G., Opsahl, C. & Bowers, M.B. (1985). Behavioural correlates of computerised tomographic (CT) changes in older psychiatric patients. *Journal of the American Geriatrics Society*, 33, 96–103.

Thomas, R.I., Cameron, D.J. & Fahs, M.C. (1988). A

prospective study of delirium and prolonged hospital stay. *Archives of General Psychiatry*, 45, 937–940.

Trzepacz, P.T. (1994). The neuropathogenesis of delirium. A need to focus our research. *Psychosomatics*, 35, 374–391.

Trzepacz, P.T., Baker, R. & Greenhouse, J. (1988). A symptom rating scale for delirium. *Psychiatric Research*, 23, 89–87.

Verslegers, W., de Deyn, P.P., Saerens, J. *et al.* (1991). Slow progressive bilateral posterior artery infarction presenting as agitated delirium, complicated by Anton's syndrome. *European Neurology*, 31, 216–219.

World Health Organization (1992). *The ICD-10 Classification of Mental and Behavioural Disorders. Clinical Descriptions and Diagnostic Guidelines.* Geneva: World Health Organization.

7   Affective disorders

Christopher Ball and Michael Philpot

Introduction

Geriatric psychiatrists vary in the extent to which they use neuroimaging in their day-to-day practice (Spear, 1993). This probably not only reflects the variable availability of scanning facilities, access to them and their cost but also varying attitudes concerning the usefulness of imaging. However, the increasing vogue for the adoption of care protocols should ensure more uniform practice in future. Weinberger (1984) recommended that CT be performed for first episodes of major depressive disorder in the elderly, yet in an audit of over 600 elderly patients referred to an old-age psychiatry service, no patient had a scan performed for this indication (Spear, 1993). This rather confirms the view that many old-age psychiatrists find routine imaging of little value in their day-to-day management of the affective disorders.

This chapter presents information from research studies in this area and considers their implications for patient management; it has been organized around a number of naive questions that might concern the clinician:

(1) Do the brain images of old people with an affective disorder differ from those without an affective disorder?

(2) Do elderly people who develop an affective disorder late in life differ from those who developed it earlier in life?

(3) Are any of the abnormalities seen on imaging related to any of the psychopathological features found in the patient?

(4) Can neuroimaging help to differentiate between an affective disorder and dementia?

(5) Are any neuroimaging changes related to treatment response or prognosis?

The focus will be primarily on depression, as there is little work on mania *per se*, and on the more familiar forms of neuroimaging as employed in studies that include substantial numbers of older people. Tables 7.1, 7.2 and 7.3 give some salient details of the subjects and techniques used in the major studies.

Table 7.1 *Some CT studies involving elderly depressed patients*

| Reference | Number | | | Mean age[a]±SD (years) | Diagnostic criteria | CT measures |
	Depressed	Demented	Controls			
Jacoby & Levy (1980); Jacoby et al. (1983)	41	40	50	72 ± 6	Inpatients with 'affective disorder'	VSR, frontal horn ratio, regional brain density
Dolan et al. (1985; 1986)	108[b]	—	52	55 ± 14	RDC major depression	Sulcal rating, VBR, regional brain density
Pearlson et al. (1989)	26[c]	13	31	70 ± 2	DSM-III major depressive episode	VBR, regional brain density
Beats (1991)	25	—	—	74	DSM-III-R major depressive episode	Volumetric analysis of lateral and ventricles, and white matter lesions, regional brain density
Alexopoulos et al. (1992)	45[d]	21	—	74	DSM-III unipolar major depressive episode	VBR, frontal horn ratio, sulcal rating, width of 3rd vehicle

Notes:
VSR, ventricular:skull ratio; BVR, ventricular:brain ratio
[a] Mean age of depressed patients.
[b] Included 40 patients over the age of 60 years.
[c] Sample subdivided into 15 patients with cognitive impairment and 11 without.
[d] Sample subdivided into 13 early-onset and 32 late-onset cases.

Table 7.2 *Some MRI studies involving elderly depressed patients*

| Reference | Number | | | Mean patient age ±SD (years) | Diagnostic criteria | MRI measures |
	Depressed	Demented	Controls			
Zubenko et al. (1990);	67	61	44	73 ± 7	DSM-IIIR major depressive episode	Prevalence of cortical and subcortical changes
Rabins et al. (1991)	21	16	14	>60	DSM-IIIR major depressive episode	Visual ratings of cortical and subcortical changes
Coffey et al. (1993)	48	—	76	62 ± 16	DSM-III major depressive episode	Visual ratings of cortical and subcortical changes Volumative measures of ROIs
O'Brien et al. (1994)	32	43	—	70 ± 7	DSM-IIIR major depressive episode	Visual ratings of cortical atrophy in ROIs
Hickie et al. (1995)	39	—	—	64	DSM-IIIR major depressive episode	Visual ratings of cortical and subcortical changes
O'Brien et al. (1996)	60	61	39	71 ± 8	DSM-IIIR major depressive episode	Deep WMHI and PVHI rated on 0–3 scale

Notes:
ROI, regions of interest; WMHI, white matter hyperintensities; PVHI, periventricular hyperintensities.

Table 7.3 *SPET studies involving elderly depressed patients*

| Reference | Number | | | Mean age ± SD (years) | Diagnostic criteria | Medication free? | SPET method | CT/MR template | Reference area[a] |
	Depressed	Demented	Controls						
Sackeim et al. (1990);	41	—	40	60 ± 12	RDC major endogenous depression	11/41	Xenon-133	No	None
Lesser et al. (1994)	39	—	20	61 ± 8	DSM-IIIR major depressive episode	39/39	Xenon-133 and HMPAO	MR	Maximal uptake of whole brain
Upadhyaya et al. (1990)	18	14	12	77 ± 9	DSM-IIIR major depressive episode	Not stated	HMPAO	No	Cerebellum
Philpot et al. (1993)	10	—	9	77 ± 8	DSM-IIIR major depressive episode	4/10	HMPAO	No	Cerebellum
Curran et al. (1993)	20	20	30	70 ± 6	DSM-IIIR major depressive episode	9/20	HMPAO	No	Occipital lobes

Notes:

[a] In HMPAO SPET rCBF is expressed as a ratio of tracer uptake in the region of interest to tracer uptake in a reference area, such as the cerebellum.

Do the brain images of old people with affective disorders differ from those without affective disorders?

Structural imaging
Ventricular size

The pioneering CT study of Jacoby & Levy (1980) was unable to demonstrate significant differences between elderly inpatients with affective disorders and age-matched controls, despite using a number of quantitative measures such as ratings of ventricular size, cortical atrophy, ventricular : skull ratio (VSR) and Evans' ratio. They did, however, identify a subgroup of patients with 'enlarged' ventricles associated with a more endogenous form of depression and greater mortality (Jacoby, Levy & Bird, 1981). In contrast, Pearlson & Veroff (1981), Shima *et al.* (1984) and Dolan, Calloway & Mann (1985) all found greater mean ventricular : brain ratio (VBR) in depressed patients than in controls. Dolan *et al.* (1985) demonstrated that the increased VBR was present even after controlling for age. Later, Pearlson *et al.* (1989) were unable to demonstrate a significant difference in the VBR between elderly depressed patients and controls, although the trend was for the patients' ventricles to be larger; depressed patients with cognitive impairment did have significantly larger ventricles than controls. Abas, Sahakian & Levy (1990) and Beats, Levy & Förstl (1991) also failed to find a significant difference between patients and controls but noted a similar trend towards larger lateral ventricles in those with affective disorders. Despite this, Beats *et al.* (1991) reported a significant enlargement of the area of the third ventricle in patients.

Using a visual scoring system and MRI, Rabins *et al.* (1991) found depressed patients had significantly larger lateral and third ventricles than age-matched controls. Coffey *et al.* (1993) performed a similar study with a younger group of patients but could not demonstrate the same effect in the lateral ventricles.

Cortical atrophy

Jacoby & Levy (1980) found no differences between patients and controls on visual measures of sulcal enlargement and, as with ventricular size, subsequent results have been conflicting. Dolan *et al.* (1986) demonstrated age-related sulcal widening in a group of depressed patients and when age was controlled for, the patients still had greater sulcal widening in frontal and temporal regions than did controls. Rabins *et al.* (1991) found that an 'overall' atrophy score (a composite measure of ratings of the sulcal appearance in a number of regions) helped to discriminate between patients and controls. Conversely, Abas *et al.* (1990) found that although the cortical atrophy score tended to be higher in the patients this difference was not statistically significant. Zubenko *et al.* (1990), in a MRI study, found no difference between the degree of cortical atrophy in elderly depressed patients and a control group. Coffey *et al.* (1993) confirmed this finding but did demonstrate that the volume of the frontal lobe in their patients was smaller than that of their controls.

Brain density studies

Jacoby *et al.* (1983) found regional brain density to be reduced in the left temporal region and the right thalamus of depressed patients compared with controls and Pearlson, Rabins & Burns (1991) demonstrated that brain density of the centrum semiovale was reduced in both the cognitively normal and the cognitively impaired depressed. Beats *et al.* (1991) found no differences in the density of either the gray or the white matter of the frontal and parietal lobes of their sample but did find decreased density in the right thalamus and increased density in both caudate nuclei.

Subcortical abnormalities

MRI has advantages over CT in its ability to distinguish gray from white matter and because of improved resolution is particularly good at identifying small lesions. Many studies have now demonstrated the presence of patchy areas of WMHI 'white matter signal hyperintensity' in healthy elderly people and those with affective disorders and/or dementia (Baldwin, 1993). Although the pathologic nature of these lesions remains controversial, there is general agreement that elderly depressed patients have a higher frequency of white and gray matter lesions in subcortical structures than controls (Churchill *et al.*, 1991; Coffey *et al.*, 1990; Krishnan *et al.*, 1993; O'Brien *et al.*, 1994; 1996; Rabins *et al.*, 1991). Harrell *et al.* (1991) and Lesser *et al.* (1991) found no difference in the prevalence of subcortical WMHI between patients and controls although Lesser *et al.* (1991) found that lesions were more extensive in the depressed group.

These phenomena may be subject to regional variation as all the depressed patients in one Japanese study had imaging evidence of previous cerebral infarction, despite having been clinically screened for cerebrovascular risk factors (Fujikawa *et al.*, 1992). Reviewing the Japanese literature, Fujikawa & Yamawaki (1994) concluded that the frequency of small deep WMHI (characterized by the authors as silent infarcts) was so high in the depressed elderly that depression could be seen as a prestroke disorder and preventative therapy for cerebrovascular disease might be considered in addition to antidepressants.

Several authors have suggested that cardiovascular risk factors, particularly hypertension, are associated with white matter changes and depressive disorders (Awad *et al.*, 1986; Coffey *et al.*, 1990; Howard *et al.*, 1993; O'Brien & Ames, 1994). However, even after controlling for differences in vascular risk factors and current blood pressure, O'Brien and colleagues (1996) still found deep WMHI to be significantly more common in depressed than in control subjects. Baldwin (1993) made further suggestions: that the lesions might develop after the onset of an affective disorder, reflecting damage associated with its treatment, or that depression and white matter lesions might both be caused by a third, and as yet unidentified, process. Baldwin's first hypothesis was not supported by the work of O'Brien *et al.* (1996) who found no correlation between the presence of deep WMHI and the length of the current depressive episode, number of previous depressive episodes or treatment with ECT in 60 patients with major depression and a mean age of 71.2 years.

Functional imaging

Global cerebral blood flow
Studies from the early 1980s and those using young subjects tended to report that global CBF was unchanged in depression (Gur *et al.*, 1984; Silfverskiold & Risberg, 1989) or even increased (Rosenberg *et al.*, 1988), while more recent studies using middle-aged to elderly subjects have shown a reduction (Lesser *et al.*, 1994; Sackeim *et al.*, 1990; Schlegel *et al.*, 1989) which appears to be greater in the nondominant hemisphere (Lesser *et al.*, 1994; Schlegel *et al.*, 1989) and in men (Lesser *et al.*, 1994; Sackeim *et al.*, 1990). The study of Lesser *et al.* (1994) combining SPET and MRI also showed that patients with the highest levels of WMHI had the lowest global CBF.

Regional cerebral blood flow
The ability of PET to localize accurately areas of reduced tracer uptake is crucial in identifying the important structures or neural circuits that are dysfunctional in any disorder. Resolution is poorer with SPET but focal reductions in rCBF have been identified in a variety of regions including frontal (Austin *et al.*, 1992; Lesser *et al.*, 1994; Sackeim *et al.*, 1990; Schlegel *et al.*, 1989), central (Kanaya & Yonekawa, 1990; Sackeim *et al.*, 1990), parietal (Austin *et al.*, 1992; Lesser *et al.*, 1994; Sackeim *et al.*, 1990; Schlegel *et al.*, 1989) and temporal lobes (Austin *et al.*, 1992; Edmondstone *et al.*, 1994; Lesser *et al.*, 1994; Kanaya & Yonekawa, 1990; Sackeim *et al.*, 1990; Schlegel *et al.*, 1989), and the basal ganglia (Austin *et al.*, 1992). In addition, increased rCBF has been demonstrated in the right temporal lobe (Amsterdam & Mozley, 1992) and the left frontal lobe (Uytdenhoef *et al.*, 1983).

To date only five studies, two using the xenon-[133]inhalation method (Lesser *et al.*, 1994; Sackeim *et al.*, 1990) and three using radioligands labeled with technetium-99m (Curran *et al.*, 1993; Philpot *et al.*, 1993; Upadhyaya *et al.*, 1990), have included substantial numbers of elderly depressed patients. Sackeim *et al.* (1990) used a novel statistical approach to determine whether an abnormal functional neural network could be identified. Reductions in rCBF were found in some frontal and central regions, the left anterior parietal and the right superior temporal regions. Unfortunately, and despite the sophistication of the analysis, the results demonstrated little more than much earlier work showing hypofrontality in depressed patients (Buschbaum *et al.*, 1986; Post *et al.*, 1987). Lesser *et al.* (1994) combined both SPET methods (i.e. xenon inhalation and [99]mTc-HMPAO) and MRI to determine rCBF against brain structure. rCBF was reduced bilaterally in orbitofrontal and inferior temporal regions and in the right high frontal, superior temporal and parietal areas. These findings generally confirm those of Sackeim *et al.* (1990). Unfortunately the tracer uptake in subcortical areas was not measured but cortical uptake correlated negatively with VBR.

Upadhyaya *et al.* (1990) found no significant differences in relative rCBF using HMPAO when comparing patients with controls, although an average measure of global CBF was lower in the depressed patients. On visual inspection, areas of impaired perfusion were found in 30–40% of depressed patients but only 10–15% of the controls.

Philpot *et al.* (1993) compared HMPAO uptake in depressed patients and age-matched controls in a split-dose paradigm measuring rCBF during a 'resting' state and during a verbal fluency task. At rest, reduced flow was found in the left parietal and temporal regions and the basal ganglia of the depressed patients. During activation, the relative rCBF in the patients increased, particularly in the frontal regions, such that differences between the depressed group and the controls were abolished. Curran *et al.* (1993) only found reductions of rCBF in elderly depressed men. These were in the right anterior cingulate, both temporal and frontal cortices, and the caudate and the thalamic nuclei.

PET studies

Reductions in frontal metabolism have been demonstrated in a number of studies of unipolar depression (Baxter *et al.*, 1989; Phelps *et al.*, 1984) as has reduced metabolism in the basal ganglia and the temporal lobes (Cohen *et al.*, 1989). Wu *et al.* (1993) found reduced callosal metabolic activity in depressed patients with thickened corpora callosum. Results from patients with obsessive–compulsive disorder (Baxter *et al.*, 1989) and Parkinson's disease (Mayberg *et al.*, 1990) suggest that the left frontal abnormalities are related to the symptom of low mood (see below).

In summary, while some measures may now be used to differentiate groups of depressed patients from groups of healthy elderly subjects, the variability of findings from study to study and the overlapping ranges of values between patient groups and controls restrict the practical use of imaging in the single case to the exclusion of other brain disorders.

Do elderly people who develop an affective disorder late in life differ from those who developed it earlier in life?

For many years the notion has persisted that depressive illnesses developing for the first time in old age are, in some way, more 'organic' than illnesses developing in youth or middle age (Post, 1962). Some evidence from autopsy studies supports this view, but large studies are difficult to conduct and small ones prone to misinterpretation. Clinical evidence of 'organicity', usually in the form of cognitive impairment, has been taken by some to indicate underlying pathologic brain change. This has not always been supported by data from imaging studies (Baldwin *et al.*, 1993). Defining the age at which a disorder is said to be of 'late' onset is fraught with difficulties as it presupposes a categorical difference between middle and old age that may be far from valid (see Macdonald, 1993, for a provocative critique of this area).

Jacoby & Levy (1980) were unable to demonstrate any differences between inpatients who had early-onset and those who had late-onset depressive disorders but they did show a trend for the late-onset group to have larger ventricles than the early-onset group. This trend has been reported in a number of other CT studies (e.g. Alexopoulos *et al.*, 1992), and Shima *et al.* (1984) found a positive correlation between age of onset and VBR in a middle-aged sample. However, Scott *et al.* (1983) found no difference in the ventricular sizes of those with early and late-onset disease, a finding replicated by many more studies (Andreason *et al.*, 1990; Beats *et al.*, 1991; Pearlson *et al.*, 1991; Schlegel & Kretzschmar, 1987) although Beats and colleagues did find that enlargement of the third ventricle was associated with an *earlier* onset of the illness. Cortical atrophy has been shown to be related to the age of onset in two studies, one using CT (Abas *et al.*, 1990) and the second using MRI (Rabins *et al.*, 1991). Krishnan *et al.* (1988) defined 'late-onset' illnesses as those occurring for the first time after the age of 45 years. MRI abnormalities occurred in 72% of their late-onset depressed patients compared with only 20% of early-onset cases matched for age at scanning. The changes were statistically associated with history of cardiovascular risk factors. In a similar study by Guze & Szuba (1992), white matter changes were found in 44% of patients with late-onset disease and 30% of those with early-onset disease and medically ill controls. Similarly, Fujikawa *et al.* (1992) found white matter lesions in all the patients with late-onset disease but in only 54% of early-onset elderly depressed patients. Hickie *et al.* (1995) found ratings of periventricular hyperintensities and deep WMHI were correlated positively with age at onset. However, other studies using MRI have failed to show differences in the prevalence of white matter lesions between early- and late-onset disease, although the trend is for lesions to occur more frequently in late-onset cases (Churchill *et al.*, 1991; Coffey *et al.*, 1989; Figiel *et al.*, 1991).

O'Brien *et al.* (1996) reported that 6 of 30 (20%) subjects aged over 65 who had first been depressed before reaching age 65 had severe deep WMHI compared to 8 of 16 (50%) subjects with late-onset (first episode coming after age 65) major depression. Only 2 of 21 (9.5%) control subjects aged above 65 had such severe lesions. However, the late-onset cases were significantly older than the early-onset subjects and, as the presence of deep WMHI was related to age, this may have confounded the results.

Functional imaging studies shed little light on this issue. Curran *et al.* (1993) reported no differences in rCBF between early- and late-onset depression in elderly patients. Other SPET and PET studies make no comment.

The evidence from structural imaging indicates that although 'soft' brain lesions may be more common in those with late-onset disorders this is not a statistically robust finding in studies using subjects from Western nations.

Are any of the abnormalities seen on imaging related to any of the psychopathologic features found?

Few CT or MRI studies in the elderly have reported either the overall severity of the depression or details of individual symptoms and their associations or otherwise with imaging measures. The notable exception is scores of cognitive performance and, by implication, brain dysfunction. However, given that the majority of studies employ hospitalized patients meeting DSM-III (American Psychiatric Association, 1980) or DSM-IIIR (American Psychiatric Association, 1987) criteria for major depressive episode the results may only relate to the severe end of the spectrum of depression.

Jacoby & Levy (1980) used the 'Newcastle' scale (Carney, Roth & Garside, 1965) to determine the degree to which their patients suffered from an endogenous type depression. Although this scale did not correlate with any of the CT variables, the subgroup of patients with enlarged ventricles did have higher Newcastle scores and lower anxiety scores. By contrast, Shima et al. (1984) found that nonmelancholics had larger ventricles than melancholics. Rabins et al. (1991) found that those patients who had received electroconvulsive therapy (ECT, a putative measure of illness severity) had greater temporal horn atrophy and more subcortical lesions than those who had received only medication. Coffey et al. (1988) reported subcortical white matter abnormalities in 66% of elderly patients referred for ECT. A number of studies of younger patients have demonstrated an association between higher VBR and 'psychotic' depression (Luchins, Lewine & Meltzer, 1984; Schlegel & Kretzschmar, 1987; Targum et al., 1983;). However, Rabins et al. (1991) found no such association.

Deficits in rCBF have been shown to correlate with the severity of the depression in some studies (Austin et al., 1992; Kanaya & Yonekawa, 1990; Sackeim et al., 1990) but not all (Lesser et al., 1994; Schlegel et al., 1989). Austin et al. (1992) found a positive correlation between scores on the Newcastle scale and rCBF in the cingulate and frontal areas, but this has not been found elsewhere (Philpot et al., 1993; Schlegel et al., 1989). Thomas et al. (1993) found reduced uptake of HMPAO in 'frontal' and 'posterior' regions of the brains of patients with a major depressive disorder compared with those with a dysthymia and a superimposed depressive episode.

Philpot et al. (1993) found no correlations between rCBF and the Newcastle scale or depression severity. This group was able to demonstrate negative correlations between rCBF and anxiety and somatic symptoms, whilst psychotic symptoms correlated in a positive way. Bench et al. (1993) also found positive correlations between anxiety and rCBF in the right posterior cingulate cortex and both inferior parietal lobes. Psychomotor retardation and depressed mood correlated negatively with rCBF in the dorsolateral prefrontal cortex.

Recently, a number of studies of the imaging correlates of depressive symptoms in other mental disorders have appeared. Lebert et al. (1994) found that patients with AD who had the symptom of 'emotionalism' or emotional lability had relatively higher left frontolateral rCBF than patients without this symptom. Conversely, Starkstein et al. (1995) reported reduced rCBF in the left superior temporal and parietal regions in AD patients with major depression compared with nondepressed AD patients. Interestingly, AD patients with dysthymia showed no additional deficits in rCBF when compared with nondepressed AD patients. Lastly, Ring et al. (1994) showed with PET that patients with Parkinson's disease with major depression had reduced rCBF in the medial frontal cortex and cingulate cortex in comparison with those with Parkinson's disease alone. The findings were similar to those found in a group of patients with major depression and no Parkinson's disease.

Although structural changes appear to have little consistent relationship to severity or subtype of depression, the discovery of more specific associations between individual symptoms and functional imaging variables is interesting from the pathophysiologic aspect. However, at present these changes have little relevance for clinical management.

Can neuroimaging help differentiate affective disorders and dementia?

Subtle cognitive impairments can be demonstrated in many elderly depressed patients. Some of these do not return to normal after recovery from the illness (Abas *et al.*, 1990). However, the clinician is often faced with the problem of patients presenting with depressive symptoms and more obvious cognitive impairment and no clear means of determining the primary diagnosis (Rabins & Pearlson, 1994). Imaging has been employed, together with other putative biological markers of depression, in attempts to improve this position.

Jacoby & Levy (1980) and Jacoby *et al.* (1983) found no associations between CT measures and scores on cognitive tests. The mean CT results for depressed patients fell between those of normal subjects and those of patients with dementia but were, on the whole, not significantly different from either. The exceptions were the findings of decreased regional density in the left temporal and right thalamic areas. Pearlson *et al.* (1989) also found that the mean VBR of a depressed group lay between those of normal and demented subjects but also that the mean VBR for cognitively impaired depressed patients (i.e. those with 'pseudodementia') was significantly greater than that of normal subjects. The same researchers demonstrated a similar pattern of results using regional brain density measures at the level of the lateral ventricles (Pearlson *et al.*, 1989) and the white matter at the level of the centrum semiovale (Pearlson *et al.*, 1991). Cognitively impaired depressed patients had significantly lower values in the right occipital and posterior central regions than did cognitively normal depressed patients (Pearlson *et al.*, 1989).

Zubenko *et al.* (1990) demonstrated that the presence of cortical atrophy was significantly more likely in patients with dementia than in those with depression, by using logistic regression analysis. Although Rabins *et al.* (1991) found composite scores of cortical and subcortical abnormalities both correlated with cognitive performance in depressed subjects, there was no difference between patients with AD and depressed patients on any MRI measure; a finding similar to that of Harrell *et al.* (1991). Similarly, Alexopoulos *et al.* (1992) were unable to distinguish between patients with late-onset depression and patients with dementia. Patients with an onset of depression before 60 years had significantly smaller lateral and third ventricles than patients with dementia.

Abas *et al.* (1990) found that VBR was correlated with psychomotor speed and information processing and these functions did not improve in about one-third of patients after recovery from depression. Failure to improve on these timed tests was associated with enlarged ventricles, and psychomotor speed was also significantly impaired in elderly depressed patients with WMHI revealed by MRI (Hickie *et al.*, 1995). Beats *et al.* (1991) found that the size of the third ventricle correlated positively with the degree of cognitive impairment when the subject was depressed. Lastly, O'Brien *et al.* (1994) present one of the few studies that attempt to use MRI ratings to discriminate between depressed and demented subjects. Using a hippocampal atrophy rating, the best cut point gave a high sensitivity (93%) and specificity (84%). The comparison of a subgroup of cognitively impaired depressed elderly patients with a group of demented patients matched for severity of impairment yielded a similarly high sensitivity and specificity. The method lost sensitivity in patients over 75 years, although the specificity improved to 100%.

There have been few studies of functional imaging directly comparing depressed patients with demented ones. Upadhyaya *et al.* (1990) found no quantitative differences in HMPAO uptake between depressed patients and AD patients, but visual analysis of scans revealed that focal deficits in uptake were more common in the dementia patients. Curran *et al.* (1993) found the mean rCBF values of a depressed elderly group were generally more like those of healthy controls than a group with AD. However, changes were largely restricted to male subjects and the impairments in tests of psychomotor speed and cognitive organization correlated with deficits in the frontal regions. The abnormalities were not related to the severity of depressive disorder but the authors concluded that they were attributable to premorbid cognitive impairment. Dolan *et al.* (1992) demonstrated decreased rCBF in the left anterior medial prefrontal cortex and increased rCBF in the cerebellar vermis in depressed patients with reversible cognitive impairment, abnormalities that were not present in age-matched cognitively normal depressed patients. These changes are distinct from the bilateral temporoparietal abnormalities found in AD (Kennedy & Frackowiak, 1994) and may help to delineate the pathophysiology of 'pseudodementia' but are unlikely to be of great practical value in themselves.

Are any imaging changes related to treatment response and prognosis?

Few imaging studies have followed depressed patients through to the recovery phase. Those which have may be divided into two groups : those that identify imaging features during the depressed phase which may be associated with good, or bad, outcome, and those that record the changes in imaging which occur after recovery or as a result of treatment. Clearly, the first is most suited to structural imaging and the latter to functional imaging.

As mentioned above, Jacoby *et al.* (1981) identified a subgroup of nine depressed elderly patients who had enlarged ventricles and, over a two year follow-up period, had a higher mortality than the other patients. The study was the first in a series that reported similar results (Shima *et al.*, 1984; Young *et al.*, 1988). Conversely, Alexopoulos *et al.* (1992) did not find any CT measures that discriminated better those who responded to medication and those who went on to have ECT.

Coffey *et al.* (1988) found that patients with WMHI on MRI had a poorer response to antidepressants; and this has recently been confirmed by Hickie *et al.* (1995).

Similarly, little is known about the specific effects of treatment on the brain or whether particular patterns of imaging abnormality have prognostic significance. Although Calloway *et al.* (1981) identified a relationship between previous exposure to ECT and enlarged VBR, this has not been supported by others (Coffey *et al.*, 1988; Devanand *et al.*, 1994; Dolan *et al.*, 1985). Goodwin *et al.* (1993) re-scanned a group of middle-aged depressed subjects following full recovery. It was possible to match 16 patients for medication status before and after treatment. Changes in rCBF were confined to the subcortex and cingulate gyrus with increases in tracer uptake occurring bilaterally in the putamen and inferior anterior cingulate, and in the right thalamus and posterior cingulate cortex. The authors suggest that while subcortical abnormalities might be state dependent cortical abnormalities might be trait dependent. The same research team has also shown that similar changes (only significant in the inferior anterior cingulate cortex) occurred following a single ECT treatment session in a group of depressed patients with a mean age of 60 years (Scott *et al.* 1994). However, Bench Frackowiak & Dolan (1995) found that while some cortical deficits in rCBF (in the left dorsolateral prefrontal cortex and anterior cingulate) did improve, reduced rCBF in the left angular gyrus did not. Curran *et al.* (1993) suggested that a good outcome was related to higher rCBF in the subcortical areas, the right parietal and the posterior cingulate cortex.

The current state of knowledge suggests that treatment should not be withheld on the basis of imaging data alone but that the patient should continue to receive treatment with the appropriate tenacity (Macdonald, 1993).

Manic disorder

Although many imaging studies of depression include some bipolar patients (e.g. Beats *et al.*, 1991; Bench *et al.*, 1992; Kellner *et al.*, 1986), there are obvious logistical difficulties in persuading drug-free manic patients to undergo scanning procedures! Studies on young adults have identified a number of abnormalities: a greater VBR (Pearlson *et al.*, 1984), an increase in periventricular and cortical regional brain density (Dewan *et al.*, 1988) and an increase in subcortical WMHI (Dupont *et al.*, 1990).

Studies of CBF have failed to show any differences between young manic and young depressed patients (Rubin *et al.*, 1995; Silfverskiold & Risberg, 1989). Baxter *et al.* (1985) found that manic patients had an increased global brain glucose metabolism and that serial measurements on a rapid-cycling patient showed a 30–40% increase in metabolism during the hypomanic phases.

Studies of elderly patients are very few in number. Broadhead & Jacoby (1990) scanned 35 manic patients over the age of 60 comparing them with 35 below the age of 40 and 20 elderly controls. CT revealed that the elderly manic group had greater cortical atrophy scores than controls but the mean VBR and third ventricle size were similar. Age of illness onset was not related to any CT measure but increased cortical atrophy was associated with decreased cognitive performance.

McDonald *et al.* (1991) studied using MRI 12 patients whose manic illness began after the age of 50. Compared with matched controls, there was no difference in VBR or periventricular WMHI. Differences, however, were revealed in the number of large subcortical lesions found in the middle third of the brain parenchyma. Similar numbers were noted in both cerebral hemispheres.

Conclusions

Indiscriminate neuroimaging of populations with psychiatric disorders is a relatively unrewarding pastime (McClellan, Eisenberg & Giyanani 1988; Zubenko *et al.*, 1990). Even when careful consideration is given to the selection of patients for scanning, the yield of abnormalities that change the management of the patients is small (Spear, 1993). This clinical finding has gone some way to answering the questions posed at the beginning of the review, to which few firm answers can yet be given.

(1) Some depressed patients do have more structural and functional brain abnormalities on scanning than controls but many do not

(2) There are few consistent differences between patients with early- and late-onset disease, although the trend is for there to be a greater number of lesions in the late-onset group. This may not be the case in some non-Western countries

(3) Functional studies are beginning to identify specific abnormalities associated with specific mental symptoms, e.g. reduced rCBF in frontal brain regions is associated with the symptom of depression in many different guises

(4) Patients with cognitive impairment probably have more structural and functional abnormalities on scan than those who do not: measures of hippocampal atrophy may help in making a more firm diagnosis of dementia, and, by exclusion, depressive illness (O'Brien, 1995)

(5) It is probable that patients with extensive lesions do not do so well with treatment, particularly medication. But even these patients can improve with ECT (Coffey *et al.*,

1988) and Macdonald (1993) is right to conclude that treatment should not be withheld on the basis of a scan result alone.

Neuroimaging studies (particularly functional studies) are expensive, time consuming and need a great deal of cooperation from the patient. Each of these factors has contributed to the small power of many studies and the limited range of clinical cases (often confined to tertiary referral centers and rarely derived from community-based surveys). Although this research has led to progress in the understanding of the striatal–frontal abnormalities that underlie severe depression (Krishnan, 1991), there has, as yet, been little clinical pay-off.

Newer forms of neuroimaging (such as fast MRI or MR spectroscopy) may provide additional answers to these questions. If studies employing representative samples of sufficient numbers of subjects and driven by hypothesis-testing continue to be undertaken, we may possibly look forward to the day when neuroimaging becomes a powerful and routine tool in the clinical management of elderly patients with an affective disorder.

References

Abas, M.A., Sahakian, B.J. & Levy, R. (1990). Neuropsychological deficits and CT scan changes in elderly depressives. *Psychological Medicine*, 20, 507–520.

Alexopoulos, G.S., Young, R.C. & Shindledecker, R.D. (1992). Brain computed tomography findings in geriatric depression and primary degenerative dementia. *Biological Psychiatry*, 31, 591–599.

American Psychiatric Association (1980). *Diagnostic and Statistical Manual of Mental Disorders*, 3rd edn. Washington DC: American Psychiatric Association.

American Psychiatric Association (1987). *Diagnostic and Statistical Manual of Mental Disorders*, 3rd edn (revised). Washington, DC: American Psychiatric Association.

Amsterdam, J.D. & Mozley, P.D. (1992). Temporal lobe asymmetry with iofetamine (IMP) SPECT imaging in patients with major depression. *Journal of Affective Disorders*, 24, 43–53.

Andreason, N.C., Swayze, V., Flaum, M., Alloger, R. & Cohen, G. (1990). Ventricular abnormalities in affective disorder: clinical and demographic correlates. *American Journal of Psychiatry*, 147, 893–900.

Austin, M.-P., Dougall, N., Ross, M. *et al.* (1992). Single photon emission tomography with ^{99m}Tc-exametazine in major depression and the pattern of brain activity underlying the psychotic/neurotic continuum. *Journal of Affective Disorders*, 26, 31–44.

Awad, I.A., Spetzler, R.F., Hodak, J.A., Awad, C.A. & Carey, R. (1986). Incidental subcortical lesions identified on magnetic resonance imaging in the elderly. 1. Correlation with age and cerebrovascular risk factors. *Stroke*, 17, 1084–1089.

Baldwin, R.C. (1993). Late life depression and structural brain changes: a review of recent magnetic resonance imaging research. *International Journal of Geriatric Psychiatry*, 8, 15–23.

Baldwin, R.C., Benbow, S.M., Marriott, B. & Tomenson, B. (1993). Depression in old age: a reconsideration of cerebral disease in relation to outcome. *British Journal of Psychiatry*, 163, 82–90.

Baxter, L.R., Phelps, M.E., Mazziotta, J.C. *et al.* (1985). Cerebral metabolic rates for glucose in mood disorders. Studies with positron emission tomography and fluorodeoxyglucose ^{18}F. *Archives of General Psychiatry*, 42, 441–447.

Baxter, L., Schwartz, J., Phelps, M. *et al.* (1989). Reduction of prefrontal cortex glucose metabolism common to three types of depression. *Archives of General Psychiatry*, 46, 243–250.

Beats, B., Levy, R. & Förstl, H. (1991). Ventricular enlargement and caudate hyperdensity in elderly depressives. *Biological Psychiatry*, 30, 452–458.

Bench, C.J., Frackowiak, R.S.J. & Dolan, R.J. (1995). Changes in regional cerebral blood flow on recovery from depression. *Psychological Medicine*, 25, 247–261.

Bench, C.J., Friston, K.J., Brown, R.G., Frackowiak, R.S.J. & Dolan, R.J. (1993). Regional cerebral blood flow in depression measured by positron emission tomography: the relationship with clinical dimensions. *Psychological Medicine*, 23, 579–590.

Bench, C.J., Friston, K.J., Brown, R.G., Scott, L.C., Frackowiak, R.S.J. & Dolan, R.J. (1992). The anatomy of melancholia – focal abnormalities of cerebral blood flow in major depression. *Psychological Medicine*, 22, 607–615.

Broadhead, J. & Jacoby, R. (1990). Mania in old age: a first prospective study. *International Journal of Geriatric Psychiatry*, 5, 215–222.

Buschbaum, M.S., Wu, J., Delisi, L.E. *et al.* (1986). Frontal, cortical and basal ganglia metabolic rates assessed by positron emission tomography with (^{18}F)2–deoxyglucose in affective illness. *Journal of Affective Disorders*, 10, 137–152.

Calloway, S.P., Dolan, R.J., Jacoby, R.J. *et al.* (1981). ECT and cerebral atrophy: a computed tomography study. *Acta Psychiatrica Scandinavica*, 64, 442–445.

Carney, M.P., Roth, M. & Garside, R.F. (1965). The diagnosis of depressive syndromes and the prediction of ECT response. *British Journal of Psychiatry*, 111, 659–674.

Churchill, C.M., Priolo, C.V., Nemeroff, C.B. *et al.* (1991). Occult subcortical magnetic resonance findings in elderly depressives. *International Journal of Geriatric Psychiatry*, 6, 213–216.

Coffey, C.E., Figiel, G.S., Djang, W.T. *et al.* (1988). Leukoencephalopathy in elderly depressed patients referred for ECT. *Biological Psychiatry*, 24, 143–161.

Coffey, C.E., Figiel, G.S., Djang, W.T. *et al.* (1989). Subcortical white matter hyperintensity on magnetic resonance imaging: clinical and neuroanatomic correlates in the depressed elderly. *Journal of Neuropsychiatry and Clinical Neuroscience*, 1, 135–144.

Coffey, C.E., Figiel, G.S., Djang, W.T. & Weiner, R.D. (1990). Subcortical hyperintensity on magnetic resonance imaging: a comparison of normal and depressed elderly subjects. *American Journal of Psychiatry*, 147, 187–189.

Coffey, C.E., Wilkinson, W.E., Weiner, R.D. *et al.* (1993). Quantitative cerebral anatomy in depression. A controlled magnetic resonance imaging study. *Archives of General Psychiatry*, 50, 7–16.

Cohen, R., Semple, W., Gross, M. *et al.* (1989). Evidence for common alterations in cerebral glucose metabolism in major affective disorders and schizophrenia. *Neuropsychopharmacology*, 2, 241–254.

Curran, S.M., Murray, C.M., van Beck, M. *et al.* (1993). A single photon emission computerised tomography study of regional brain function in elderly patients with major depression and with Alzheimer-type dementia. *British Journal of Psychiatry*, 163, 155–165.

Devanand, D.P., Dwork, A.J., Hutchinson, E.R., Bolwig, T.G. & Sackeim, H.A. (1994). Does ECT alter brain structure? *American Journal of Psychiatry*, 151, 957–970.

Dewan, M.J., Haldipur, C.V., Lane, E.E., Ispahani, A., Boucher, M.F. & Major, L.F. (1988). Bipolar affective disorder 1. Comprehensive quantitative computed tomography. *Acta Psychiatrica Scandinavica*, 77, 670–676.

Dolan, R.J., Bench, C.J., Brown, R.G., Scott, L.C., Friston, K.J. & Frackowiak, R.S.J. (1992). Regional cerebral blood flow in depressed patients with cognitive impairment. *Journal of Neurology, Neurosurgery and Psychiatry*, 55, 768–773.

Dolan, R.J., Calloway, S.P. & Mann, A.H. (1985). Cerebral ventricular size in depressed subjects. *Psychological Medicine*, 15, 873–878.

Dolan, R.J., Calloway, S.P., Thacker, P.F. & Mann, A.H. (1986). The cortical appearance of depressed subjects. *Psychological Medicine*, 16, 775–779.

Dupont, R.M., Jernigan, T.L., Butters, N. *et al.* (1990). Subcortical abnormalities detected in bipolar affective disorder using magnetic resonance imaging: clinical and neuropsychological significance. *Archives of General Psychiatry*, 47, 55–60.

Edmondstone, Y., Austin, M.-P., Prentice, N. *et al.* (1994). Uptake of 99mTc-exametazine shown by single photon emission tomography in obsessive–compulsive disorder compared with major depression and normal controls. *Acta Psychiatrica Scandinavica*, 90, 298–303.

Figiel, G.S., Krishna, K.R.R., Doraiswamy, P.M., Rao, V.P., Nemeroff, C.B. & Boyko, O.B. (1991). Subcortical hyperintensities on brain magnetic resonance imaging: a comparison between late age onset and early age onset elderly depressed subjects. *Neurobiology of Aging*, 26, 245–247.

Fujikawa, T. & Yamawaki, S. (1994). Magnetic resonance imaging in patients with affective disorder: relationship to silent cerebral infarction. *Nippon Rinsho – Japanese Journal of Clinical Medicine*, 52, 1175–1179.

Fujikawa, T., Yamawaki, S., Fujita, Y., Shibata, Y. & Touhouda, Y. (1992). Clinical study of correlation presenile, senile depressive states with silent cerebral infarction – MRI findings and its distribution. *Seishin Shinkeigaku Zasshi – Psychiatrica et Neurologica Japanica*, 94, 851–863.

Goodwin, G.M., Austin, M.-P., Dougall, N. *et al.* (1993). State changes in brain activity shown by the uptake of ^{99m}Tc-exametazine with single photon emission tomography in major depression before and after treatment. *Journal of Affective Disorders*, 29, 243–253.

Gur, R.E., Skolnik, B.E., Gur, R.C. *et al.* (1984). Brain function in psychiatric disorders. II. Regional cerebral blood flow in medicated unipolar depressives. *Archives of General Psychiatry*, 41, 695–699.

Guze, B.H. & Szuba, M.P. (1992). Leukoencephalopathy and major depression: a preliminary report. *Psychiatry Research: Neuroimaging*, 45, 169–175.

Harrell, L.E., Duvall, E., Folks, D.G. *et al.* (1991). The relationship of high intensity signals on magnetic resonance images to cognitive and psychiatric state in Alzheimer disease. *Archives of Neurology*, 48, 1136–1140.

Hickie, I., Scott, E., Mitchell, P., Wilhelm, K., Austin, M.-P. & Bennett, B. (1995). Subcortical hyperintensities on magnetic resonance imaging: clinical correlates and prognostic significance in patients with severe depression. *Biological Psychiatry*, 37, 151–160.

Howard, R.J., Beats, B., Förstl, H., Graves, P., Bingham, J. & Levy, R. (1993). White matter changes in late onset depression: a magnetic resonance imaging study. *International Journal of Geriatric Psychiatry*, 8, 183–185.

Jacoby, R.J., Dolan, R.J., Levy, R. & Baldy, R. (1983). Quantitative computed tomography in elderly depressed patients. *British Journal of Psychiatry*, 143, 124–127.

Jacoby, R.J. & Levy, R. (1980). Computed tomography in the elderly 3. Affective disorder. *British Journal of Psychiatry*, 136, 270–275.

Jacoby, R.J., Levy, R. & Bird, J.M. (1981). Computed tomography and the outcome of affective disorder: a follow up study. *British Journal of Psychiatry*, 139, 288–292.

Kanaya, T. & Yonekawa, M. (1990). Regional cerebral blood flow in depression. *Japanese Journal of Psychiatry and Neurology*, 44, 571–576.

Kellner, C.H., Rubinow, D.R. & Post, R.M. (1986). Cerebral ventricular size and cognitive impairment in depression. *Journal of Affective Disorders*, 10, 215–219.

Kennedy, A.M. & Frackowiak, R.S.J. (1994). Positron emission tomography. In *Dementia*, ed. A. Burns & R. Levy, pp. 457–474. London: Chapman & Hall.

Krishnan, K.R.R. (1991). Organic basis of depression in the elderly. *Annual Review of Medicine*, 42, 261–266.

Krishnan, K.R.R., Goli, V., Ellinwood, E.H., France, R.D., Blazer, D.G. & Nemeroff, C.B. (1988). Leukoencephalopathy in patients diagnosed as major depressive. *Biological Psychiatry*, 23, 519–522.

Krishnan, K.R., McDonald, W.M., Doriaiswamy, P.M. *et al.* (1993). Neuroanatomical substrates of depression in the elderly. *European Archives of Psychiatry and Clinical Neuroscience*, 243, 41–46.

Lebert, F., Pasquier, F., Steinling, M. & Petit, H. (1994). Affective disorders related to SPECT patterns in Alzheimer's disease: a study of emotionalism. *International Journal of Geriatric Psychiatry*, 9, 327–329.

Lesser, I.M., Miller, B.L., Boone, K.B. *et al.* (1991). Brain injury and cognitive function in late onset psychotic depression. *Journal of Neuropsychiatry and Clinical Neuroscience*, 3, 33–40.

Lesser, I.M., Mena, I., Boone, K.B., Miller, B.L., Mehringer, C.M. & Wohl, M. (1994). Reduction in cerebral blood flow in older depressed patients. *Archives of General Psychiatry*, 51, 667–686.

Luchins, D.J., Lewine, R.R.J. & Meltzer, H.Y. (1984). Lateral ventricular size, psychopathology and medication response in psychosis. *Biological Psychiatry*, 19, 29–44.

Macdonald, A.J.D. (1993). Old age depression and organic brain change. In *Recent Advances in Psychogeriatrics*, ed. T. Arie, pp. 45–58. London: Longman.

McClellan, R.L., Eisenberg, R.L., Giyanani, V.L. (1988). Routine CT scanning of psychiatry inpatients. *Radiology*, 169, 99–100.

McDonald, W.M., Krishnan, K.R., Doraiswamy, P.N. & Blazer, D.G. (1991). Occurrence of subcortical hyperintensities in elderly subjects with mania. *Psychiatric Research*, 40, 211–220.

Mayberg, H.S., Starkstein, S.E., Sazdot, B. *et al.* (1990). Selective hypometabolism in the inferior frontal lobe in depressed patients with Parkinson's disease. *Annals of Neurology*, 28, 57–64.

O'Brien, J.T. (1995). Is hippocampal atrophy on magnetic resonance imaging a marker for Alzheimer's disease? *International Journal of Geriatric Psychiatry*, 10, 431–436.

O'Brien, T.J. & Ames, D. (1994). Why do the depressed elderly die? *International Journal of Geriatric Psychiatry*, 9, 689–693.

O'Brien, J.T., Desmond, P., Ames, D., Schweitzer, I., Harrigan, S. & Tress, B. (1996). A magnetic resonance imaging study of white matter lesions in depression and Alzheimer's disease. *British Journal of Psychiatry*, 168, 477–485.

O'Brien, J.T., Desmond, P., Ames, D., Schweitzer, I., Tuckwell, V. & Tress, B. (1994). The differentiation of depression from dementia by temporal lobe imaging. *Psychological Medicine*, 24, 633–640.

Pearlson, G.D., Garbacz, D.J., Tompkins, R.H. *et al.* (1984). Clinical correlates of lateral ventricular enlargement in bipolar affective disorder. *American Journal of Psychiatry*, 141, 253–256.

Pearlson, G.D., Rabins, P.V. & Burns, A. (1991). Centrum semiovale white matter changes associated with normal ageing, Alzheimer disease and late life depression with and without reversible dementia. *Psychological Medicine*, 21, 321–328.

Pearlson, G.D., Rabins, P.V., Kim, W.S. *et al.* (1989). Structural brain CT changes and cognitive deficits in elderly depressives with and without reversible dementia (pseudodementia). *Psychological Medicine*, 19, 573–584.

Pearlson, G.D. & Veroff, A.E. (1981). Computerized tomographic scan changes in manic-depressive illness. *Lancet*, ii, 470.

Phelps, M.E., Mazziotta, M., Baxter, L. & Gerner, R. (1984). Positron emission tomographic study of affective disorders. Problems and strategies. *Annals of Neurology*, 15 (Suppl. 1), S149–S156.

Philpot, M.P., Banerjee, S., Needham-Bennett, H., Costa, D.C. & Ell, P.J. (1993). ^{99m}Tc-HMPAO single photon emission tomography in late life depression: a pilot study of regional cerebral blood flow at rest and during a verbal fluency task. *Journal of Affective Disorders*, 28, 233–240.

Post, F. (1962). *The Significance of Affective Symptoms in Old*

Age. Maudsley Monograph No. 10. London: Oxford University Press.

Post, R.M., Delisi, L.E., Holcomb, H.H. et al. (1987). Glucose utilization in the temporal cortex of affectively ill patients: positron emission tomography. Biological Psychiatry, 22, 545–553.

Rabins, P.V. & Pearlson, G.D. (1994). Depression induced cognitive impairment. In Dementia, ed. A. Burns & R. Levy, pp. 667–679. London: Chapman & Hall.

Rabins, P.V., Pearlson, G.D., Aylward, E., Kumar, A.J. & Dowell, K. (1991). Cortical magnetic resonance imaging changes in elderly inpatients with major depression. American Journal of Psychiatry, 148, 617–620.

Ring, H.A., Bench, C.J., Trimble, M.R., Brooks R.S., Frackowiak, R.S.J. & Dolan, R.J. (1994). Depression in Parkinson's disease. A positron emission study. British Journal of Psychiatry, 165, 333–339.

Rosenberg, R., Vorstrup, S., Anderson, A. & Bolwig, T. (1988). Effects of ECT on cerebral blood flow in melancholia assessed with SPECT. Convulsive Therapy, 4, 62–73.

Rubin, E., Sackeim, H.A., Prohovnik, I., Moeller, J.R., Schnur, D.B. & Mukherjee, S. (1995). Regional cerebral blood flow in mood disorders: IV. Comparison of mania and depression. Psychiatry Research: Neuroimaging, 61, 1–10.

Sackeim, H.A. Prohovnik, I., Moeller, J.R. et al. (1990). Regional cerebral blood flow in mood disorders I: Comparison of major depressives and normal controls at rest. Archives of General Psychiatry, 47, 60–70.

Schlegel, S., Aldenhoff, J.B., Eissner, D., Lindner, P. & Nickel, O. (1989). Regional cerebral blood flow in depression: association with psychopathology. Journal of Affective Disorders, 17, 211–218.

Schlegel, S. & Kretzschmar, K. (1987). Computed tomography in affective disorders. Part 1. Ventricular and sulcal measurements. Biological Psychiatry, 22, 4–14.

Scott, A.I.F., Dougall, N., Ross, M. et al. (1994). Short-term effects of electroconvulsive treatment on the uptake of ⁹⁹ᵐTc-exametazine in brain in major depression shown with single photon emission tomography. Journal of Affective Disorders, 30, 27–34.

Scott, M.L., Golden, C.J., Ruedrich, S.L. et al. (1983). Ventricular enlargement in major depression. Psychiatry Research, 8, 91–93.

Shima, S., Shikano, T., Kitamura, T. et al. (1984). Depression and ventricular enlargement. Acta Psychiatrica Scandinavica, 70, 275–277.

Silfverskiold, P. & Risberg, J. (1989). Regional cerebral blood flow in depression and mania. Archives of General Psychiatry, 46, 253–259.

Spear, J. (1993). The quality of computerised tomography use in two psychogeriatric services. Psychiatric Bulletin, 17, 536–537.

Starkstein, S.E., Vazquez, S., Migliorelli, R., Teson, A., Petracca, G. & Leiguarda, R. (1995). A SPECT study of depression in Alzheimer's disease. Neuropsychiatry, Neuropsychology and Behavioural Neurology, 8, 38–41.

Targum, S.D., Rosen, L.N., DeLisi, L.E. et al. (1983). Cerebral ventricular size in major depressive disorders: association with delusional symptoms. Biological Psychiatry, 18, 329–336.

Thomas, P., Vaiva, G., Samaille, E. et al. (1993). Cerebral blood flow in major depression and dysthymia. Journal of Affective Disorders, 29, 235–242.

Upadhyaya, A.K., Abou-Saleh, M.T., Wilson, K., Grime, S.J., & Critchley, M. (1990). A study of depression in old age using single-photon emission computerised tomography. British Journal of Psychiatry, 157 (Suppl. 9), 76–81.

Uytdenhoef, P., Portelange, P., Jacquy, J., Charles, G., Linkowski, P. & Mendelwicz, J. (1983). Regional cerebral blood flow and lateralised hemispheric dysfunction in depression. British Journal of Psychiatry, 143, 128–132.

Weinberger, D.R. (1984). Brain disease and psychiatric illness: when should a psychiatrist order a CAT scan. American Journal of Psychiatry, 141, 1521–1527.

Wu, J.C., Buschbaum, M.S., Johnson, J.C. et al. (1993). Magnetic resonance and positron emission tomography imaging of the corpus callosum: size shape and metabolic rate in unipolar depression. Journal of Affective Disorders, 28, 15–25.

Young, R.C., Nambudiri, D., Alexopoulos, G.S. et al. (1988). VBR and response to nortriptyline in geriatric depression (abstract). Annual Meeting, Society for Neuroscience.

Zubenko, G. S., Sullivan, P., Nelson, J.P., Belle, S.H., Huff, J. & Wolf, G.L. (1990). Brain imaging abnormalities in mental disorder of late life. Archives of Neurology, 47, 1107–1111.

8   Paranoid and schizophrenic disorders of late life

Robert Howard and John O'Brien

Introduction

Since the early 1970s, the application of successive advances in brain imaging techniques to schizophrenia has contributed more than any other area of investigation to the current view that abnormalities of brain structure and function underpin the illness. Until the late 1950s all psychoses arising in later life were regarded as manifestations of organic brain pathology, so it is ironic that brain imaging studies of such patients have had a tendency to appear in the literature at least five years after those involving younger subjects with schizophrenia. Despite these delays and the relative paucity of studies, what appears to be emerging from the literature is that the brain imaging findings from populations of patients with an onset of schizophrenia, or a paranoid state, in late life parallel those from younger-onset cases. This chapter reviews the findings of those structural and functional brain imaging studies that have examined patients with schizophrenic or paranoid symptomatology that has onset in old age.

The classification of paranoid and schizophrenic disorders of late life remains controversial. Undoubtedly disagreement over nosology has hindered research, including neuroimaging studies of these conditions. It also makes direct comparison between the studies that do exist difficult, as not all researchers have used the same diagnostic groupings. The following terms have been proposed and, as they will be used in this chapter, brief definitions are provided here.

Late onset schizophrenia
This refers to patients who satisfy diagnostic criteria for schizophrenia but who have an illness onset after a certain age, though the age cut-off chosen does vary. Many researchers adopt the age of 45 because in DSM-III (American Psychiatric Association, 1980) diagnosis of schizophrenia was precluded above this age. DSM-IV (American Psychiatric Association, 1994) and ICD-10 (World Health Organization, 1992) do not have an exclusion on the basis of age, though neither contains a specific category or code for late-onset schizophrenia.

Late paraphrenia

This refers to any nonaffective, nonorganic, psychosis that has onset after the age of 55 or 60. It was never intended to be more than a descriptive term (Roth & Morrisey, 1952) and it is not incorporated in DSM-IV or ICD-10. Included under this label would be patients with late-onset schizophrenia, delusional disorder and schizoaffective disorder.

Late life psychosis

This is a rather loose term that often includes all psychotic illnesses with onset after a certain age, usually 45 or 60. Sometimes affective psychoses are excluded but organic psychoses often are included, leading to difficulties in interpreting the results of studies that adopt this term.

Structural brain imaging

Pneumoencephalography

From a series of 278 psychiatric patients with a variety of diagnoses, Haug (1962) reported pneumoencephalographic findings from seven schizophrenics who had an illness onset after the age of 45 years. All of these patients had highly abnormal pneumoencephalograms; five showed dilatation of the ventricular system and four had cortical atrophy. As a result of these findings, Haug suggested that the term 'involutional psychosis' should be reserved for such patients and that they should be classed separately from those schizophrenics who had experienced an illness onset early in life. He believed that these late-onset cases were closer to the organic psychoses than to schizophrenia, but had a degree of structural brain abnormality that was intermediate between young-onset functional patients and cases of senile dementia. On an optimistic note, he was also able to report that '. . . the finding of an abnormal encephalogram (ventricular dilatation, cortical atrophy) in a mental patient at the involutional age need not imply that a malignant presenile psychosis is present'.

CT

The first CT study specifically to examine patients with schizophrenic symptoms that had an onset in late life was by Miller *et al.* (1986). Five females, whose age at onset of symptoms ranged from 58 to 81 years' were scanned. Three of the patients had extensive cortical and subcortical infarcts and one had normal pressure hydrocephalus. The scan appearances were so abnormal that the authors chose to entitle their paper *Late life paraphrenia: an organic delusional syndrome*. It has to be said that better selection of

patients with scrupulous exclusion of those with a history or clinical signs of neurological disease or dementia has not confirmed this dramatic conclusion.

Rabins *et al.* (1987) determined VBRs (ventricle:brain ratios) with CT in 29 patients
whose onset of schizophrenia had been over the age of 44 years. This was a retrospective study and involved patients who had undergone CT scanning identified from
admissions over a three year period. Mean VBR was 13.3% in patients, significantly
greater than in a group of 23 age-matched controls (8.6%). Among a further comparison group of 23 age-matched patients with AD, who scored below 24 on the MMSE
(Folstein, Folstein & McHugh, 1975) and who had experienced hallucinations and delusions, mean VBR was 17.5%. Pearlson *et al.* (1987) reported the results of VBR estimations on a group of eight patients with 'late paraphrenia' who represented a subgroup
of the patients of Rabins *et al.* (1987), but who had their illness onset after the age of 60.
VBR was (not unexpectedly) increased in these patients compared with a group of 14
age-matched normal controls.

Naguib & Levy (1987) prospectively identified and CT scanned 45 patients with late
paraphrenia and reported an increase in VBR measurements that was strikingly similar
to that of the late-onset schizophrenic patients examined by Rabins *et al.* (1987). Mean
VBR in patients was 13.09% compared with 9.75% in controls. Since larger values of VBR
were not associated with length of illness or any measured cognitive parameters, the
authors suggested that the observed structural abnormality might have preceded the
appearance of psychosis. Burns *et al.* (1989) performed visual ratings of sulcal widening
on most of Naguib & Levy's (1987) patients and reported no differences in sulcal appearance between patients and controls, despite the presence of enlarged ventricles in
patients.

A reexamination of lateral ventricular size on the scans of Naguib & Levy's (1987)
patients, using a visual rating scale, and planimetric measurements made on CT scans of
14 prospectively recruited late paraphrenics failed to confirm the presence of ventricular
enlargement but demonstrated less well-preserved cerebral cortices in patients who had
not experienced Schneiderian first-rank symptoms (Howard *et al.*, 1992a, b).

Förstl and his coworkers (1994) have reported the results of quantitative CT measurements of the third and lateral ventricles, right and left Sylvian and anterior fissures in 14
patients with 'late paranoid psychosis' (onset after 50 years), 14 patients with AD and 14
age- and sex-matched 'undemented controls'. All of the measurements from the paranoid patients yielded values that were intermediate between those from the controls and
the AD patients. For example, VBR was 7.83% in controls, 12.22% in paranoid psychosis
and 16.90% in patients with AD. Length of illness came close to being inversely correlated
with the areas of the third ($r = -0.46$) and lateral ($r = -0.43$) ventricles. Small vascular
lesions were seen in six patients and basal ganglia calcification was present in three.
Paranoid psychosis patients who had first-rank symptoms had significantly smaller VBR
estimations than those who did not (10.6% compared with 14.7%).

Exclusion from CT studies of patients with obvious neurological signs or history of
stroke, alcohol abuse or dementia has shown that structural abnormalities other than
large ventricles on CT in patients with late paraphrenia are probably no more common

than in controls. However, despite apparently adhering to these exclusions, Flint, Rifat & Eastwood (1991) found areas of clinically unsuspected cerebral infarction on the scans of 5 out of 16 late paraphrenic patients. Most of these infarcts were subcortical or frontal and they were more likely to occur in patients with delusions but no hallucinations. The results of this study need to be interpreted with some caution, since only 16 of a collected sample of 33 patients had actually undergone CT scanning. It is possible that these represented the more 'organic' cases, or at least those that were thought most likely to have some underlying structural abnormality.

MRI

The superiority of MRI over CT, both in terms of gray/white matter resolution and visualization of deep white matter regions is undoubted. A large number of MRI studies of the brains of elderly patients with depression and schizophrenia-like illnesses have taken advantage of this feature specifically to examine changes in periventricular and deep white matter. The results need to be interpreted with some caution, since few studies have assessed abnormalities in the white matter in a standardized manner and appropriate control populations matched for cerebrovascular disease risk factors are rarely used.

MRI studies of WMHI

Among populations of elderly subjects examined with MRI, areas of signal hyperintensity within white matter are a common finding. WMHI are reported to occur in from 30% (Bradley et al., 1984) to 90% (Awad et al., 1987) of the nonpsychiatric elderly population. They appear to be associated with increasing age (Bondareff et al., 1990; Deicken et al., 1991; Kobari, Meyer & Ichijo, 1990; Zubenko et al., 1990) and hypertension (Bondareff et al., 1990; Deicken et al., 1991). There are further reports of associations with a late onset of depression (Churchill et al., 1991; Coffey et al., 1989; 1990; Howard et al., 1993a; Krishnan et al., 1988; Lesser et al., 1991; Rabins et al., 1991; Zubenko et al., 1990) and schizophrenic symptoms (Breitner et al., 1990; Jeste et al., 1991; Lesser et al., 1991; Miller et al., 1989; 1991; 1992).

The precise clinical significance and underlying neuropathological nature of such WMHI remain unclear. 'Caps' of signal hyperintensity anterior to the frontal horns of the lateral ventricles, together with patches of white matter signal abnormality that are distinct from periventricular changes are more common in patients who have sustained cerebral infarction than among elderly controls whose indication for MRI was evaluation of headache or dizziness (Kertesz et al., 1988). However, 'rims' of hyperintensity around the lateral ventricles are seen in 74% of such elderly controls (Kertesz et al., 1988) and have been dubbed 'pseudolesions', regarded as normal phenomena in the elderly (Baldwin, 1993; Bondareff et al., 1990; Sze et al., 1986). Demonstration of the presence of extensive WMHI for up to 7 years in the brains of subjects without neurological or cognitive deficit (Fein et al., 1990) further suggests that even quite large patches of WMHI do not necessarily indicate clinically significant central nervous system disease. In the absence of studies of the prevalence of WMHI in normal elderly people living in the community, no true normative data for these phenomena have been available (Baldwin, 1993).

Exactly what such areas of signal hyperintensity represent in neuropathologic terms has still to be established. Since WMHI are found in association with a variety of neuropsychiatric conditions including AD (Fazekas *et al.*, 1987; Mirsen *et al.*, 1991) and vascular dementia (Hershey *et al.*, 1987; Kinkel *et al.*, 1985), they may indicate the presence of several types of pathology. Attempts to correlate both ante- and postmortem MRI images with neuropathologic examination of brains have demonstrated that each of the recognized types of hyperintense signal lesion (rims, caps, punctate and patchy lesions) have their own distinct neuropathologic correlates. Rims are characterized by subependymal gliosis and loss of ependymal lining, caps and punctate lesions by dilated perivascular spaces and gliosis, and large patches by myelin pallor and dilated perivascular spaces (Chimowitz *et al.*, 1992). The results of MRI studies of white matter abnormality in patients with a late-life onset of schizophrenic symptoms have been interpreted by their authors as evidence for organic etiology. In a series of eight patients without focal neurological signs (Breitner *et al.*, 1990), all showed significant white matter abnormality or vascular pathology on MRI. Temporoparietal and occipital lesions were particularly prevalent and little such pathology was evident on the scans of normal controls.

Miller and colleagues (1989; 1991; 1992) have reported the results of structural MRI investigations in patients with what they have termed 'late life psychosis'. If their results are taken at face value, then 42% of nondemented patients with an onset of psychosis after the age of 45 (mean age at scanning 60.1 years) were found to have white matter abnormalities on MRI, compared with only 8% of a healthy age-matched control group. The appearance of large patchy WMHI was six times more likely in the temporal lobes and four times more likely in the frontal lobes of patients than in controls (Miller *et al.*, 1991). These authors have hypothesized that, while insufficient to give rise to focal neurological signs, WMHI might produce dysfunction in the overlying frontal and temporal cortex which could contribute to psychotic symptomatology. They acknowledge that, since WMHI in the occipital lobes could also be implicated, it might not be possible to pinpoint an isolated anatomical site of white matter lesion that may predispose to psychosis. When comparisons were made between those patients who had structural brain abnormalities on MRI (10) with those who did not (7), there were no significant differences on age, educational level, IQ or performance on a wide battery of neuropsychological tests. Measurements of VBR indicated a nonsignificant increase in patients (10.6%) compared with controls (8.8%).

Although the DSM-IIIR (American Psychiatric Association, 1987) diagnoses of the 24 patients used by Miller *et al.* (1991) were given as schizophrenic disorder (late-onset type) (ten), delusional disorder (seven), schizophreniform psychosis (two) and psychosis not otherwise specified (five), these diagnoses were based upon an assessment made at the time of initial patient referral. The authors conceded that 'at the completion of the examinations, some diagnoses would have been changed to either organic delusional syndromes or to organic hallucinosis'. In fact, two patients were said to have gait disturbances suggestive of previous stroke, one had a history of transient ischemic attacks, five had Binswanger's disease, two had severe cognitive and memory difficulties and were given later diagnoses of AD and Pick's disease, one had a brain tumor and one had evidence of previous traumatic brain injury. Thus, 12 of the original cases of 'late life psychosis' had clear organic psychoses (even without the benefit of cognitive follow-up) and would not have been considered to have late-onset schizophrenia or late paraphrenia by most workers in the field.

In a comparison of T_2-weighted axial images taken from 38 late paraphrenic patients (age at psychosis onset >60 years), from which group cases of dementia or previous stroke had been carefully excluded, with images from 31 healthy age-matched community controls, areas of periventricular WHMI were found in about 96% of both patients and controls (Howard et al., 1995a). Deep WMHI were almost as common in both groups, with no significant differences between patients and controls. Severity of white matter change on all scans was significantly associated with subject age and the presence of hypertension.

Volumetric MRI studies

Pearlson et al. (1993) have reported the results of an MRI study of late-onset schizophrenic patients based on a sample of 11 individuals with illness onset after the age of 55 years. The volume of the third ventricle was derived from its measured area on two contiguous 3 mm coronal images and VBR was calculated from the T_2-weighted axial cut on which the lateral ventricles had their maximal area. Third ventricle volume was significantly greater in the late-onset schizophrenics (mean 561 mm³) than in an age-matched control group (mean 386 mm³). VBR estimations were greater among the late-onset schizophrenics (mean 9.0%) than the controls (mean 7.1%), but this difference did not reach accepted levels of statistical significance. Whole brain and CSF volumes were ascertained from 5 mm axial T_2 images using a semiautomated technique. Mean percentage CSF volume, compared with whole brain volume, was 11.8% in normal controls and 15.5% in late-onset schizophrenics. Once again, this difference did not reach accepted levels of statistical significance.

Howard et al. (1994; 1995b) have reported quantitative volumetric brain measurements from a sample of 50 patients with late paraphrenia. Measures of brain, extracerebral CSF, third and lateral ventricles were made from 5 mm thick coronal T_1-weighted images. When measurements from the late paraphrenics as a whole were compared with those from 35 healthy aged controls, lateral and third ventricular volumes were modestly increased among patients. Those patients whose scans were suitable for volumetric analysis were divided into schizophrenic (31) and delusional disorder (16) subjects. While the schizophrenics had larger right (mean patient volume 13.02 cm³, mean control volume 12.21 cm³) and left (mean patient volume 13.73 cm³, mean control volume 12.25 cm³) lateral and third (mean patient volume 1.27 cm³, mean control volume 1.00 cm³) ventricular volumes than controls, these differences were not statistically significant. Delusional disorder patients, however, had significantly greater right (mean volume 21.32cm^3) and left (mean volume 23.70cm^3) lateral and third (1.55cm^3) ventricular volumes than controls and there was a trend, which just failed to reach statistical significance, for them to have smaller left temporal lobe volumes (63.64cm^3) than control subjects (69.09cm^3) ($p = 0.15$). The volumes of a number of other brain regions, reported as abnormal in previous MRI studies of younger patients with schizophrenia, such as the hippocampus, parahippocampal gyrus, superior temporal gyrus, thalamus and basal ganglia structures were not significantly different between patients and controls.

Summary of structural imaging studies

What is very clear from these studies is that the results obtained strongly reflect the nature of the patients included. If psychotic individuals with a history and clinical signs of neurological disease or marked cognitive impairment are scanned, then workers should not be suprised when they acquire images that reveal both localized and more widespread gross abnormalities of brain structure. Careful selection of patients, with exclusion of those likely to have dementia or neurological disease, together with inclusion of appropriate normal elderly control populations in imaging studies appears to indicate changes in the appearance of the brains of late-onset schizophrenics that are directly analogous to those seen in younger patients. The structural imaging data also suggest that degrees of abnormality of cerebral structure may underly clinical subtypes of late-onset psychosis.

Functional brain imaging

Functional brain imaging includes SPET, PET, MR spectroscopy and functional MRI (see Chapter 1). As the MR techniques have not yet been applied to psychotic disorders in late life, they will not be discussed in this chapter. Although there have been many SPET and PET studies of younger patients with schizophrenia, there is a dearth of studies assessing those with late-onset schizophrenia or late paraphrenia. Because of this, a brief review of findings from those with early-onset schizophrenia is presented first, to allow some comparison with the few studies of the elderly yet reported.

Functional imaging in early-onset schizophrenia

Studies of regional perfusion and metabolism
The first study of CBF in schizophrenia was by Kety *et al.* (1948) who, using a nitrous oxide inhalation method that could only measure *total* CBF, found no differences

between control subjects and those with schizophrenia. Subsequently it became possible to measure rCBF and, using xenon-133 inhalation, Ingvar & Franzen (1974) described a relative hypofrontal pattern of perfusion in schizophrenia. Since then a substantial literature has developed examining the issue of hypofrontality in schizophrenia. A variety of techniques have been used including SPET with xenon-133 or ^{99m}Tc-HMPAO and PET with oxygen-15-labeled water (to measure perfusion) or [^{18}F]FDG (to measure glucose metabolism). Blood flow and/or metabolism was initially measured under resting conditions but, because of the potential variation between individuals under resting conditions, the use of cognitive challenge tasks has become popular (Weinberger, Berman & Zec, 1986). Although conflicting results have been reported, Andreasen *et al.* (1992) reviewed 28 SPET and 19 PET studies in early-onset schizophrenia and concluded that the majority clearly support a dysfunction of the prefrontal cortex in at least some patients with schizophrenia.

However, several uncertainties remain. The observation of hypofrontality in other disorders such as depression (Bench *et al.*, 1992) questions the specificity of this finding for schizophrenia. Other factors such as illness duration, the possible heterogeneity of schizophrenia, symptom profile at time of investigation and exposure to antipsychotic medication might also have effects on rCBF that should be examined (Andreasen *et al.*, 1992). This is particularly so as most blood flow studies have only investigated medicated subjects with chronic schizophrenia. Reports of hypofrontality in subjects who had not received antipsychotic drugs (Andreasen *et al.*, 1992; Buchsbaum *et al.*, 1992) suggest that exposure to such drugs cannot be the sole explanation for hypofrontality in schizophrenia. In an important study, Berman *et al.* (1992) measured rCBF with xenon-133 inhalation in eight pairs of monozygotic twins who were concordant for schizophrenia, ten pairs who were discordant for schizophrenia and three pairs in which neither twin had schizophrenia. Subjects were studied under three conditions: rest, a number matching test (a control task) and the Wisconsin card sorting test (a task linked to prefrontal function). During the Wisconsin card sorting test alone, all of the schizophrenic twins were hypofrontal compared with their unaffected co-twin. Unaffected co-twins were no different to twins who were both normal. The authors concluded, first, that when appropriate controls were used hypofrontality could be demonstrated in most, if not all, schizophrenics and, second, that nongenetic factors were the cause of hypofrontality in schizophrenia. Among twins concordant for schizophrenia, greater antipsychotic drug exposure was not associated with more pronounced hypofrontality, suggesting that rCBF changes were the result of underlying illness rather than drug treatment.

Might hypofrontality in schizophrenia be linked to subtypes of the disorder or reflect specific symptom profiles? Some studies have found a correlation between hypofrontality and the presence of negative, but not positive, symptoms (Andreasen *et al.*, 1992; Gur, Resnick & Gur, 1989; Ingvar & Franzen, 1974; Lewis *et al.*, 1992; Tamminga *et al.*, 1992; Wolkin *et al.*, 1992). This interesting finding has clear parallels with the type I (acute, positive symptoms) and type II (chronic, negative symptoms) dichotomy proposed by Crow (1980). On the basis of symptoms and neuropsychological profiles, Liddle (1987) has proposed that three specific syndromes may be recognized: psychomotor poverty (flatness of affect, poverty of speech), disorganization (thought disorder, inappropriate affect) and reality distortion (delusions and hallucinations). In a PET study of 30 schizophrenic subjects, Liddle et al. (1992) demonstrated that each of the three syndromes was associated with a specific pattern of cerebral perfusion. Psychomotor poverty correlated with hypoperfusion of the left prefrontal cortex, disorganization with hypoperfusion of the right ventral and medial prefrontal cortex and reality distortion with increased perfusion of the left parahippocampal region. Using unmedicated subjects, Ebmeier et al. (1993) replicated some features of each of the blood flow patterns reported by Liddle et al. (1992), though they did not find a positive correlation between reality distortion and left temporal lobe blood flow. McGuire, Shah & Murray (1993) found that blood flow was increased in Broca's area during auditory hallucinations, suggesting that the production of auditory hallucinations in schizophrenia is associated with increased activity in cortical areas specialized for language.

In summary, such work clearly indicates that specific CBF patterns may be related to certain symptoms or syndromes. However, further clarification is required before any firm conclusions can be drawn.

As well as hypofrontality, other regional changes in perfusion and/or metabolism have been described in schizophrenia, most particularly increased perfusion in temporal lobes and basal ganglia (Woods, 1992). Such changes are less consistent and less clearly defined than frontal lobe changes and their significance remains uncertain. Current evidence suggests that increased perfusion and metabolism of basal ganglia in schizophrenia may be the result of antipsychotic medication (Woods, 1992).

Receptor changes

The dopamine hypothesis of schizophrenia has led to the application of specific ligands for dopamine receptors to the study of the syndrome. Using [^{11}C]methylspiperone and PET, Wong et al. (1986) reported increased binding in patients with schizophrenia compared with controls. They interpreted this as evidence of increased dopamine D_2 receptor density, consistent with the dopamine overactivity hypothesis of schizophrenia and the postulated mechanism of antipsychotic drug action at the D_2 receptors. However, Farde et al. (1987) could not replicate this finding using the ligand [^{3}H]raclopride. This discrepancy may be explained by the findings of a recent postmortem study that there is a sixfold increase in dopamine D_4 receptors in schizophrenia, while D_2 receptors were only increased by 10% (Seeman, Guan & Van Toi, 1993). As [^{11}C]methylspiperone binds D_4 receptors as well as D_2 and D_3 receptors, while [^{3}H]raclopride binds only D_2 and D_3 receptors (Seeman et al., 1993), the increase in binding observed by Wong et al. (1986) may reflect an increase in D_4 rather than D_2 receptors. In support of this, Pilowsky et al. (1994) found no overall increase in dopamine D_2 receptors in the basal ganglia with SPET using the D_2 ligand [^{123}I]IBZM. This study did find that subtle changes in D_2 receptors may occur, as there was a left lateralized asymmetry of striatal D_2 receptors (in male patients only) and an absence in schizophrenic subjects of the expected decline in D_2 receptors with age. In summary, in vivo confirmation of in vitro changes in dopamine receptor density in schizophrenia has been limited. This may be partly because of the lack of specificity of some of the ligands used. Convincing and consistent *in vivo* changes in dopamine receptors in schizophrenia remain to be demonstrated.

Functional imaging in late-onset schizophrenia

Using some of the subjects that had taken part in the structural imaging studies reported above, Miller *et al.* (1992) reported SPET findings from 18 subjects with late life psychosis, 12 with late life psychotic depression and 30 age-matched controls. Clearly the caveats outlined above with regard to subject selection and diagnostic accuracy apply equally to this study. Using ^{99m}Tc-HMPAO and a rotating gamma camera, SPET scans acquired were rated visually, and hypoperfusion was defined as blood flow less than 66% of maximal cerebral uptake. Quantification of results was not possible. In 83% of those with late life psychosis and 83% of those with late life psychotic depression there was at least one area of hypoperfusion, significantly more than the 27% of controls with similar deficits. Frontal hypoperfusion was seen in 39% of subjects with late life psychosis, 66% of those with depression and 13% of controls. The most common pattern of hypoperfusion was patchy and multifocal, resembling that seen in subjects with vascular dementia. Areas of hypoperfusion on SPET tended to be associated with MRI lesions, although no absolute association was seen. Some anecdotal associations were noted between perfusion deficits and symptoms, as three out of four subjects with occipital perfusion deficits had visual hallucinations. The authors concluded that SPET changes in late life psychosis were heterogeneous but tended to support clinical and structural imaging changes, though the results did not support the notion of a single brain region in the pathogenesis of late life psychosis or late life psychotic depression. A recent pilot study of ^{99m}Tc-HMPAO SPET in late-onset schizophrenia supports this view (Huang, 1994). Of four subjects studied, two had normal scans on visual inspection, one a clear area of left frontal hypoperfusion while the remaining subject demonstrated right temporoparietal hypoperfusion.

Dopamine receptor changes have also been examined in late-onset psychotic disorders. Pearlson *et al.* (1993) report findings from a PET study with the ligand [^{11}C]methylspiperone that included 13 patients with late-onset (onset after age 55) schizophrenia never treated with antipsychotic drugs and 17 controls. Unfortunately, the controls were not matched with patients for either age or sex (mean (SD) age: controls 39 years (25), patients 74 years (13); proportion women: controls 29%, patients 77%), both of which are known to influence dopamine receptor density. In an attempt to overcome this problem, a predicted neuroreceptor concentration (B_{max}) for each patient was computed by regression of control values with age and sex as predictors. The B_{max} residuals were significantly higher in those with schizophrenia compared with controls, a finding interpreted by the authors as indicating increased dopamine D_2 receptor density in late-onset schizophrenia, mirroring the results obtained by the same group in younger subjects (Wong *et al.*, 1986). However, as previously discussed, [^{11}C]methylspiperone may not be a specific D_2 receptor ligand and may bind to D_3 and D_4 receptors as well

(Seeman *et al.*, 1993). Howard, Cluckie & Levy (1993b) examined six never-medicated female subjects with late paraphrenia who also fulfilled DSM-IIIR criteria for late-onset schizophrenia and five age-matched female controls. No rise in basal ganglia D_2 receptor binding was found with the $[^{123}I]$iodobenzamide D_2 ligand, similar to the negative findings in younger patients using this ligand reported by Pilowsky *et al.* (1994).

Summary of functional imaging studies

Functional brain imaging studies of late-onset schizophrenia and late paraphrenia are still in their infancy. From the preliminary data available it appears that hypofrontality does occur in some cases of late-onset schizophrenia, but that it is not a universal finding, nor does it appear to occur more often in late-onset schizophrenia than in late-onset psychotic depression (Miller *et al.*, 1992). Studies using dopamine receptor ligands mirror results obtained with younger subjects. As hypofrontality correlates with negative symptoms, at least in younger subjects, such a finding might be expected to be less frequent in the elderly, whose illness is characterized by positive, not negative, symptoms. Conversely, the clear heterogeneity of patients presenting with late paraphrenia (Holden, 1987) suggests that a variety of CBF patterns might be seen, with some patients presenting with a pattern more characteristic of an organic disorder (e.g. Charlesworth *et al.*, 1993). Further functional imaging studies of late-onset schizophrenia and late paraphrenia are required. These must include quantification of data in addition to visual inspection, rigorous definition of cases, careful selection of controls and validation of diagnosis by follow-up.

Conclusion

Studies showing gross structural brain changes in elderly subjects with psychotic disorders are nearly always methodologically flawed by the use of unrepresentative patient samples, the inclusion of subjects with organic disorders or other medical illnesses and the absence of appropriate control groups. While the study of more carefully selected and representative subjects has not confirmed a high prevalence of cerebral pathology in such patients, more subtle changes of ventricular enlargement are seen. The etiology and significance of this is unknown, though ventricular enlargement may be more marked in those with delusional disorder than in those with late-onset schizophrenia. Although there are few functional imaging studies of late-onset psychotic disorders, they generally mirror results with younger patients with schizophrenia. However, it is not known how changes revealed by structural and functional imaging are related to each other, nor whether they predate illness, progress over time or carry any prognostic significance in terms of relapse of cognitive decline. There is a clear need for further research, which should include rigorous clinical assessment of patients using a variety of diagnostic criteria, the use (preferably combined) of structural and functional imaging techniques as well as long-term follow-up of subjects.

References

American Psychiatric Association (1980). *Diagnostic and Statistical Manual of Mental Disorders*, 3rd edn. Washington DC: American Psychiatric Association.

American Psychiatric Association (1987). *Diagnostic and Statistical Manual of Mental Disorders*, 3rd edn (revised). Washington, DC: American Psychiatric Association.

American Psychiatric Association (1994). *Diagnostic and Statistical Manual of Mental Disorders*, 4th edn. Washington DC: American Psychiatric Association.

Andreasen, N.C., Rezai, K., Alliger, R. *et al.* (1992). Hypofrontality in neuroleptic-naive patients and in patients with chronic schizophrenia. *Archives of General Psychiatry*, 49, 943–958.

Awad, I.A., Spetzler, R.F., Hodak, J.A., Awad, C.A., Williams, F. & Carey, R. (1987). Incidental lesions noted on magnetic resonance imaging of the brain: prevalence and clinical significance in various age groups. *Neurosurgery*, 20, 222–226.

Baldwin, R.C. (1993). Late life depression and structural brain changes: a review of recent magnetic resonance imaging research. *International Journal of Geriatric Psychiatry*, 8, 115–123.

Bench, C.J., Friston, K.J., Brown, R.G., Scott, L.C., Frackowiak, R.S.J. & Dolan, R.J. (1992). The anatomy of melancholia – focal abnormalities of cerebral blood flow in major depression. *Psychological Medicine*, 22, 607–615.

Berman, K.F., Torrey, E.F., Daniel, D.G. & Weinberger, D.R. (1992). Regional cerebral blood flow in monozygotic twins discordant and concordant for schizophrenia. *Archives of General Psychiatry*, 49, 927–934.

Bondareff, W., Raval, J., Woo, B., Hauser, D.L. & Colletti, P.M. (1990). Magnetic resonance imaging and the severity of dementia in older adults. *Archives of General Psychiatry*, 47, 47–51.

Bradley, W.G., Waluch, V., Brant-Zawadzki, M., Yadley, R.A. & Wyckoff, R.R. (1984). Patchy periventricular white matter lesions in the elderly: a common observation during NMR imaging. *Noninvasive Imaging*, 1, 35–41.

Breitner, J.C., Husain, M., Krishnan, K., Figiel, G. & Boyko, O. (1990). Cerebral white matter disease in late-onset paranoid psychosis. *Biological Psychiatry*, 28, 266–274.

Buchsbaum, M.S., Haier, R.J., Potkin, S.G. *et al.* (1992). Frontostriatal disorder of cerebral metabolism in never-medicated schizophrenics. *Archives of General Psychiatry*, 49, 935–942.

Burns, A., Carrick, J., Ames, D., Naguib, M. & Levy, R. (1989). The cerebral cortical appearance in late paraphrenia. *International Journal of Geriatric Psychiatry*, 4, 31–34.

Charlesworth, G.M., Hymas, N., Wischik, C.M., Hodges, J.R. & Sahakian, B. (1993). Late paraphrenia, advanced schizophrenic deterioration and dementia. *International Journal of Geriatric Psychiatry*, 8, 765–773.

Chimowitz, M.I., Estes, M.L., Furlan, A.J. & Awad, I.A. (1992). Further observations on the pathology of subcortical lesions identified on magnetic resonance imaging. *Archives of Neurology*, 49, 747–752.

Churchill, C.M., Priolo, C.V., Nemeroff, C.B., Krishnan, K. & Breitner, J.C. (1991). Occult subcortical magnetic resonance findings in elderly depressives. *International Journal of Geriatric Psychiatry*, 6, 213–216.

Coffey, C.E., Figiel, G.S., Djang, W.T., Saunders, W.B. & Weiner, R.D. (1989). White matter hyperintensity on magnetic resonance imaging: clinical and neuroanatomic correlates in the depressed elderly. *Journal of Neuropsychiatry*, 2, 135–144.

Coffey, C.E., Figiel, G.S., Djang, W.T. & Weiner, R.D. (1990). Subcortical hyperintensity on magnetic resonance imaging: a comparison of normal and depressed elderly subjects. *American Journal of Psychiatry*, 147, 187–189.

Crow, T.J. (1980). Molecular pathology of schizophrenia: more than one disease process? *British Medical Journal*, 280, 1–9.

Deicken, R.F., Reus, V.I., Manfredi, L. & Wolkowitz, O.M. (1991). MRI deep white matter hyperintensity in a psychiatric population. *Biological Psychiatry*, 29, 918–922.

Ebmeier, K.P., Blackwood, D.H.R., Murray, C. *et al.* (1993). Single photon emission tomography with 99m Tc-exametazime in unmedicated schizophrenic patients. *Biological Psychiatry*, 33, 487–495.

Farde, L., Wiesel, F.A., Hall, H., Stone-Elander, S. & Sedvall, G. (1987). No D_2 receptor increase in PET study of schizophrenia. *Archives of General Psychiatry*, 44, 671–672.

Fazekas, F., Chawluck, J.B., Alavi, A., Hurtig, H.I. & Zimmerman, R. (1987). MR signal abnormalities at 1.5T in Alzheimer's dementia and normal aging. *American Journal of Neuroradiology*, 8, 421–426.

Fein, G., van Dyke, C., Davenport, L. *et al.* (1990). Preservation of normal cognitive functioning in elderly subjects with extensive white-matter lesions of long duration. *Archives of General Psychiatry*, 47, 220–223.

Flint, A., Rifat, S. & Eastwood, M. (1991). Late-onset paranoia: distinct from paraphrenia? *International Journal of Geriatric Psychiatry*, 6, 103–109.

Folstein, M.F., Folstein, S.E. & McHugh, P.R. (1975). 'Mini-mental state', a practical method of grading the cognitive state of patients for the clinician. *Journal of Psychiatric Research*, 12, 189–198.

Förstl, H., Dalgalarrondo, P., Riecher-Rossler, A., Lotz, M., Geiger-Kabisch, C. & Hentschel, F. (1994). Organic factors and the clinical features of late paranoid psychosis: a comparison with Alzheimer's disease and normal ageing. *Acta Psychiatrica Scandinavica*, 89, 335–340.

Gur, R.E., Resnick, S.M. & Gur, R.C. (1989). Laterality and frontality of cerebral blood flow and metabolism in schizophrenia: relationship to symptom specificity. *Psychiatric Research*, 27, 325–334.

Haug, J.O. (1962). Pneumoencephalographic studies in mental disease. *Acta Psychiatrica Scandinavica*, 38 (Suppl.), 165.

Hershey, L.A., Modic, M.T., Greeough, P.G. & Jaffe, D.F. (1987). Magnetic resonance imaging in vascular dementia. *Neurology*, 37, 29–36.

Holden, N.L. (1987). Late paraphrenia or the paraphrenias? A descriptive study with a 10-year follow-up. *British Journal of Psychiatry*, 150, 635–639.

Howard, R., Almeida, O., Levy, R., Graves, P. & Graves, M. (1994). Quantitative magnetic resonance imaging volumetry distinguishes delusional disorder from late-onset schizophrenia. *British Journal of Psychiatry*, 165, 474–480.

Howard, R., Beats, B., Förstl, H., Graves, P., Bingham, J. & Levy, R. (1993a). White matter changes in late-onset depression: a magnetic resonance imaging study. *International Journal of Geriatric Psychiatry*, 8, 183–185.

Howard, R., Cluckie, A. & Levy, R. (1993b). Striatal-D$_2$ receptor binding in late paraphrenia. *Lancet*, 342, 562.

Howard, R., Cox, T., Almeida, O. *et al.* (1995a). White matter signal hyperintensities in the brains of patients with late paraphrenia and the normal community living elderly. *Biological Psychiatry*, 38, 86–91.

Howard, R., Förstl, H., Almeida, O., Burns, A. & Levy, R. (1992a). Computer assisted CT measurements in late paraphrenics with and without Schneiderian first rank symptoms: a preliminary report. *International Journal of Geriatric Psychiatry*, 7, 35–38.

Howard, R., Förstl, H., Naguib, M., Burns, A. & Levy, R. (1992b). First rank symptoms in late paraphrenia: cortical structural correlates. *British Journal of Psychiatry*, 160, 108–109.

Howard, R., Mellers, J., Petty, R. *et al.* (1995b). Magnetic resonance imaging volumetric measurements of the superior temporal gyrus, hippocampus, parahippocampal gyrus, frontal and temporal lobes in late paraphrenia. *Psychological Medicine*, 25, 495–503.

Huang, C.Y. (1994). Schizophrenia and Schizophrenia like Illnesses in the Elderly. A Study of Risk Factors, Phenomenology and Neuroimaging Findings. Dissertation for Part II of Fellowship of RANZCP. Melbourne: Royal Australian and New Zealand College of Psychiatrists.

Ingvar, D.H. & Franzen, G. (1974). Abnormalities of cerebral blood flow distribution in patients with chronic schizophrenia. *Acta Psychiatrica Scandinavica*, 50, 425–462.

Jeste, D.V., Dupont, R., Jernigan, T., Sewell, D., Heindel, W. & Harris, M.J. (1991). Clinical and brain-imaging studies of late-onset schizophrenia. Abstract in *American College of Neuropsychopharmacology, 30th Annual Meeting*, San Juan, Puerto Rico, 9–13 December, p. 55.

Kertesz, A., Black, S.E., Tokar, G., Benke T., Carr, T. & Nicholson, L. (1988). Periventricular and subcortical hyperintensities on magnetic resonance imaging: 'rims, caps and unidentified bright objects'. *Archives of Neurology*, 45, 404–408.

Kety, S.S., Woodford, R.B., Harmel, M.H., Freyhan, F.A., Appel, K.E. & Schmidt, C.F. (1948). Cerebral blood flow and metabolism in schizophrenia: the effects of barbiturate seminarcosis, insulin coma and electroshock. *American Journal of Psychiatry*, 104, 765–770.

Kinkel, W.R., Jacobs, L., Polachini, I. & Bates, V. (1985). Subcortical arteriosclerotic encephalopathy (Binswanger's disease): computed tomographic, nuclear magnetic resonance and clinical correlations. *Archives of Neurology*, 42, 951–959.

Kobari, M., Meyer, J.S. & Ichijo, M. (1990). Leuko-araiosis, cerebral atrophy and cerebral perfusion in normal aging. *Archives of Neurology*, 47, 161–165.

Krishnan, K., Goli, V., Ellinwood, E.H., France, R.D., Blazer, D.G. & Nemeroff, C.B. (1988). Leukoencephalopathy in patients diagnosed as major depressive. *Biological Psychiatry*, 23, 519–522.

Lesser, I.M., Miller, B.L., Boone, K.B. *et al.* (1991). Brain injury and cognitive function in late-onset psychotic depression. *Journal of Neuropsychiatry and Clinical Neuroscience*, 3, 33–40.

Lewis, S.W., Ford, R.A., Syed, G.M., Reveley, A.M. & Toone, B.K. (1992). A controlled study of ^{99m}Tc-HMPAO single-photon emission imaging in chronic schizophrenia. *Psychological Medicine*, 22, 27–35.

Liddle, P.F. (1987). The symptoms of chronic schizophrenia: a re-examination of the positive–negative dichotomy. *British Journal of Psychiatry*, 151, 145–151.

Liddle, P.F., Friston, K.J., Frith, C.D., Hirsch, S.R., Jones, T. & Frackowiak, R.S.J. (1992). Patterns of cerebral blood flow in schizophrenia. *British Journal of Psychiatry*, 169, 179–186.

McGuire, P.K., Shah, G.M.S. & Murray, R.M. (1993). Increased blood flow in Broca's area during auditory hallucinations in schizophrenia. *Lancet*, 342, 703–706.

Miller, B., Benson, F., Cummings, J.L. & Neshkes, R. (1986). Late-life paraphrenia: an organic delusional syndrome. *Journal of Clinical Psychiatry*, 47, 204–207.

Miller, B.L., Lesser, I.M., Boone, K. *et al.* (1989). Brain white matter lesions and psychosis. *British Journal of Psychiatry*, 155, 73–78.

Miller, B.L., Lesser, I., Boone, K., Hill, E., Mehringer, C. & Wong, K. (1991). Brain lesions and cognitive function in late-life psychosis. *British Journal of Psychiatry*, 158, 76–82.

Miller, B.L., Lesser, I.M., Mena, I. *et al.* (1992). Regional cerebral blood flow in late-life-onset psychosis. *Neuropsychiatry, Neuropsychology, and Behavioral Neurology*, 5, 132–137.

Mirsen, T.R., Lee, D.H., Wong, C.J. *et al.* (1991). Clinical correlates of white matter changes on magnetic resonance imaging scans of the brain. *Archives of Neurology*, 48, 1015–1021.

Naguib, M. & Levy, R. (1987). Late paraphrenia: neuropsychological impairment and structural brain abnormalities on computed tomography. *International Journal of Geriatric Psychiatry*, 2, 83–90.

Pearlson, G.D., Garbacz, D., Tompkins, R.H., Ahn, H.O. & Rabins, P.V. (1987). Lateral cerebral ventricular size in late-onset schizophrenia. In *Schizophrenia and Aging*, ed. N.E. Miller & G.D. Cohen, pp. 246–248. New York: Guildford Press.

Pearlson, G.D., Tune, L.E., Wong, D.F. *et al.* (1993). Quantitative D_2 dopamine receptor PET and structural MRI changes in late-onset schizophrenia. *Schizophrenia Bulletin*, 19, 783–795.

Pilowsky, L.S., Costa, D.C., Ell, P.J., Verhoeff, N.P.L.G., Murray, R.M. & Kerwin, R.W. (1994). D_2 dopamine receptor binding in the basal ganglia of antipsychotic-free schizophrenic patients. *British Journal of Psychiatry*, 164, 16–26.

Rabins, P.V., Pearlson, G.D., Aylward, E., Kumar, A.J. & Dowell, K. (1991). Cortical magnetic resonance imaging changes in elderly inpatients with major depression. *American Journal of Psychiatry*, 148, 617–620.

Rabins, P.V., Pearlson, G.D., Jayaram, G., Steele, C. & Tune, L.E. (1987). Ventricle-to-brain ratio in late-onset schizophrenia. *American Journal of Psychiatry*, 144, 1216–1218.

Roth, M. & Morrisey, J. (1952). Problems in the diagnosis and classification of mental disorders in old age. *Journal of Mental Science*, 98, 66–80.

Seeman, P., Guan, H.C. & van Toi, H.H.M. (1993). Dopamine D_4 receptors elevated in schizophrenia. *Nature*, 365, 441–445.

Sze, G., de Armond, S.J., Brant-Zawadzki, M., Davis, R.L., Norman, D. & Newton, T. (1986). Foci of MRI signal (pseudolesions) anterior to the frontal horns: histologic correlations of a normal finding. *American Journal of Radiology*, 147, 331–337.

Tamminga, C.A., Thaker, G.K., Buchanan, R. *et al.* (1992). Limbic system abnormalities identified in schizophrenia using positron emission tomography with fluoro-deoxyglucose and neocortical alterations with deficit syndrome. *Archives of General Psychiatry*, 49, 522–530.

Weinberger, D.R., Berman, K.F. & Zec, R.F. (1986). Physiological dysfunction of dorsolateral prefrontal cortex in schizophrenia, I: regional cerebral blood flow (rCBF) evidence. *Archives of General Psychiatry*, 43, 114–124.

Wolkin, A., Sanflipo, M., Wolf, A.P., Angrist, B., Brodie, J.D. & Rotrosen, J. (1992). Negative symptoms and hypofrontality in chronic schizophrenia. *Archives of General Psychiatry*, 49, 959–965.

Wong, D.F., Wagner, H.N. Jr, Tune, L.E. *et al.* (1986). Positron emission tomography reveals elevated D_2 dopamine receptors in drug-naive schizophrenics. *Science*, 234, 1558–1563.

Woods, S.W. (1992). Regional cerebral blood flow imaging with SPECT in psychiatric disease: focus on schizophrenia, anxiety disorders, and substance abuse. *Journal of Clinical Psychiatry*, 53 (Suppl. 11), 20–25.

World Health Organization (1992). The *ICD10 Classification of Mental and Behavioural Disorders. Clinical Descriptions and Diagnostic Guidelines*. Geneva: World Health Organization.

Zubenko, G.S., Sullivan, P., Nelson, J.P., Belle, S.H., Huff, J. & Wolf, G. (1990). Brain imaging abnormalities in mental disorders of late life. *Archives of Neurology*, 47, 1107–1111.

Part 3
Clinical guidelines

9(a) Indications for neuroimaging

Andrew Leuchter

Introduction

Recent research into late life mental disorders has revealed a host of structural and functional changes in the brains of elderly psychiatric patients. It now is clear that those with structural changes (such as increased atrophy on CT or WMHI on MRI) have a different prognosis from depressed or demented patients without such changes. Several studies also have established that patients with late life depression have characteristic global decreases in cerebral perfusion and metabolism that may distinguish them from those with dementia.

These research findings help to elucidate the pathophysiology of late-life mental disorders and may explain some of the heterogeneity in presentation and prognosis. Our ability to image the brain, however, has in some cases outpaced our ability to understand the clinical implications of the structural and functional findings seen using modern neuroimaging techniques.

Clinical application of neuroimaging techniques has flourished since the early 1970s, seemingly under the basic principle of 'the more we know, the better care will be'. With increasing emphasis on medical cost containment, the utilization of these technologies and usefulness of their results must be scrutinized more carefully. Which of the structural and functional findings seen with modern neuroimaging techniques have clinical utility?

CT and MRI scanning

Structural imaging using CT or MRI commonly is performed to screen for reversible mass lesions (meningiomas, subdural hematomas) or irreversible lesions (deep tumors, strokes) that could be contributing to or causing a psychiatric illness. A structural imaging study should, in most cases, be a component of the evaluation of new-onset cognitive losses.

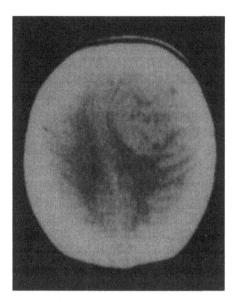

Figure 9.1 *Noncontrast CT scan on a 55-year-old woman with mental status changes but no other focal neurologic signs. The scan shows a large left frontal mass with a large shift with low-density areas in the center, probably representing areas of necrosis.*

The detection of a treatable structural lesion causing reversible cognitive impairment is the most definitive benefit of performing a structural imaging study (Jacoby, Levy & Dawson, 1980). Some physicians claim that a careful neurological examination is adequate to detect any significant mass lesion. While this statement may be true in most cases, it is possible for a slowly developing mass lesion to present with mental status changes in the absence of any peripheral neurologic signs or symptoms. This situation is illustrated by the case of a 55-year-old female who was in good health until she developed the insidious onset of memory deficits and word finding difficulties. These were gradually progressive over a span of eight months, until the deficits became so severe that she was forced to seek medical attention by her family. A scan revealed a large left frontal mass (Fig. 9.1), originally thought to be a glioma because of the size and the low-density necrotic areas seen centrally. A scan with contrast, however, revealed the mass to be a meningioma impinging on the left frontal convexity, apparently starting to herniate across the falx cerebri (Fig. 9.2). This mass was resected, and the patient immediately recovered her cognitive functions without incident. Careful neurological examinations had revealed no focal signs and no papilledema.

The advantage of detecting reversible lesions is clear, since these may be corrected. The advantage of detecting irreversible lesions or other brain features is primarily related to increasing diagnostic certainty, since findings such as stroke, leukoaraiosis or atrophy are not directly amenable to treatment. Such findings may alter the diagnostic formulation: for example, findings of widespread leukoaraiosis or focal atrophy may support a diagnosis of vascular dementia (see Chapter 4). The absence of lacunae or strokes may help to rule out a diagnosis of vascular or mixed dementia and support a diagnosis of AD. The presence of atrophy alone, even using quantitative measures, has not yet been shown to be a strong indicator of dementia (see Chapter 3).

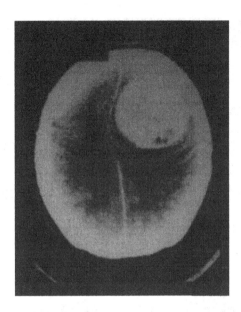

Figure 9.2 *The CT scan with contrast of the patient scanned in Fig. 9.1 shows that the mass is clearly extraaxial, representing a large meningioma.*

The advantages of MRI

In general, significantly more information about brain structure is gained from MRI than from CT scanning (Lufkin, 1990). MRI has superior spatial resolution, can image small brain areas surrounded by bone, can resolve differences between gray and white matter, can detect small areas of white matter demyelination and provides more complete characterization of the nature of lesions than CT scanning (see Chapter 1(b)). The superiority of MRI is illustrated by Figs. 9.3 and 9.4, which show a comparable transaxial image obtained from one patient on a single day. The CT scan (Fig. 9.3) shows a single small area of low density in the left temporal lobe, consistent with an old area of infarction. The contralateral temporal lobe appears normal. The MRI scan (Fig. 9.4) reveals an area of high signal in the area of the old infarction, as well as an extensive area of high signal in the contralateral temporal area, most consistent with a subacute infarction that was isodense with brain tissue by CT. In addition, the MRI shows much greater anatomical detail.

Apart from the example of subacute infarction, there are other clinical situations in which the advantages of MRI militate for its selection over CT. These include evaluation of the following conditions.

New-onset seizures
New-onset seizures may be caused by a small astrocytoma or glioblastoma that may be below the spatial resolution of CT. MRI with gadolinium contrast has a spatial resolution that is far superior to CT.

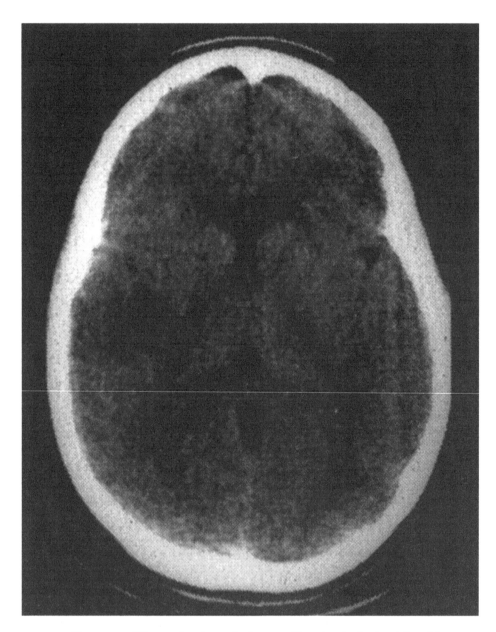

Figure 9.3 *CT scan showing a single area of low density in the right midtemporal region, consistent with loss of brain tissue in the area of an old infarct. The contralateral temporal lobe appears to be normal, with no loss of density or apparent lesions.*

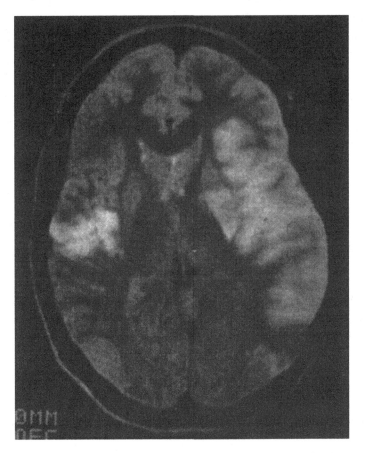

Figure 9.4 *T_2-weighted MRI scan on the same subject as in Fig. 9.3; the scan was performed on the same day and shows a comparable transaxial section. The image shows an area of high signal in the right temporal region, in the same area as the loss of density on the CT scan. In addition, the contralateral temporal lobe shows a large area of high signal, consistent with an area of subacute infarction. Because there has not yet been a loss of tissue density, this area appeared normal on CT.*

Hydrocephalus

Although either CT or MRI can detect the ventricular enlargement of hydrocephalus, MRI is superior for detecting the increased water content in the periventricular region (seen as hyperintensity on T_2-weighted images) that is characteristic of normal-pressure hydrocephalus. Furthermore, the spatial resolution of MRI is essential for evaluation of small obstructions of the aqueductal system, which may differentiate communicating from noncommunicating hydrocephalus.

White matter lesions

Since MRI visualizes proton density rather than electron density, it is superior to CT for the detection of increased water content in the white matter that may be indicative of demyelination. Such demyelination in the elderly commonly results from hypertension, hypotension or the effects of cerebrovascular disease, but it also may be caused by other processes including multiple sclerosis.

Posterior fossa or spinal cord lesions

Lesions in the posterior fossa or spinal cord usually cannot be adequately visualized by CT because of beam hardening artifact. MRI is unaffected by bone surrounding the structure of interest.

Detection of blood brain barrier breakdown

When the integrity of the blood brain barrier is in question (commonly as a result of inflammation, tumor or stroke), a structural imaging study is often indicated. MRI scans with gadolinium contrast generally are preferred to CT scans with iodinated contrast material. Not only is the resolution superior, but gadolinium is more easily eliminated from the body, has a much lower prevalence of allergic reactions and is better tolerated by the patient than iodinated contrast materials.

The advantages of CT

There also are several situations in which CT scanning is preferable to MRI.

Acute hemorrhagic infarct

Acute hemorrhage is better visualized initially on CT scanning, owing to the high protein content of blood and the density difference from brain tissue. The detection of these hemorrhages may be a major reason to perform a structural imaging study. Not until 72–90 hours after hemorrhage, when blood breakdown products such as methemoglobin appear, does MRI become superior for the detection of an infarct.

Calcification

CT retains advantages over MRI for the detection of calcification, because of the sensitivity of X-ray techniques for the visualization of calcium in soft tissues.

Patients with metal, medical or electronic implants

Magnetic metals may be heated, dislodged or ripped from the body by the intense magnetic fields of MRI. Nonmagnetic metals, although they may not pose a danger to the patient, may cause adjacent image distortion. Medical implants (e.g. penile prostheses) or electronic implants (e.g. pacemakers) may be damaged by the magnetic field.

Patients who cannot tolerate MRI

A number of patients have strong negative reactions to confinement in MRI scanners, because of confinement in a narrow space, the noise of the scanner or other factors. MRI may be a particular problem for patients with confusional states, who may become agitated by confinement and may have difficulty remaining still in one position for long periods of time. For these individuals, CT scanning commonly is preferred since machines are more open to the environment and quieter, and the time required to complete a scan is usually shorter.

Accessibility of equipment

In most major metropolitan areas in the USA, MRI scanners are plentiful. Many scanners have extended hours of operation, sometimes 24 hours a day. However, there still is a broader installed base of CT scanners in most American communities and there are many locations and/or times of day when MRI is not readily available. Under these conditions, CT is the logical alternative.

Functional findings

The indications for the use of functional imaging in elderly psychiatric patients are unclear at present. It is clear that there are marked functional disturbances in patients with depression as well as dementia. Patients with either condition have comparable global decreases in perfusion or metabolism, but the topographic distribution of the suppressed activity differs: those with depression show hypoperfusion or hypometabolism primarily over the frontotemporal regions bilaterally or over the right, while those with dementia show decreased activity primarily in the parietal regions bilaterally (Kumar *et al.*, 1993; Lesser *et al.*, 1994).

The diagnostic usefulness of these findings has not been studied extensively. While some studies have suggested that biparietal hypoperfusion on SPET or hypometabolism on PET examination is useful for identifying patients with dementia caused by AD, the sensitivity and specificity of this finding has not been established. Differing patterns of regional hypoperfusion or hypometabolism have been reported in different forms of dementia; for example, frontotemporal perfusion or metabolic deficits have been reported in frontotemporal dementias and may distinguish these patients from those with AD. There have not been large-scale studies, however, comparing specificity of functional findings in patients with different types of dementia (Miller *et al.*, 1994).

The few studies that have compared metabolic and perfusion findings in subjects with dementia and depression show significant differences between the groups (Curran *et al.*, 1993; Kumar *et al.*, 1993), but the clinical usefulness of these findings has not been established (see Chapter 7). One potential exciting use of functional imaging in depressed patients could be the prediction of antidepressant treatment response, since these functional abnormalities appear to resolve during the course of successful antidepressant treatment. There are not adequate data to be certain, however, that the resolution of these changes consistently occurs or is predictive of response (Sackeim & Prohovnik, 1993).

The EEG has been in use as a functional imaging technique for many more years than PET or SPET, and some clinical indications for this technique have been established. It is clear that the EEG is almost invariably abnormal in patients with delirium, and that the degree of abnormality is comparable to the degree of cognitive impairment. EEG, therefore, is useful in establishing or confirming the diagnosis of delirium and in monitoring the treatment offered for this syndrome. QEEG has significantly enhanced the usefulness of EEG for confirming the diagnosis and monitoring the course of delirium, since it more accurately and reproducibly quantifies slowing (Jacobson, Leuchter & Walter, 1993; Leuchter & Jacobson, 1991; see also Chapters 1(d) and 6).

For other applications, such as aiding in the diagnosis of dementia, the applications of EEG are less definitive. The EEG is sensitive for detecting the excessive slowing seen in patients with dementia, but this is a nonspecific finding and may be seen in subjects with delirium or even depression. Focal or asymmetric slowing may indicate cerebrovascular damage and suggest a diagnosis of vascular dementia, but this finding is seen only in a minority of patients with that diagnosis. QEEG has greater applicability than conventional EEG to the assessment of patients with dementia. It is more sensitive to subtle generalized or focal abnormalities and, therefore, may detect brain dysfunction that is not apparent on conventional EEG. Furthermore, QEEG coherence and cordance appear to detect patterns of dysfunction that may be more specific for particular diagnoses (such as AD, vascular dementia or depression).

Conclusion

It is possible to set forth only very broad guidelines regarding the indications for neuroimaging tests in elderly psychiatric patients. The clearest guideline is that for most patients undergoing evaluation of cognitive losses, particularly losses of new onset, a structural imaging study of the brain is advised. Whether this study should be a CT or MRI scan is a matter for the judgment of the individual clinician. It is clear that MRI provides greater detail about brain structure than CT, can detect small lesions and is particularly sensitive for detecting the presence of white matter disease. It provides this information at slightly greater inconvenience to the patient and generally at greater economic cost.

Whether functional imaging studies should be performed also is a matter for clinician judgment. These tests invariably provide additional information about brain physiology and, in contrast to neuropsychologic testing and rating scales, are not likely to give spurious results because of poor motivation or cooperation on the part of the patient. The value of this information must be weighed against the costs of the procedure and the additional exposure of the patient to ionizing radiation.

Clinicians sometimes believe that the additional information from functional studies is likely to be helpful in cases where the presentation is unusual or the diagnosis is unclear. For example, in a patient with an unusual pattern of cognitive losses, if a PET scan revealed a pattern of biparietal hypometabolism consistent with AD, this could clarify the diagnosis. There is little evidence to suggest, however, that complicated clinical presentations are accompanied by clear-cut clinical findings; clinical experience indicates that unusual clusters of symptoms are reflected in unusual findings in brain physiology. No study has established that functional imaging tests systematically clarify diagnostic issues in these difficult cases.

The usefulness of the most advanced imaging technology is in part dependent upon the practice patterns of the clinician and the setting in which they practice. The primary care provider performing evaluations for dementia in the community commonly will order solely a CT scan; a specialist in an academic medical center will frequently order an MRI and at least one functional imaging study in an effort to perform a definitive diagnostic evaluation. Questions which may be asked by the clinician ordering tests include the following:

- What is likely to be the increase in diagnostic certainty as a result of this test?
- Will the increase in diagnostic certainty be of practical benefit to the patient and/or the family?
- Is an increase in diagnostic certainty likely to affect management of the patient?

In many individual cases, the information gained from more in-depth testing will be of comfort and benefit to patients and their families, be it in planning for the future, decreasing anxiety or assessing familial risks for disease. Increases in diagnostic certainty are most likely to affect management in the academic medical center, where more thorough assessment may lead to innovative treatments or advances in understanding of disease.

It is likely that the application of advanced imaging techniques in the clinical setting drives medical research. As clinicians find previously unobserved perturbations in brain function or alterations in brain structure, they frequently pose research questions that otherwise could not be formulated. In addition, clinical application of imaging techniques drives advances in medical imaging. As new technologies find clinical acceptance, the resulting demand for medical equipment fuels research and development in the medical device industry. Clinicians cannot advocate an unofficial 'subsidy' of medical research by government health programs or private insurance. It is important to recognize, however, that advances in clinical knowledge and medical technology may be 'spinoff' benefits from the clinical application of imaging techniques.

The current latitude that clinicians have in ordering neuroimaging tests has both costs and benefits for the health care system, patients and the advance of knowledge. For the health care system, which must pay for millions of CT scans, reduction in the number of tests ordered would appear to be desirable: cost savings from the reduction of diagnostic tests could, for example, subsidize life-saving surgery. For the patient with a frontal meningioma who would herniate without a CT scan to detect the tumor, the brain imaging test is a life-saving procedure of incalculable value. For medical science, the clinical application of neuroimaging techniques leads to new discoveries and technologic advances that may improve health care. We should not substitute strict guidelines for clinician judgment in the selection of neuroimaging tests without a comprehensive assessment of the effects of current physician practices. Short-term cost savings through systematic restriction of the use of neuroimaging tests may have deleterious effects on our patients and the health care system, now and in the future.

Which scan, for whom, when and why

Robin Jacoby

Why these questions?

A Grand Round was taking place at a well-known London medical school.
The registrar (resident) presenting the case began by giving the results of the
patient's investigations and asked for comments as to the diagnosis. No one
in the audience knew what it was and further test results were given. Still the
cause remained obscure. A number of consultants expressed their opinions:
certainly a puzzling case. One senior physician remained silent. When asked
by the chairman if he had anything to say, he replied 'I couldn't possibly
comment. We haven't been given any of the history or findings on examina-
tion, nor even his age. This is not life as we should know it'.

Hounsfield's invention (Hounsfield, 1973) of CT was so exciting and miraculous, especially because it permitted examination of the brain *in vivo* for the first time, that for some
it seemed to be the beginning and the end of diagnosis. Of course, there is little doubt that
it was a turning point in medicine and arguably the most important discovery in imaging
since Roentgen first used X-rays. The benefits to patients were immediate, not least in the
virtual disappearance of pneumoencephalography (PEG), an unpleasant procedure not
without hazard and frequently causing severe headache. With the installation of their first
EMI scanner at the Massachusetts General Hospital, there was an estimated reduction of
73% in PEG over 17 days (Fineberg, Bauman & Sosman, 1977). There was also an estimated
reduction in cerebral angiography and radionuclide scanning of 52% and 41%, respectively. In London at the National Hospital for Neurology and Neurosurgery, the monthly
total of PEG fell from 50 to less than 10 (Gawler *et al.*, 1976). By now PEG has been consigned to history. EMI and later scanners of other manufacture were of course very expensive and their aficionados appreciated, even before the imposition of strict health care
budgets in developed countries in the 1980s, that financial justification for such new
super-technology would be required. Although it is almost invariably possible to mount
a financial case for or against a project from virtually any perspective, there were soon

those who asserted that CT was cost effective or cheaper than the alternatives (Jacobsen, Kragsholm & Holm, 1976; Thomson, 1977).

The immediate appeal of cranial CT, and later of CT below the foramen magnum, was in the diagnosis of space-occupying lesions, principally neoplastic or vascular, with no more invasiveness than a little intravenous contrast medium. Furthermore, the crucial innovation was visualization of the brain substance as opposed to the CSF spaces or vascular tree. It was this factor that clearly brought neuroimaging well into the domain of psychiatry from the margins where it had hitherto been camped. Certainly, some patients with suspected dementia had been subjected to PEG in the past, but air studies had generally been reserved for the minority of younger (presenile) cases. The majority were consigned to large mental hospitals or long-stay geriatric wards without investigation. Not that subjecting the latter to PEG would have necessarily been fruitful or accurate. Nott & Fleminger (1975) had shown that air studies could give a very high rate of misdiagnosis; a finding replicated by Ron et al. (1979). These two studies are almost more important in the history of affective disorder than of dementia, since Ron and her colleagues showed that it was depression which was being missed, and that failure to take account of anamnestic factors and mental state phenomena were major contributors to error. Where neuroimaging – in this case PEG – was concerned, the errors could be reduced if all clinical findings and investigation results were weighted in context. Therefore, enlarged ventricles certainly increased the chance of a diagnosis of dementia; whereas a past history of depression reduced it. Why, however, did some patients whose air encephalograms showed enlarged lateral ventricles, prove not to have dementia? Part of the answer was given later by CT research (e.g. Jacoby et al., 1980), namely that some nondemented individuals simply have enlarged ventricles as part of a distribution which overlaps with that of demented patients. Another reason is that dehydration and possibly other factors to do with the procedure of PEG itself, such as hypocapnia associated with anesthesia, might result in temporary ventricular enlargement (Jacoby & Cohen, 1981).

CT is nearly 25 years old and much has been achieved over this time. In clinical practice for the diagnosis of intracranial space-occupying and many vascular lesions, its preeminence is threatened only by MRI. Even so, routine use of CT after strokes has been challenged on grounds, inter alia, of cost over benefit (Allison, 1994). In psychiatric research, too, advances in knowledge have been largely a result of transmission and emission tomographies. (CT is a transmission tomography because the computed output is derived after X-rays have been *transmitted through* tissue whereas in MRI, SPET and PET output is derived from radiation *emitted from* tissue (see Chapter 1).) These advances are the subject of the other chapters of this book and there is no need to repeat or summarize what readers may find there for themselves. The benefits of neuroimaging are not called into question for the clinical detection of intracranial space-occupying lesions or for research. For the clinical diagnosis and management of functional and neurodegenerative disorders their value is less clear cut. The consequences of uncertainty are not lost on paymasters and budget holders. In the UK, charges to National Health Service (i.e. state-funded) budgets vary somewhat not only between hospital trusts but also according to whether the patient comes from within or outwith the catchment area, and whether or not block contracts are negotiated. However, 1995/96 prices of the following uncomplicated scans in Oxford are in the order of: CT £170, MRI £200, and SPET £250. The routine CT scanning of all patients undergoing investigation for a condition as common as dementia in old age would involve the expenditure of very large sums of money. Setting aside the considerations of intellectual clinical curiosity, the financial factor alone requires us to be clear for whom, when and why we request a scan.

For whom, when and why?

One of the curious phenomena of modern neuroimaging is the discrepancy between the technological sophistication of the various techniques themselves and the relatively unsophisticated way in which their output is used in everyday clinical life. A simple example is enough to illustrate the point. A single image from a CT scan requires the computer to resolve thousands of simultaneous equations in an instant. In the world today, the great majority of CT images, perhaps over 99%, are subjected to nothing more than the eye of a radiologist. There is no doubt that such an eye is highly sophisticated but, although trained to look at new images, the level of sophistication is no different to that of the pre-CT era. When CT was first invented there were those (this author was one) who predicted that in the near future radiology technicians would, at the flick of a switch, obtain pre-programed data such as total ventricular volume, total CSF volume and so on. Clinicians would then have been able to compare results for individual patients with population norms. Why this has not happened provides some answers to the questions posed by this chapter. Three reasons may be suggested, but there are probably more. First, there are technical problems in programing the scanner's computer for accurate output, one of the more serious of which is partial volume artefact; in plain language the accurate differentiation between brain/bone or brain/CSF interfaces (Jacoby *et al.*, 1980). Second, very few (neuro)radiologists are committed to other than 'eyeball' techniques. Third, clinicians as a group have not indicated that they would find it useful. In practice, therefore, they still order scans on which they receive descriptive reports and clinical judgements. We have to recognize this fact in deciding when and whom to scan and should perhaps start to answer the questions by defining three categories of scan: (i) definitive, (ii) informative and (iii) inappropriate.

Definitive scans

Definitive scans are those that are necessary to confirm or refute a diagnosis and, therefore, to determine management.

Space-occupying lesions

By and large the majority of patients in whom an intracranial space-occupying lesion is suspected should undergo CT scanning. CT is the cheapest of the modern neuroimaging techniques and is noninvasive. It is less oppressive than MRI, where the patient has to lie still in a tunnel cut off from the outside world – not an investigation for the claustrophobic. MRI, however, is preferred for lesions suspected in areas where CT yields less satisfactory images. Pituitary and hypothalamic tumors are cases in point. Even if active intervention would be unlikely in, say, the case of a primary cerebral tumor, knowledge of the diagnosis can help patients and their families to plan for the future and clinicians to undertake proper palliative management.

Huntington's disease

A CT scan is indicated if Huntington's disease is suspected. Flattening of the normally rounded heads of the caudate nuclei as they project into the anterior horns of the lateral ventricles is characteristic but not invariable. The importance of making the diagnosis in this devastating condition in a patient who consents to be investigated outweighs any cost considerations.

Informative scans

Informative scans are those that contribute to the probability of a diagnosis. Dementia is the prime example of a condition where scans are informative.

Dementia

Chapters 3, 4 and 5 of this book have discussed the possibilities for and accuracy of diagnosis by neuroimaging in dementia. Without wishing to traduce what the authors have written, the findings could be summarized in highly compressed form as follows. For CT and MRI in AD overall, i.e. in early-, middle- and late-onset disease, significant cerebral atrophy and ventricular enlargement are found. But overlap between AD and the unaffected elderly populations is around 20%. Furthermore, CT and MRI accuracy is more or less of the same order as that of clinical criteria such as those of the NINCDS/ADRDA (McKhann et al., 1984). CT can also be used to demonstrate focal medial temporal atrophy, said to be characteristic of AD and for which higher predictive value has been claimed (Jobst et al., 1992). With MRI of medial temporal structures, sensitivity and specificity of 85–90% have been shown in separating patients with AD from controls (see review by O'Brien, 1995). For vascular dementia, CT and MRI scans will demonstrate abnormalities resulting from vascular lesions such as the discrete lucencies of infarcts and lacunes, and leukoaraiosis. But the diagnosis of vascular dementia has to be based on clinical grounds, namely global cognitive impairment in the context of hypertension or vascular events, such as strokes or transient ischemic attacks. For frontal dementias (Pick's disease or frontal lobe dementia) it is not possible on the basis of research to give the predictive ability of CT or MRI, but suspicion of the diagnosis can be raised by the finding of focal frontotemporal changes. For other dementias, such as prion diseases or Lewy body dementia, there is no evidence that the transmission tomographies differentiate them from, for example, AD. As to other emission tomographies, PET is not effectively a clinical resource and can be discounted from this discussion. SPET, which is more readily available, can show temporoparietal perfusion deficits in AD as well as other focal, e.g. frontal, deficits.

If these are the possibilities offered to clinicians by modern neuroimaging, what is their practical clinical value in the diagnosis and management of dementia? Dementia is above all a *clinical* diagnosis. Does one need to go any further than that in an individual patient for whom there might not be any specific treatment available? Even where specific prophylactic therapy, such as aspirin in cerebrovascular disease, is indicated, is a CT scan necessary before prescribing the tablets? There are those for whom the answer to both questions would be negative on clinical and economic grounds, but this is not a view to support. In opposing it, one must admit that from here onwards science cedes some ground to personal opinion. A diagnosis that is as accurate in life as possible is surely of value to clinicians because it enables them to give a more accurate prognosis and treat intercurrent problems in a more rational and considered way. If future developments in the treatment of dementia, especially AD, are to make progress, it will be vital to differentiate pathological types as far as possible. The question should not, therefore, be whether it is reasonable to try and make an accurate pathologic diagnosis in life, but whether neuroimaging adds accuracy to clinical findings. In the opinion of this author, it does, but not as an either/or entity, which is how the case is too often argued. In other words, it is not a matter whether clinical criteria are better than a scan for making a diagnosis of AD. The one enhances the other. In real life, the clinician faced with a patient whose history and mental state are characteristic of dementia and with a CT or MRI scan that shows enlarged ventricles and dilated sulci is unlikely to think that there is an approximately 20% chance that this scan is that of a normal person. Quite correctly, he or she will make a clinical judgement that the most likely diagnosis is AD and that all the evidence – clinical, laboratory and radiological – tends to support this opinion. Given the same patient but a normal scan, he or she should not fall into the trap of thinking that the diagnosis of dementia *must* be incorrect. In such a case the scan should play a useful role in raising the possibility that some other condition, such as a depressive illness, could be accounting for all or part of the picture. This is the art of medicine which is as important as science. It is also true that in everyday clinical practice there are fewer patients who would fit NINCDS/ADRDA clinical criteria of *probable* AD than *possible* cases. In the author's view, a so-called positive scan may justify its expense by adding confidence to clinical judgement. Although not an exclusive reason for undertaking a scan, because the pick-up rate is low, there is nevertheless the added advantage of detecting hitherto unsuspected space-occupying lesions (Jacoby *et al.*, 1980).

The reader might be forgiven here for asking whether the questions in the title are ever to be given straightforward answers where dementia is concerned. They are, but with the caveat that they must inevitably be to some extent personal to the author. If budget constraints permit, a CT scan is desirable as part of the routine investigation of dementia in patients referred to a specialist service. It is doubtful that scanning all patients in primary care can be justified either on financial or clinical grounds. It has to be said, however, that routine scans in specialist services are a waste of money if clinicians do not take a greater interest in them than simply reading a report, and especially if the radiologists who compose the reports state nothing more than 'normal for the patient's age'. The latter is a judgement of highly dubious validity and one that should not be accepted. If comments relating to age are to be made, it should be on the basis of measurements that can be compared with centiles in appropriately matched control populations. Thus, if the local department of radiology will do it, temporal lobe orientated sections should be requested for the routine investigation of cases of suspected AD. With them, linear measurements of temporal lobe width can be made and compared with age-matched norms. Using this technique, Jobst *et al.* (1992) found a detection rate of 91% with only a 4% false-positive rate in controls; giving expected rates of 92% and 5.7% after fitting a Gaussian model to the distribution. It is worth repeating that any sort of CT scan in this context should not be seen as a make or break diagnostic test but as an enhancement to clinical judgement. MRI scans are generally comparable with CT in the clinical investigation of dementia. In favour of MRI is a higher quality of image and better visualization of white matter, of smaller structures and of areas near brain bone interfaces. MRI images are usually more readily obtainable in planes other than the customary transverse one, e.g. coronal. This enables even better visualization of medial temporal structures (de Leon, 1994). Against MRI is the slightly greater expense, the lesser availability and the relatively oppressive nature of the technique, notably for claustrophobic patients and those whose dementia makes it difficult for them to understand the need to lie still in the scanner. At this time, therefore, it would be difficult to recommend the routine use of MRI in the investigation of dementia. In some early cases where cognitive impairment is borderline and as accurate a diagnosis as possible is felt to be needed, MRI may be of greater value than CT. Figure 9.5 shows temporal lobe CT and Fig. 9.6 MRI views of a 59-year-old university professor, which helped him to decide whether he should try a course of tacrine. A SPET scan is not part of routine investigation. In the clinical setting, the author has found SPET very useful in adding confidence to a diagnosis of frontal dementia where focal perfusion deficits may be clearly defined. Similarly, in cases where the clinical distinction is not clear between a frontal dementia and AD with frontal mental state phenomena, a scan showing diffuse hypoperfusion especially in the posterior parietal area can help to decide in favor of AD. However, a negative scan (i.e. without clear cut perfusion deficits) should not be taken as evidence of absent pathologic changes.

Inappropriate scans

Inappropriate scans in the clinical as opposed to research setting are those that make no contribution to diagnosis and therefore none to management. In this context, an example would be routine scanning of patients with paranoid and schizophrenic disorders. Holden (1987) demonstrated that patients assigned a clinical diagnosis of late life schizophrenia or late paraphrenia constitute a heterogeneous group. In this book (see Chapter 8) Howard and O'Brien correctly point out that if such patients have histories of neurological disease or neurological signs and/or cognitive impairment on examination, neuroimaging is likely to reflect it. It is more rational, therefore, not to ask what the indications are for ordering a scan, be it CT, MRI or SPET, for a patient with late paraphrenia, but what the indications are for scanning a patient with suspected cerebrovascular disease or dementia who happens to have presented with a paraphrenic psychosis. Late paraphrenia is neither common nor rare but within that diagnostic group patients with cognitive impairment are common. As described above, a scan may enhance

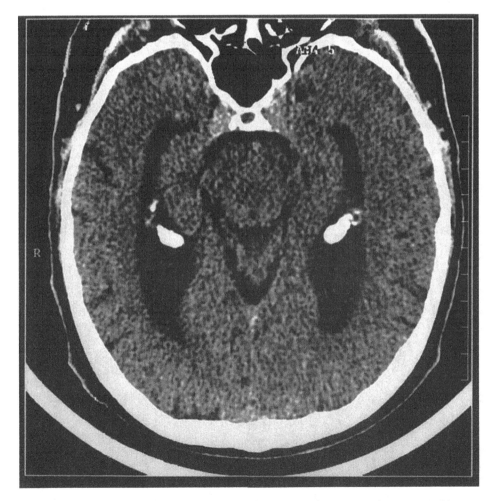

Figure 9.5 *Temporal lobe orientated CT scan of the brain of a 59-year-old university professor completing a course of tacrine for the treatment of AD. Temporal lobe width was below the 5th centile for the patient's age.*

confidence in assigning a second diagnosis when years of medical training in applying Occam's razor inhibit it.

There are specific circumstances in which it would not be appropriate to scan even though a condition is suspected in which it would generally be correct to do so. An example is the patient with metastatic cerebral carcinomatosis for whom the investigation would not affect treatment. Another is the very old patient in a state of advanced dementia for whom the disturbance of being transported to a scanner would be considerable if not cruel and for whom the scan is not going to alter clinical management.

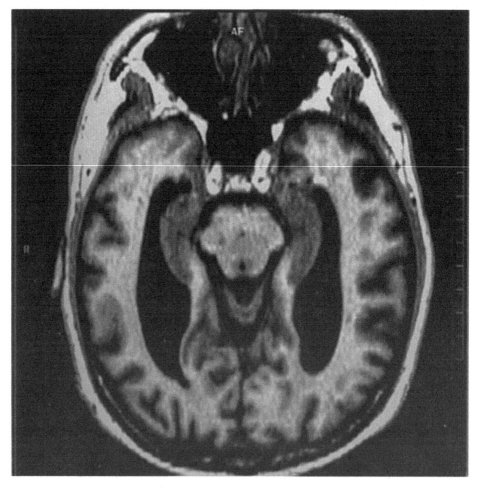

Figure 9.6 *Temporal lobe orientated MRI scan of the brain of a 59-year-old patient whose CT scan at the equivalent level was depicted in Fig. 9.5. Temporal lobe width was below the 5th centile for the patient's age.*

Conclusion

In the clinical setting of old age psychiatry, neuroimaging can neither be equated with biochemical tests nor considered an alternative route to diagnosis. It is unusual, or indeed rare, that a scan, say CT, is the *sine qua non* for a diagnosis, such as in revealing a brain tumor. More commonly, a scan can be considered as the piece in a jigsaw puzzle the subject of which can probably be determined in many cases without it. However, when it is added, the picture is completed, allowing the viewer to determine much better what is going on. Of course, it is possible to mount an economic argument that the majority of scans ordered by old-age psychiatrists do not affect patient management and that the money could be spent more usefully elsewhere. In crude terms this may be correct, but how can a price be put on good clinical practice or improving diagnostic accuracy? It might be a matter of dispute as to how far neuroimaging does in fact increase diagnostic accuracy, but if patients (as opposed to research subjects) are not scanned, King Lear's retort to Cordelia that 'nothing will come of nothing' will apply. There is also a need to look to the future. Advances in understanding the pathogenesis of AD are highly likely to lead to specific treatments in the near or medium term. When they arrive it will be essential that clinicians, not just researchers, are able to define those to be treated. The task of researchers in the field of neuroimaging is to inform clinical practice. In the words of Coiera (1995):

> *Any attempt to use information technology will fail dramatically when the motivation is the application of technology for its own sake rather than the solution of clinical problems.*

References

Allison, S.P. (1994). Is routine computed tomography in strokes unnecessary? Costs outweigh benefits. *British Medical Journal*, 309, 1499–1500.

Coiera, E. (1995). Recent advances: medical informatics. *British Medical Journal*, 310, 1381–1387.

Curran, S.M., Murray, S.M., van Beck, M. *et al.* (1993). A single photon emission computed tomography study of regional brain function in elderly patients with major depression and with Alzheimer-type dementia. *British Journal of Psychiatry*, 163, 155–165.

de Leon, M.J. (1994). Hippocampal formation atrophy in ageing and the prediction of Alzheimer's disease. In *Ageing and Dementia: A Methodological Approach*, ed. A. Burns, pp. 103–124. London: Edward Arnold.

Fineberg, H.V., Bauman, R. & Sosman, M. (1977). Computerized cranial tomography: effect on diagnostic and therapeutic plans. *Journal of the American Medical Association*, 238, 224–227.

Gawler, J., Du Boulay, G.H., Bull, J.W.D. & Marshall, J. (1976). Computerized tomography (the EMI scanner): a comparison with pneumoencephalography and ventriculography. *Journal of Neurology, Neurosurgery and Psychiatry*, 39, 203–211.

Holden, N. (1987). Late paraphrenia or the paraphrenias? *British Journal of Psychiatry*, 150, 635–639.

Hounsfield, G.N. (1973). Computerized transverse axial scanning (tomography): part 1. Description of the system. *British Journal of Radiology*, 46, 1016–1022.

Jacobsen, H.H., Kragsholm, M., & Holm, C. (1976). The economy of the EMI scanner. *Neuroradiology*, 11, 183–184.

Jacobson, S.A., Leuchter, A.F. & Walter, D.O. (1993). Conventional and quantitative EEG in the diagnosis of delirium among the elderly. *Journal of Neurology, Neurosurgery and Psychiatry*, 56, 153–158.

Jacoby, R.J. & Cohen, S.I. (1981). Assessment of cerebral atrophy: discrepancy between pneumoencephalography and computed tomography. *Journal of Neurology, Neurosurgery and Psychiatry*, 44, 654–655.

Jacoby, R.J., Levy, R. & Dawson, J.M. (1980). Computed tomography in the elderly: I. The normal population. *British Journal of Psychiatry*, 136, 249–255.

Jobst, K., Smith, A.D., Szatmari, M. *et al.* (1992). Detection in life of confirmed Alzheimer's disease using a simple measurement of medial temporal lobe atrophy by computed tomography. *Lancet*, 340, 1179–1183.

Kumar, A., Newberg, A., Alavi, A., Berlin, J., Smith, R. & Reivich, M. (1993). Regional cerebral glucose metabolism in late-life depression and Alzheimer disease; a preliminary positron emission tomography study. *Proceedings of the National Academy of Sciences, USA*, 90, 7019–7023.

Lesser, I.M., Mena, I., Boone, K.B. *et al.* (1994). Reduction in cerebral blood flow in older depressed patients. *Archives of General Psychiatry*, 51, 667–686.

Leuchter, A.F. & Jacobson, S.A. (1991). Quantitative measurement of brain electrical activity in delirium. *International Psychogeriatrics*, 3, 231–247.

Lufkin, R.B. (1990). *The MRI Handbook*. St. Louis, MO: Mosby.

McKhann, G., Drachman, D., Folstein, M., Katzman, R., Price, D. & Stadlan, E. (1984). Clinical diagnosis of Alzheimer's disease: report of the NINCDS/ADRDA work group under the auspices of the Department of Health and Human Task Force in Alzheimer's disease. *Neurology*, 34, 939–944.

Miller, B.L., Chang, L., Oropilla, G. & Mena, I. (1994). Alzheimer's disease and frontal lobe dementias. In *Textbook of Geriatric Neuropsychiatry*, ed. C.E. Coffey & J.L. Cummings, pp. 389–404. Washington: American Psychiatric Press.

Nott, P.N., & Fleminger, J.J. (1975). Presenile dementia: the difficulties of early diagnosis. *Acta Psychiatrica Scandinavica*, 51, 210–217.

O'Brien, J.T. (1995). Is hippocampal atrophy on magnetic resonance imaging a marker for Alzheimer's disease? *International Journal of Geriatric Psychiatry*, 10, 431–435.

Ron, M.A., Toone, B.K., Garralda, M.E. & Lishman, W.A. (1979). Diagnostic accuracy in presenile dementia. *British Journal of Psychiatry*, 134, 161–168.

Sackeim, H.A. & Prohovnik, I. (1993). Studies of brain imaging in mood disorders. In *The Biology of Depressive Disorders: Part A: A Systems Perspective*, ed. J.J. Mann & D.J. Kupfer, pp. 205–258. New York: Plenum Press.

Thomson, J.L.G. (1977). Cost effectiveness of an EMI brain scanner: a review of a 2-year experience. *Health Trends*, 9, 16–19.

Index

Note: page numbers in *italics* refer to figures and tables. Pl indicates plate.